PSYCHIATRY
WITHOUT DRUGS

SAFE HOLISTIC SOLUTIONS TO STRUGGLES OF THE MIND AND SPIRIT

By Keith Scott-Mumby MD, MB ChB, HMD, PhD

Printed in the United States of America
First Printing, 2018
ISBN 978-0-9913188-9-6

Mother Whale Inc.
8550 W Charleston Blvd, Ste 102-160
Las Vegas
NV 89117

www.Alternative-Doctor.com

For further information, or to contact the author via email, please send to:
scottmumbywellness@gmail.com

Cover Illustration Copyright © 2018 by Mother Whale Inc.
Cover design and layout and by Dragos Balasoiu: www.beepixeled.com
Illustrations by Oliver Scott-Mumby Citizen Moose: www.citizenmoose.com

DISCLAIMER

This book is for information only and is not intended as a substitute for the medical advice of physicians. The reader should regularly consult a suitable healthcare worker or physician in matters relating to his/her health and particularly with respect to any symptoms that may require proper diagnosis or medical attention.

Although the author and publisher have made every effort to ensure that the information in this book was correct at press time, the author and publisher do not assume and hereby disclaim any liability to any party for any loss, damage, or disruption caused by errors or omissions, whether such errors or omissions result from negligence, accident, or any other cause.

A book can only remain a source of information. It cannot make recommendations for you, or order suitable treatment, since the author knows nothing about you and your lifestyle.

Under no circumstances can Dr. Keith Scott-Mumby accept responsibility for you, your health or your state of mind.

"I have long said that only one percent of psychiatrists are sane. Here is the most sane one I know. Indeed, this critical work is beyond The Myth of Madness, bringing the potential of healing to the multitude poisoned by the PharmacoMafia. This is the most important books in the entire history of psychiatry!"

C. Norman Shealy MD, PhD
neurosurgeon and founder of the former American Holistic Medicine Association, now the International Institute of Holistic Medicine.

"*The public is in the middle of a psychiatric plague.*

Learning the truth is the first step forward."

Jon Rappoport
investigative reporter, www.nomorefakenews.com

"A critical requirement for every diagnosis in mental health is that the condition is NOT caused by a medical condition, drug or medication. That's in the Diagnostic and Statistical Manual, the so-called "Bible" of psychiatry. And yet, as the author points out, the biological components and interactions of food, nutrition, pathogens, hormonal imbalances, vitamins and minerals which would seem to part of that biological piece are often ignored in the pursuit and understanding of psychiatric diagnoses. Dr. Keith provides an enlightening view of brain function based upon these basic building blocks of life, and opens the door to exciting new possibilities of healing. This text should be required reading for all medical students."

Gregory P. Brown MD
Board Certified Forensic Psychiatrist, Associate Professor of Psychiatry and the Residency Program Training Director at University of Nevada Las Vegas Medical School and expert psychiatric witness called in the O J Simpson trial.

Contents

PART 6 WEIRD STUFF   409

VALUABLE RESOURCES   439

REFERENCES   445

"*Pleasure is short-lived, happiness is long-lived; pleasure is visceral, happiness is ethereal; pleasure is taking, happiness is giving; pleasure can be achieved with substances; happiness cannot be achieved with substances; pleasure is experienced alone; happiness is experienced in social groups. The extremes of pleasure all lead to addiction, whether they be substances or behaviors, yet there's no such thing as being addicted to too much happiness.*"

\- **Dr. Robert Lustig,** *The Hacking of the American Mind.*

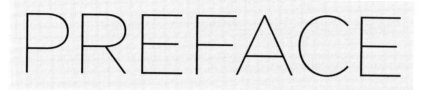

Broken People Hidden Truths

The calling of a physician:

To cure, sometimes; to heal, often; to comfort always.

I have been moved to write this book because of the suffering I have seen in struggling and unhappy people, who cannot find themselves and live to BE themselves. In other words, those who are confused or hurting in mind. People who are categorized as mentally ill get a very raw deal; they are ostracized by family, friends and society, they suffer in isolation; they are not properly understood; and the medical profession—psychiatry specifically—offers little real help and often causes irretrievable damage to the soul or being.

Moreover this is the only medical specialty in which you could lose your freedom; in which you may be incarcerated against your will and at times against your own best interests. In no sense is locking up a patient "for his or her own good" analogous to treatment or healing.

For the doctor, it is considered sufficient to shut the patient up—to quieten his or her complaints, squeeze the spark out of him or her—in the grotesque pretense that now he or she can no longer complain, that somehow counts as a cure. There are drugs in abundance which can perform this "chemical lobotomy" as it has been called. It does not serve truth or justice and is a travesty of healing care.

To me this is on a level with closing down the customer service department of a troubled business: no more complaints heard... problem fixed! But you can see right away that nothing is solved; if the products being sold are inferior then refusing to admit requests for assistance does not rectify any of the shortcomings.

As someone who believes that humans are spiritual beings—meaning non-material mind entities—I look beyond the brain for the real nature of experience, thought and desires. The brain is simply the physical relay point, via which we make our world come to life. Our real life is deeper within. Fooling around with brain mechanics and the biochemistry is not addressing any of the deeper issues that a human being might have.

Sure, brains do malfunction and this needs to be attended to. I totally agree with this. But suppressing all feelings and experience is not what is needed. For one thing, it's not addressing the brain's physical problem at all, merely overriding it. Secondly, it does not reach as far as the inner experience the patient is having. On the contrary, suppressing all interaction and responses means that he or she cannot be reached in any meaningful sense. We don't know *really* what the person is experiencing within, once he or she has been drugged up to the eyeballs.

Therefore this kind of approach is to be deplored because it puts a block on real solutions and real recovery.

Physical Factors in Mental Disease

Most so-called "mental illness" (call it psychological distress, psychiatric disorder or whatever you will) has simple but undetected physical causes. The person is not really mentally deranged; just behaving strangely and feeling upset, because the mind is disordered by the physical problem.

The truth is, being sick makes you feel bad, act differently and experience unpleasant, sometimes disabling thoughts. We all experience this from time to time: there is not a person alive who hasn't felt tired, mopey, out of sorts and maybe grumpy, because of a nasty virus illness. These symptoms are not the problem; *the symptoms are the result of the problem.*

The path forward then, with any mental disorder, is to vigorously explore the possibility of physical problems and get them corrected. If someone is bloated, lethargic and depressed because of low thyroid function, what fool doctor would suppose that the "correct" or accepted treatment is to prescribe an antidepressant?

You wouldn't even offer psychotherapy to cheer the person up. You would, of course, prescribe the missing thyroid hormones! Yet some doctors have had their license revoked for doing just that.

If a woman has outrageous and demanding PMS (PMT in Europe), meaning she behaves like a borderline psychotic at certain times of the month, would you diagnose a brain chemistry disease and load her with toxic antipsychotic medicines? Or would you address the estrogen imbalance and correct anything found (progesterone—real natural progesterone, not the Big Pharma fake substitutes—works wonders for PMS).

If a patient is chronically depressed because his irritable bowel condition has not been successfully relieved for many decades, leading to a restricted life, would you use a psychotropic drug to offer him relief? Or would you get to work investigating food allergies, leaky gut syndrome and dysbiosis? One does not solve the problem but the patient has to pretend he now "feels better"; the other route offers the likelihood of a permanent cure.

This book sets out to teach the layman and practitioner alike just what enormous mental impact hidden physical factors like these might have and how they might underlie what is simply assumed to be a psychiatric problem.

Is Mental Illness a Myth?

We might need to question whether there even is such a thing as mental illness or whether people are just broken by living, as Thomas Szasz called it. Szasz's book *The Myth of Mental Illness: Foundations of a Theory of Personal Conduct* (1961) questions psychiatry's foundations and argues against the tendency of psychiatrists to label people who are "disabled by living" as mentally ill. It received much publicity when it was published, and has become a classic, but also made Szasz an enemy of many doctors. Along with R D Laing (*The Divided Self*, 1960) Szasz helped found what has since been called the anti-psychiatry popular movement.

According to thinkers like Szasz (and I concur), almost all so-called mental illness is a delusion of the doctors, not of the patients! The assumption is made that some neurological or biochemical defect, perhaps a very subtle one, will ultimately be found for any of the currently recognized disorders of thinking and behavior.

"Mental illness" is thus regarded as basically no different than all other diseases (that is, of the body). The only difference, in this view, between mental and bodily diseases is that the former, affecting the brain, manifest themselves by means of mental symptoms; whereas the latter, affecting other organ systems (for example, the skin, liver, etc.), manifest themselves by means of symptoms referable to those parts of the body.

Many contemporary psychiatrists, physicians, and other scientists hold the "physical brain dysfunction" position. This view rejects the idea that people can have mental troubles because of experiences or trauma, or because of differences in personal needs, opinions, social aspirations, values, and so on. Instead, all abnormalities of thought and behavior are attributed to physico-biological processes which will eventually surrender to medical research.

Well, so far nothing has surfaced. In fact, all current decent research, as we shall see, is pointing in the opposite direction: there are NO consistent biochemical disorders that can be linked to specific diseases.

British science philosopher Karl Popper admired Szasz' work and in a 1961 letter to him, praised the book as admirable and fascinating, adding that, "It is a most important book, and it marks a real revolution."[1]

Psychiatrist David Cooper writes that *The Myth of Mental Illness*, like R. D. Laing's *The Divided Self*, proved stimulating in the development of anti-psychiatry, though he notes that neither book is in and of itself an anti-psychiatric work. He describes Szasz's work as "a decisive, carefully documented demystification of psychiatric diagnostic labeling in general."

Too bad most of the editors of the infamous Diagnostic and Statistical Manual never read it, or apparently did not. All 300 diagnoses listed in this infamous manual have no objective tests. No blood tests, x-rays, scans or any other way of confirming the diagnosis of a mental illness. Just pure opinion.

The concept of illness, whether bodily or mental, implies deviation from some clearly defined norm. In the case of physical illness, the norm is the structural and functional integrity of the human body. But what is the norm for mental health? This question cannot be easily answered.

The term "mental illness" is widely used to describe something which is very different to a disease of the brain. Many people today take it· for granted that living is an arduous process. Its hardship for modern man, moreover, derives not so much from a struggle for biological survival as from the stresses and strains inherent in the social intercourse of complex human personalities.

In that sense, we all suffer stress and, indeed, Part 3 is about the forces that influence us all—everyone—not just those reacting poorly and supposed to be mentally ill.

So the model that claims unusual or dysfunctional responses to these stresses is, *ipso facto*, a mental illness is quite frankly a grotesque distortion. It is implicit in this view that social intercourse between people is regarded as something inherently harmonious, its disturbance being due solely to the presence of "mental illness" in many people.

This is obviously fallacious reasoning, for there is little evidence of harmony and balance anywhere in human life. Some of the world's top performers are often identifiably crazy. Professors and "clever people" often do insane things. Doctors and psychiatrists themselves are a weird bunch, in many respects. So who is to choose what is normal behavior?

Put another way: "What kinds of behavior are regarded as indicative of mental illness, and by whom?"

Big Pharma and The Myth Of Psychiatric Drugs

Of course we are up against relentless and dishonest propaganda from the pharmaceutical industry, which time and again has been shown to put profits above patient concerns; and elevate tawdry scientific fraud above the quest for truth.

Make no mistake: pharmaceutical drugs are big business. Such medications are not only expensive; they are the most expensive class of drugs. Data from the USA, where the annual budget for such drugs is over $200 billion, suggest that several types of psychiatric drug, notably antipsychotics, antidepressants and drugs for attention-deficit hyperactivity disorder (ADHD), have consistently ranked among the most costly classes of prescription drugs in the past few years and that costs of psychotropic medications have risen faster than costs of other drugs (and much faster than inflation, incidentally).

Moreover, as you will read later, here is evidence that some psychiatric medications like antipsychotics are frequently prescribed 'off-label', for indications for which they have not had regulatory approval. In the USA, *antidepressants are frequently prescribed to people who have no diagnosable mental disorder.*[2]

If that's not enough, Big Pharma is pushing relentlessly to expand its market. It's winning. Here is the current state of play:

- Approximately 1 in 5 adults in the U.S. are said to experience mental illness in a given year.

- Approximately 1 in 25 adults in the U.S.—9.8 million, or 4%—experiences a serious mental illness in a given year that substantially interferes with or limits one or more major life activities.

- Approximately 1 in 5 youths aged 13–18 (21.4%) experiences a severe mental disorder at some point during their life. For children aged 8–15, the estimate is 13%.

- 1.1% of adults in the U.S. live with schizophrenia.

- 2.6% of adults in the U.S. live with bipolar disorder.

- 6.9% of adults in the U.S.—16 million—had at least one major depressive episode in the past year.

- 18.1% of adults in the U.S. experienced an anxiety disorder such as posttraumatic stress disorder, obsessive-compulsive disorder and specific phobias.

These are just claims, of course. It's absurd to state that 1 in 5 adults experiences a mental illness episode in a given year. That's propaganda (lies). As you will be reading over and over in this book, *almost nobody has real mental illness.* They are just being manipulated and lied to while the true cause of their distress is (deliberately) ignored.

Let's face it, as in all of medicine, finding the real cause of the problem and curing the patient is very bad for business.

Europe and Other Centers

The WHO European Division has similar miserable stats to report, based on the same misapprehensions and nonsense:

- About a quarter to a third of the population suffer from mental disorders every year, depending on what disorders are included (most commonly depression and anxiety).

- Only about 50% of people suffering from mental disorders receive professional help; far fewer receive adequate help.

- Mental disorders account for 44% of social welfare benefits and disability pensions in Denmark, 43% in Finland and the United Kingdom (including Scotland), and 37% in Romania and 25% in the Republic of Moldova, one of Europe's poorest countries.

- Almost 9 out of 10 of people suffering from mental health problems say they have been affected by stigma and discrimination.

- The annual suicide rate is 13.9 per 100 000 on average in the European Region, but varies widely between countries. In several countries, suicide is the number-one cause of death in adolescents.

- In Europe, men are almost five times more likely to commit suicide than women.

- An estimated 20% of people who commit suicide had been in contact with their general practitioners (GPs) or psychiatric services within one week of their deaths, and 40% in the preceding month.

- About half of all mental disorders start before the age of 14. Cost-effective interventions exist, but less than 1% of mental health budgets are spent on prevention.[3]

The Myth Of Brain "Science"

Researchers today have a great many fancy tools at their disposal. But don't let that fool you into thinking they know anything about the mind at all. They simply don't. They study brain and perception but not thought and consciousness.

Moreover, the usual science dogma is rife in this field. For all the last century and the first few years of this one, it was considered proven science that brain cells cannot be replaced; they have no power of regeneration; once you lose brain cells they are gone forever. The brain never grows; it simply ages and gets poorer and poorer in function. Not that anyone ever tested this theory. They just passed it around as "fact".

But it wasn't factual at all. It was stupid ignorance and blind acceptance of the status quo. "That's what we have always said; we'll go on saying it, so that it's believed to be true," kind of logic.

Unfortunately for these dodos, someone finally checked to see if it was true... and it wasn't. Brain cells were caught in the act of dividing, multiplying and replacing themselves.

So logically, there is no real reason that brain tissue cannot recover, the same as with any other diseased element within the body. Nature can fix a sprain, a cut or a broken bone. Recovery is natural. The body knows what to do.

Yet the sad truth is that, once entered into the system, an individual is destined to remain part of the "broken people hidden truths" machinery of greed and profit. Cures are not expected. Recovery is not sought. The patient is encouraged in the belief they are busted and there is no further hope of a normal life.

The terrible side-effects when trying to stop highly addictive drugs make it very difficult indeed for the person to escape the trap, once they are caught within it. Of course the medical attendants echo the Big Pharma mantra that the resurgence of frightening symptoms is proof that he or she really is VERY sick and cannot therefore discontinue the "treatment".

How I Have Organized the Book

OK, we need to tackle this nightmare of exploitation, head on. There is a way out for most and I am going to draw a detailed map to help you or anyone else who is involved with mental health care find that escape.

Part 1. I start out from a highly critical perspective on current psychiatric ignorance, disinformation and misguided methods. If what you read doesn't destroy your whole faith in the psychiatric profession, so that you would never consider asking for help from its practitioners, then I will have failed!

Part 2. Then comes what I have called "The Suffering Seven"—seven major topics of interest that cover a HUGE range of conditions and will introduce a great deal of general knowledge on the topic.

These 7 are:

1. Depression

2. Schizophrenia

3. Bipolar

4. Anxiety States and Phobias

5. Dementia

6. Children's Brain Dysfunction (ADD, ADHD, hyperkinetic syndrome, etc.)

7. Alcoholism and Drug Addictions

If there was to be a number 8, I think I would choose crime and delinquency, so I have introduced a short section on that, just for completeness.

There are some difficulties in attempting a classification of this type. For example ADD/ADHD and autism spectrum disorder (ASD) linger on into adult life and don't affect only children.

Depression is a common complicating factor in many other conditions, including anxiety, dementia and schizophrenia. Bipolar is really just a scaled up version of mood swings, depression... and so on. Alcoholism and addictions are obviously a bracket that includes the same or similar phenomenon throughout, which is non-psychogenic in origin (I will reveal the big secret later).

But this classification has worked for me and remains the foundation of this book.

Part 3. Covers holistic aspects of mind function and issues of genuine psychological distress that apply to us all. These are principles and techniques that anyone can benefit from. I have called this part Everyman Psychology (no gender bias intended).

Part 4. Explains general principles of holistic healing which, of course, apply full to mental and spiritual distress states.

Part 5. Consists of a comprehensive listing of holistic testing, investigation and treatment methods that can be applied widely across the board, to many types of psychiatric (and general health) dysfunction.

Part 6. Finally I present several unfamiliar ideas, known only to a few but which are enormously relevant, in that these are models of health and disease which offer the final breakthrough treatment for sufferers of various strange and misunderstood maladies.

Some of it you will find weird, for sure! But I ask you to journey with me, into adventurous territory, in the hope you will learn something new and exciting.

PREFACE 2

THE PSYCHIATRIC CHATBOT WILL SEE YOU NOW!

Here's a quick note on a new development in the madness.

In a creepy advancement on psychiatry's inability to truly diagnose anything, we are now faced with artificial intelligence "bots", which purport to diagnose and help mental conditions. This is a double menace: firstly encoding such a tool with the incompetence and inability of psychiatry to do anything worthwhile in the truly holistic domain—whether by electronic interaction or any other approach—and, secondly, the apparent veneer of being scientifically validated in the minds of many people; "Well, there's an app. So they must know what they are doing," kind of faulty reasoning.[4]

I find myself alarmed by the dreary and dangerous future this supposed "development" lays out before us.

It's a new field of exploration called, would you believe, "computational psychiatry", which blends technologies like artificial intelligence, virtual reality, and deep learning for the diagnosis and treatment of mental illnesses. Computational it may be; just remember the key geek's saying: GIGO. If you put garbage in, you get garbage out! There is no way that computers can improve on the programming they were given, if it is faulty in the first place.

However, since Facebook opened its Messenger platform to developers, there's been an explosion of chatbots, and several of them are explicitly marketed as mental health tools. Those who espouse this alarming new idea (the short-term or long-term effects of which have not been explored in any degree), resort to the term a "virtual therapist." A very dangerous simplification.

There is the delusory suggestion that advancements in deep learning, virtual reality (VR), and artificial intelligence (AI) may bring an end to issues engrained within the practice of clinical psychology — such as subjectivity and the difficulty of conducting large-scale studies—perhaps leading us into a new era of diagnosing and treating mental disorders.

This is naïve, as all such bots and apps have to be programmed by the same old inept psychiatrists and therapists who are failing in the first place. It will simply enshrine folly, ignorance and prejudice into the electronic domain.

Switching to an electronic interaction isn't going to suddenly bring about magical new skills; it will only perpetuate the old, failing lack-of-skills. The gloss of electronic gadgetry will just make the dogma LOOK more attractive.

Computational psychiatry is operated on the unproven tenet that researchers can better understand and treat mental illnesses using the aforementioned technologies. Applications vary, but some researchers in the field apply mathematical theories of cognition to data mined from long-standing observations to effectively diagnose and predict cognition, while others use virtual experiments to enable the pure study of human behavior.

Sarah Fineburg of Yale University in New Haven has recently published a study that used computational psychiatry to explore borderline personality disorder (BPD), a condition that the National Institute of Mental Health (NIMH) reports includes symptoms such as "ongoing instability in moods, behaviors, self-image, and functioning," as well as "impulsive actions and unstable relationships."[5]

What the NIMH isn't admitting is that we are, all of us, unstable in our moods, often shifting several times an hour. Now it risks being elevated to a disease state. Only in extreme degrees is this instability a problem to the patient. But the apps or "bots" are only trained to look for frequency of changes.

To add to the ridiculousness of this investigation, Fineburg observed only the responses of people with BPD to events in virtual environments. She used a game called Cyberball in which avatars pass a ball to one another, with the patient in control of one avatar. Though they believe the remaining avatars are controlled by other people, their actions are actually determined by computer systems.[6]

So people are now judged by their reactions to something that doesn't even exist and is capable of deceiving the target person. Is anyone else alarmed about this? It gives me the medical creeps!

Fineburg found that BPD sufferers experienced greater feelings of rejection than non-sufferers when they did not receive the ball, and they also experienced more negative feelings than non-sufferers even when they received the ball more often than the other avatars.

Yes... so what? I'm waiting for the completion of that remark.

Outrageous and Unproven Claims

Not only can computational psychiatry be used to study the emotions of BPD patients, it is claimed, it can also help researchers understand their language use, which some have posited was different from that of non-sufferers. However, the data was previously too vast to analyze. "We and others have identified language features that mark psychological states and traits," Fineberg told MIT Technology Review. "Computational models based on word-use patterns can predict which writers have psychosis or will progress to psychosis."[7]

I utterly refuse to believe this nonsense conclusion, which is opinion and NOT BASED ON FACT.

But Fineberg is not alone, it seems. These two strands of computation psychiatry (language and instability) are being used by other researchers to study other disorders, using virtual environments as clinical spaces and using AI to find patterns in large swathes of data.

The use of AI to diagnose disorders and recommend treatments has gained traction in the world of apps, which are supposedly acting as "virtual psychotherapists" to treat a variety of mental disorders.

So now we have the cheesily-named "Woebot" (woe bot, or robot spoken with a lisp, get it?), a chatbot that claims to use cognitive behavioral therapy principles to help combat depression. The results from a small test of the app were said to be promising, with the majority of users reporting a significant reduction in depression symptoms. Alison Darcy, a lecturer at Stanford who pioneered the app, told Business Insider, "The data blew us away. We were like, this is it."

Again, just an opinion, delivered with silly childspeak.

Due to the novelty of such systems, no one has yet studied whether or not psychiatric interactions with a computer over an extended period of time are beneficial for patients. Darcy's study only had 70 total participants and lasted just two weeks, which is too short a time period to produce any certainty about the app's impact.

I mean: is that science? If we studied the potential harmful effects of smoking on a group of smokers for just 2 weeks, what would that tell us?

In the end, it's all about deception... and they admit that! The whole idea of psychology is to study how a person's perception colors empirical data, so if the senses are sufficiently fooled into believing a virtual scenario is "real," the results of a VR supported study are just as valid as one conducted in the real world.

This is an arrogant and ignorant assumption, not based on any fact. Where is the proof that experiencing virtual reality is identical to normal everyday living and engagement with fellow human beings? There isn't any.

I'm sorry, but I don't buy into this. Not because I am a Luddite and hate technology. But because I am a humanist and holistic expert in mental symptoms and moods—and I despise modern psychiatry and its pretensions.

Conflicts of Interest (be warned): The lead author of the study (Alison M. Darcy) is the founder of a commercial entity Woebot Labs Inc. (formerly, the Life Ninja Project) which created the intervention that is the subject of this trial and therefore has financial interest in that company.

INTRODUCTION

A PROFESSION "WANTING IN HUMANITY"

Let's face it; life can seem very difficult when you don't have full control over your own mind. It's scary when thoughts, feelings and behavior patterns you don't want can force themselves into your head, against your wishes.

This is all made far worse when a profession—or should I say industry—tries to tell you you're busted and it can't be helped; the only solution is to suppress the unwanted symptoms by shutting down all or part of your mind, in an attempt to tune out the problem. Moreover, if you don't comply with their dictates, you could find yourself locked up, with the status of a prisoner. Even dead. That's modern psychiatry.

It's supposed to help. Heck, it's considered the only proper help!

Well, this book has a powerful message that's worth shouting from the rooftops: *almost all mentally ill people are NOT mentally ill*. Over 95% of them have one or more physical disorders capable of causing brain function abnormalities and significant changes in thought processing and expression of feelings. It's just not being diagnosed correctly.

Instead they are being told they have a "mental illness", such as depression, bipolar disorder, ADD, autism, OCD or schizophrenia.

The psychiatric profession has grabbed a field which it does not understand, cannot control and in which it is worse than ineffective: it is damaging. Psychiatry hurts people who trust it and turn to it for help. That has a hideous historical perspective which goes back a long way. As we all know, the old-fashioned treatment was to chain up, flog, starve and grotesquely abuse suffering individuals considered mad. The London hospital of St Mary Of Bethlehem gave us our terrible word bedlam, for the nightmare conditions which befell luckless victims, once inside.

In June 1816 Thomas Monro, Principal Physician at Bedlam, resigned as a result of scandal when he was accused of 'wanting in humanity' towards his patients.[8]

Well, I've got news for those who are not keeping up to speed in this field: NOTHING HAS CHANGED. It's all done by prescription today, that's all. The locks are still in place. The jailers and torturers are licensed incompetents, many of who, to their shame, are trained MDs who should be able to recognize the signs of physical disease.

You might argue that hitting people over the head with a chemical cosh is kinder than physical pain; a moot point. What is unarguable is that most modern psychiatric drugs are worthless and most are greatly damaging. The multi-billion dollar fraud of drugs used to treat non-existent medical diagnoses must be stopped urgently and at all costs, before more patients are injured and perhaps permanently damaged.

Plus it's the real "wanting of humanity" of the majority of psychiatrists towards the sick and miserable that is so dreadful to bear. 20th century mental hospitals (now 21st century, of course) are little different from the St Mary Of Bethlehem precedent. As brave psychiatrist Peter Breggin tells use so poignantly in his book *Toxic Psychiatry*: "The first and most lasting impression was the stench. It reminded me of my Uncle Dutch's reaction to liberating a concentration camp: nausea... Many of these people actually looked like concentration camp inmates—undernourished, silent, stone-faced with sunken eyes. They would sit around in corners or pace about...."[9]

Breggin recalls coming upon attendants beating up a patient and simply bore witness to their inhuman acts, until the institutional bullies felt shamed into stopping.

"During the day, the patients were locked out of the barracks-like sleeping quarters. Dozens of them were herded together in grey squalor with nothing to occupy their time. Many wasted a lifetime in this place."

Breggin dared to think the unthinkable thought: that the treatments being meted out were perhaps making the patients worse!

"Sharing the anguish of the patients and their intolerable living conditions took a toll on most of us [students]. A single afternoon in the hospital was more than most of us could survive unscathed. We returned to Harvard and Radcliffe with headaches, upset stomachs, a stench embedded in our nostrils, and nightmares."

It's Bad News Being A Psychiatric Patient

Not only will you be mis-managed, maybe imprisoned, with a torrent of chemical profiteering "treatments" which ruin your life. The psychiatric label can mean dying 25 years or more earlier.

A sixteen-state study has revealed increased morbidity and mortality of those diagnosed with serious mental disorders. That is, people with certain psychiatric diagnoses die 25 years or more earlier than others! The study, conducted by the National Association of State Mental Health Program Directors (NASMHPD) and published in October, 2012, attributes the increased mortality of mental health clients to preventable conditions, ranging from smoking, prescription medications and substance abuse, to diabetes, obesity, homelessness and suicide.

The study authors note that atypical antipsychotics, in particular, are increasingly associated with preventable conditions that contribute to increased mortality (i.e., weight gain, diabetes, insulin resistance, and metabolic syndrome).[10]

Furthermore, among a host of health service quality issues, access to health care is typically hindered by systemic flaws, under-funding, and discrimination against mental health consumers.

Notice these coy figures take no account of the likelihood of dying BECAUSE of your medications.

Unnatural Deaths

To state the obvious, psychiatric "care" is not supposed to kill patients, and no one expects patients to die in psychiatric hospitals. At least not die *because* of being in hospital. Yet this is what quietly happens under the watchful eye of psychiatrists every day in psychiatric institutions around the world.

The Citizen's Commission for Human Rights (CCHR) has tried to document the horror that is going on (yes, don't bother to write to me, I do know CCHR is a front group for The Church of Scientology).

Get this, from their website (cchr.org)...

Nine-year-old Randy Steele didn't feel like taking a bath in the psychiatric facility to which he had been admitted. He launched into a toy-tossing temper tantrum after refusing to take a bath and in the scuffle that ensued Randy vomited and then stopped breathing, while staff forcibly restrained him. After being revived, Randy was quickly transferred to another hospital where he died the next day (February 2000).

Hospital records later showed that Randy had been restrained 25 times in the 28 days prior to his death. Despite the evidence of blood discharging from his nose, mouth, eyes and anus, and bruises on his face and abdomen, no criminal charges were filed against his carers. It's beyond belief. At state legislative hearings, Randy's mother, Holly, held up her son's autopsy photos, pleading: "I hope that no other child has to die like this." She was ignored.[11]

Psychiatric staff forced 13-year-old Canadian Stephanie Jobin (already dosed with five different psychiatric drugs) to lie face down on the floor, shoved a beanbag chair on top of her, sat on the chair to pin her down and held her feet. After struggling for 20 minutes, Stephanie stopped breathing. Her death was ruled an accident. Again, beyond belief they could get away with this.

Eleven-year-old Andrew McClain was killed for being disobedient. He died of traumatic asphyxia (suffocation) and chest compression four days after being admitted to a Connecticut psychiatric facility. Andrew had disobeyed an instruction from a psychiatric aide to move to another table at breakfast. Two staff members subsequently restrained him, one by lying on top of him in a padded seclusion room. That's basically torture in the quiet room, where nobody can hear the screams.

I couldn't quite believe these stories. The CCHR is notoriously belligerent. So I Googled the Randy Steele incident. It's right there, investigated by staffers at *American Statesman*, published May 18, 2003. On that same page, there are several other harrowing stories of kids who were killed in restraints by their sadistic adult carers.[12]

Just children.

So you see, little has changed from medieval times. The spirit of Bedlam has not gone away. The idea that psychiatry is now humane and has "modernized" is a lie. Drugs have solved nothing. Chemicals just de-humanize patients so they can be treated in this way. Perhaps you may share my view that the psychiatric profession attracts a certain type of person with a cruel psychopathic streak?

Then there are the "unexplained" deaths in California's Camarillo and Metropolitan State hospitals. One 36-year-old man was found dead face down in a bed where he had been restrained with leather straps. A grandmother was found dead in a hospital closet two weeks after the staff informed the family that she was missing.

CCHR claims to have exposed the fact that "up to" 150 restraint deaths occur without accountability every year in the United States alone. At least thirteen of the deaths over a two-year period were children as young as 6 years old. Young children should NOT be in psychiatric care, never mind tied or strapped down.

Bear in mind, if you please, that these deaths are not in some third-world country or some down-beaten dictatorial territory, like Myanmar under the generals. This is the world's greatest and richest country, with almost unlimited resources, and a medical budget that can only leave others gasping with envy. But the worst part, for me, is the hypocrisy: the USA effects to lead the world in medical science and skills.

I don't think so.

It's not all institutions that are bad, of course; it's not all attendant staff. Some are kind and caring. And need I say, it's not just in the USA.

In Japan, Dr. Masami Houki, head of the Houki psychiatric clinic in Japan, was convicted of manslaughter after he plugged a 31-year-old female patient's mouth with tissue, then covered it with adhesive, injected her with a tranquilizer, tied her hands and feet, and forced her to lay on the back seat of a car while transferring her to the clinic. She was dead on arrival.

One might wonder what kind of a life this unfortunate woman would have suffered at the hands of her physician, had she survived. Rape? Torture? Mutilation? I doubt she would ever be released. Houki cannot be considered sane.

Yet he remains one of the very few psychiatrists—indeed, any psychiatric staff—who has been criminally charged because of deaths resulting from violent bondage procedures, euphemistically called "humane restraint therapy."

One can extrapolate and suppose that thousands of people of all ages continue to die from what is basically physical assault in psychiatric facilities across the globe. Psychiatry has placed itself above the law, from where it can assault and batter its unfortunate victims with a complete lack of accountability, all in the name of "treatment."

If all this shocks or horrifies you (it should) you might consider joining the push at Mind-Freedom International. MindFreedom International is an international coalition of over one hundred grassroots groups and thousands of individual members from fourteen nations. Based in the United States, it was founded in 1990 to advocate against forced medication, medical restraints, and involuntary electroconvulsive therapy.

MindFreedom has been recognized by the United Nations Economic and Social Council as a human rights NGO with Consultative Roster Status.[13] You can find links to the books and websites mentioned here in the **Valuable Resources** section in the back of the book!

Maybe Psychiatrists Are The Real Screwballs

The plight of patients troubles me but really: *psychiatrists are the crazy ones, out of control!*

They have a fantasy diagnosis system that is not based on any real-world objective test. Not one. Not any! It's shocking to grasp this but you need to know... it's true.

The so-called "bible" of psychiatry, the *Diagnostic and Statistical Manual* or DSM (currently number 5 or V), lists over 300 conditions, not one of which exists in reality.

OK, I'm kidding slightly. But not one of those diagnoses can be proved and therefore in a sense they are not real. It's all opinion. There is no definitive blood test, x-ray, scan result, urine change or microscope visual that can definitively establish any of the 300 conditions.

That's why you can visit one psychiatrist, who says you're depressed; another says you have anxiety neurosis; and a third (if you are unlucky) will try to tell you that you have signs of schizophrenia. But none of these experts will look at some lab work and say, "This shows you have XYZ condition." I repeat: *there are no such tests*.

Yet these people are dishing out some of the heaviest, most destructive "therapies" known: toxic chemicals, including SSRIs, electroshock convulsion treatment, and in some barbaric places they are still doing lobotomies! Great Britain and The United States of America for example.

British psychiatrist Maurice Partridge, who conducted a follow-up study of 300 lobotomy patients, said that the treatment achieved its effects by "reducing the complexity of psychic life". Following the operation, spontaneity, responsiveness, self-awareness and self-control were reduced. Activity was replaced by inertia, and people were left emotionally blunted and restricted in their intellectual range.

In other words the patients are wrecked but complain less. For "reducing the complexity of psychic life" read: *vegetative state*.[14]

Based on the fact that they have no workable diagnostic system, they have no entitlement to treat anything. Yet they subsume the right to destroy brain tissue permanently and blunt the whole purpose of living.

Holistic Psychiatry?

I complain that they do not have any lab work available. But in fact they do! It is my assertion that over 95% of so-called "mental illness" is caused by undiagnosed and untreated physical disorders, namely **food allergies, heavy metal inflammation, nutritional deficiencies, hormonal imbalances, hidden stealth pathogens and so on.**

That being so, the real treatment becomes obvious: fix the physical problem. Do not label the person as a mental case and treat him or her with frightful chemicals under the guise of medicines.

The point is that we do not need a *Diagnostic and Statistical Manual* of supposed disorders (symptoms). What we really need is a book of causes.

An effective manual of psychiatry would list food allergies as probably the main condition; there would be a chapter on hormones; another chapter on nutritional deficiencies (very common, even in the overfed West); and a chapter on parasites and stealth pathogens.

There would also be a chapter on sound procedures to pull people out of psychic trauma. Trauma and abuse does exist, of course. But:

1. Is not a mental illness, even when incapacitating (see 2.)

2. Need not be permanent, if dealt with properly

3. Should not be treated with addictive chemicals that create ongoing dysfunctionality

Of course someone may feel grief if a loved one dies; angry if a spouse is caught cheating; depressed if there is no employment month after month. But is that a disease? Really?

Let's do what the math teacher calls factorization. The treatment of depression due to food allergies (I've cured over a thousand such) is change the diet; the treatment of depression due to low thyroid function is to supplement (replace) the thyroid hormones; the treatment of depression due to B vitamin deficiency is to supply the missing vitamins; the treatment of depression due to Lyme's is antibiotics to kill the spirochete (I'm talking real Lyme's: an infection with the spirochete bacterium *Borrelia burgdorferi*).

Take out the common factor, which is "depression", and you are left with a series of proper diagnoses and we do not need the word depression at all!

Can't Diagnose Sanity, Never Mind Mental Illness

OK, let's lighten up and have some fun. Late last year I was sitting on the beach in Waikiki, Hawaii, reading a book called *Shrinks: The Untold Story of Psychiatry* by Jeffrey A. Lieberman, MD. He's obviously a shrink and takes the orthodox point of view. Not a vitamin or whole food in the entire book![15]

But the fun part was that Lieberman referenced a whacky experiment that took place in 1973 (long before I came to the States). It was published in the prestigious journal *Science* and was titled "On Being Sane In Insane Places." The author was David Rosenhan, a lawyer, not an MD (he had a degree in psychology though).[16]

The opening sentence of Rosenhan's article was "If sanity and insanity exist, how shall we know them?" Good question! As I said: psychiatry has no available tests to tell them apart.

Rosenhan proposed to investigate psychiatry's take on this important issue by sending sane, well-balanced and otherwise "normal" individuals into mental hospitals, to see if they were spotted as sane and sent home.

Unbeknownst to the hospital staffs, Rosenhan engineered the secret admission of eight totally normal individuals. They used fake identities and varied their profession from the real ones. At each hospital, they telephoned ahead for an appointment and when they arrived they complained of hearing voices and had been primed to say three words: "empty", "hollow" and "thud".

Each of the fake patients was a voluntary admission, by the way. Each was instructed to say they no longer heard voices and to start behaving totally normally, once they reached the psychiatric ward. The result?

All but one of the planted cases were diagnosed as schizophrenic! They were locked up from 7 – 52 days (brave fellows!)

Rosenhan's conclusion: *We cannot distinguish the sane from the insane in mental hospitals.*

Predictably there was widespread outrage and derision from the public at large. Some of my older subscribers may even remember this outcry (1973).

But Rosenhan wasn't done yet! The furore that he evoked suggested a further chance to humiliate the psychiatrists! He issued a new challenge to one of the hospitals, which unwisely accepted: "Over the coming year, I will send in another round of imposters into your hospital. You try to detect them, knowing full well that they will be coming, and at the end of the year, we will see how many you catch."

From a total intake of 193 patients over the subsequent year, the staff identified 41 possible fake patients. To which Rosenhan gleefully announced that he had not sent in a single imposter! So he declared that, given psychiatry's inability to tell sane from insane individuals, they were clearly incompetent.

It resulted in the medical insurance companies, like Aetna and Blue Cross, slashing the mental health benefits in their policies. Their complaint, apart from the absurdity of being unable to identify true mental illness, was that in this one specialty, only the patient and psychiatrist could ever know what medical services were provided and why.

I laughed so much, I nearly spilled my Mai Tai!

It may seem I am being harsh but in my view the discipline of psychiatry is a danger to the community and an embarrassment to the medical profession.

Now remember, as you read, I'm not claiming to be an expert in all of these healing mind modalities I will be introducing. I am just an all-rounder who knows the models and knows where to look and what to look for!

I'm a man of logic and method. A no-nonsense teacher (which is what the word doctor actually means). There's a right way to do things and many wrong ways. The only right way, with something as alarming and demoralizing as mental problems, is to go through every single possible correctable cause or reason and treat whatever is found.

Somewhere along the line, it is to be hoped, there will be a resolution, or at least a lightening of the burden. To crush the mind and spirit of the patient with toxic drugs is not the way to do this.

The ultimate purpose in writing this book is two-fold:

1. To wipe out the undeserved reputation of psychiatrists as experts in mental health and help the world at large stop trusting them and their unscientific opinions

2. To get real, effective help for patients who are struggling with the way their mind works; treatment which can change how they feel in the direction of how they would rather feel. It's possible.

OK, let's get started...

PART 1

YOU MUST BE KIDDING ME

1.1 Still Believe In Science?
We'll Fix That Problem For You!

I don't want you to read this book with the idea that the science is all done in the fields of psychology, psychiatry, medicine and biology. It isn't. In fact it's horribly corrupted by fraud, dishonesty and distorting influences from vested interests, such as the pharmaceutical industry. I trust nothing. Let me explain...

According to a famous scientific paper, listening to *When I'm Sixty-Four* by The Beatles can make you younger. This miraculous effect, dubbed "chronological rejuvenation", was revealed in the journal *Psychological Science* in 2011. It wasn't a hoax, the scientists who published the paper were well aware that this "finding" was nonsense but they wanted to make an important point, which was *to show how easy it is to generate phoney statistical evidence for pretty much anything,* simply by picking and choosing methods and data in ways that scientific researchers do every day.[17]

That paper has become the most cited in the history of the journal *Psychological Science.* But worse was to come: the following year, Nobel prizewinning psychologist Daniel

Kahneman published an open email to social psychologists warning of a "train wreck" if they didn't clean up their act.

Then came another nail in the coffin of credibility, a paper in the journal *Science* described a major effort to replicate 100 psychology experiments that had been published in top journals. The attempt was a signal failure: the replication success rate was little more than a third, *meaning that two thirds of all published papers in the field of psychology were worthless* in the kindest estimation—and fake in the most cynical judgment.

People began to talk of a "crisis" in the integrity of psychology science papers.

In fact, this problem is recognized far beyond psychology – dubious results are alarmingly common in most fields of science. But the problem seems to be worst in areas that require judgment and quantification of human well-being; in other words, the science underpinning everyday political, economic and healthcare decisions.

Science is supposed to be a dispassionate search for the truth. But, long ago, we began to suspect that it had hidden agendas, mostly political. We all looked on as scientist after scientist who reported on climate change was fired and replaced by shills who didn't see any problem with global warming.

There was the fiasco of government scientists telling us what to eat for optimum health and then it emerging that the science was deliberately manipulated by the food industry and that people became catastrophically sick as a result.

So where is the objectivity of science today? Does it still exist?

This is a scary concern and it is necessary to ask the question: is fake science being generated deliberately, to justify human population control measures? Are we being subjected to a massive psy op (psychic mass mind control operation) or propaganda campaign, to soften us up for domination, as the Nazis did under Joseph Goebbels?

Some people are angry and think this is so.

The Argument for Naivety

Of course, we are all only human and it is tempting for some to dismiss these widening gulfs in scientific credibility as mere mistakes or investigators being "overambitious". Most people want to climb the professional ladder. The main way to do that if you're a scientist is to publish lots of papers in reputable journals.

The problem is that journals don't like articles proving that something didn't work! They have a clear preference for research showing strong, positive relationships – between a particular medical treatment and improved health, for example. This means researchers often try to find those sorts of results. A few go as far as making things up. But a huge number tinker with their research in ways they justify as harmless, but which can bias the outcome. That means danger for the public and danger for patients, caught in this crosswind of fake findings.

Distorting the results can take many forms. You peek at the results (no longer "blind") and stop an experiment when it shows what you were expecting, before there is a risk the numbers will start to level out and may eventually disprove your pet theory.

Another trick commonly employed, especially by the pharmaceutical companies, is to run several different statistical approaches and select for publication the one that best shows what you are trying to prove, even if all the others contradict that one position.

Or you throw out data points that don't fit your hypothesis, telling yourself that something must be wrong with those particular results.

Then there is "p-hacking. The p-value in statistics tells you how reliable or "significant" the results are. But how reliable is the p-value?

Research published last year by Megan Head and her colleagues at the Australian National University in Canberra scrutinized results from a wide range of scientific disciplines for evidence for "p-hacking" – collecting or selecting data or statistical analyses until non-significant results start to become "significant". They found it to be particularly common in biological sciences. "A lot of biologists go into biology because they don't want to do maths, and then they get a rude shock when they learn they have to do statistics," says Head.[18]

"There's no nefarious motive," Roger Peng at Johns Hopkins University in Baltimore, Maryland, told *New Scientist*. It's just natural to assume these results are likely to be "wrong". That's Peng's opinion. But he's assuming no researchers are influenced by the lure of money and status. I believe they are.

Come on! How bad does it have to be before people start to admit this is a crooked and dishonest path that is corrupting knowledge for self-gain? This is *altogether nefarious*.

Peer Review Not Effective at Spotting Fraud or Bias

You might think that journals, which get peers from the same scientific field to review papers prior to publication, would pick up on such practices. But, say the critics, the system doesn't work like that. "The vast majority don't require that you make any data available beyond a brief description of the methods," says apologist Peng.

Moreover, peer-reviewers don't usually get to see the raw data or a full explanation of the methods. And even if they did, they might not have the time, ability or inclination to check them. Refereeing is unpaid and anonymous work, so there's no reward and no recognition in doing an extra thorough job of it.

All this helps explain why so many studies don't hold up when others try to replicate them. But it doesn't explain why psychology in particular is faced with a plague of dishonesty in its scientific publications.

There's nothing new about researchers being subconsciously committed to proving their own theories, or journals favoring headline-grabbing research. Sure, the pressure on researchers to publish is ever greater, however, what's really new is the scrutiny being given to their published findings. So, is the problem really getting worse, or is it that the dross is beginning to surface for the first time?

Time will tell. Meanwhile, a dark shadow is cast on all such research. Who has the time to check the quality of research of others?

Other Disciplines

Psychology may have borne the brunt of the controversy so far, but statistician John Ioannidis of Stanford University in California has for a long time argued that the problem is widespread in science. In a 2005 paper, he claimed that *sloppy methods could mean more than half of all published scientific results are flawed.*[19]

Some fields of research are less susceptible than others, though. In astronomy, chemistry and physics, for instance, "people have a very strong tradition of sharing data, and of using common databases like big telescopes or high energy physical experiments", Ioannidis says. "They are very cautious about making claims that eventually will be refuted."

But in fields where such checks and balances are absent, irreproducible results are rife and that includes psychology, social sciences, medicine and the pharmaceutical industry.

Take the case of cancer researcher Anil Potti when he was at Duke University in Durham, North Carolina. In 2006, staff at the MD Anderson Cancer Center in Houston, Texas, wanted to investigate treatments based on Potti's published work on gene expression. Before pressing ahead, they asked their colleagues, biostatisticians Keith Baggerly and Kevin Coombes, to look over the findings. It took them almost 2000 hours to disentangle the data and reveal a catalogue of errors. Their efforts illustrate how hard it can be for peer reviewers to pick up on mistakes.[20]

It later transpired that Potti had actually falsified data intentionally, but in the meantime, three clinical trials had been started on the basis of his research.

Evidence is mounting that medical research is particularly prone to "irreproducibility" (meaning it's faked). In 2012, Glenn Begley, a biotech consultant, showed that just 11 percent of the preclinical cancer studies coming out of the academic pipeline that he sampled were replicatable. Another study estimates that irreproducible preclinical research costs the US alone $28 billion a year and slows down the development of life-saving drugs.

"The truth is everyone knew that this was a problem," says Begley. "No one really knew the magnitude of the problem."[21]

The trouble was, the cat was now out of the bag. In 2013 the *Economist* ran a headline proclaiming "Trouble at the lab: Scientists like to think of science as self-correcting. To an alarming degree, it is not".[22] Cleaning Up Their Act

So, what can be done? There has already been a rapid response in one area of research where irreproducible results can have life-or-death consequences. Since 2005, a group of major medical journals has required researchers to publicly register clinical trials, and the methods they intend to use, before recruiting patients. That means researchers can no longer switch tracks to get better results.

John Ioannidis estimates that about half of all clinical trials now are pre-registered, vastly reducing the possibility of flawed work.

Psychologists have also taken matters into their own hands. In 2011, the authors of the *When I'm Sixty-Four* paper – Joseph Simmons and Uri Simonsohn of the University of Pennsylvania and Leif Nelson of the University of California, Berkeley – met with Eric Eich, the newly appointed editor of *Psychological Science*, to discuss the problems facing their discipline. "That was really eye-opening for me," says Eich. "There were a lot of things that were essentially broken."

In January 2014, as a result of its embarrassment, *Psychological Science* began asking researchers more questions about their methods and giving them more space to explain them. It also introduced a "nudge" to reward good practice by displaying badges on papers to recognize those who made data and methods available or pre-registered their study.

The result? Submissions almost vanished overnight! That's how corrupt the industry had become. However, after many months, submission rates started back up again and now some 40 percent of new *Psychological Science* papers have open data – up from 3 percent before the badges were introduced.

Now the idea is gaining legs. In 2015, Nosek and his colleagues came up with guidelines that journals could follow to increase transparency and reproducibility. These have since been endorsed by the US National Institutes of Health, and adopted by more than 500 journals, including *Science*, and 50 organisations. *Nature* has its own guidelines.

Universities may join the movement too. Ioannidis and others are working to create a "coalition of university leaders" to address the problem. "Universities are the gatekeepers of promotion and tenure," he says. "I hope that we will be moving pretty soon on that front." One obvious solution is to stop rewarding scientists on the basis of how much they have published – to consider quality not quantity when making academic promotions.

"It will take years to play out," says Eich. "But hopefully at the end of it, you get more replicable, high-quality science." Given that we fund academic research through our taxes and rely on it to improve our lives, that will be good for everybody.[23]

1.2 Do You Believe In Psychiatry? We Can Cure That Too!

Jon Rappoport is a brilliant investigating journalist and for decades he has been hacking away at the foundation of the fraudulent edifice of modern "evidence-based" medicine. Psychiatry in particular, and the over-arching pharmaceutical industry backing it, comes under his withering scrutiny...

Rappoport describes psychiatry as a fraud, a pseudoscience.

Yet, this "science" is accorded special treatment and licensure and favored status by governments around the world. Why? Because untold numbers of patients can be diagnosed and drugged with highly toxic substances, and even held against their will in closed wards. Dissidents can be contained, using psychiatric justifications, as was done in former Soviet Russia (USSR). Whole populations can be convinced they are either "mentally healthy" or "mentally ill," as if those two fictional categories described some highly significant status.

If psychiatry were merely recognized as an experimental hypothesis, and so-called professionals diagnosed one another and applied labels to one another and drugged one another, in order to assess the outcome, as any scientist would, before subjecting the public to his idiosyncratic notions...well, fine. Anyone could understand that.

But of course, this is not where we find ourselves. Psychiatrists are considered lofty authorities. They are called as expert witnesses in criminal trials. They can, in many cases, arbitrarily force their will on patients. They are called upon by media to render their analyses. They occupy sanctified chairs at universities.

The bible of the psychiatric profession, the DSM (Diagnostic and Statistical Manual of Mental Disorders), published by the American Psychiatric Association, lists some 300 official mental disorders by name, as well as the criteria which allow licensed psychiatrists to diagnose these disorders in patients.

Yet, as I have already pointed out, in the DSM there is not one defining laboratory test for any of those 300 disorders. No blood test, no saliva test, no urine test, no antibody test, no brain scan, no genetic assay... nada... zilch.

This is supposed to be a science.

What we have left are groupings and clusters of behaviors, which committees of psychiatrists have decided constitute specific mental disorders.

Does this seem outrageous? Impossible? Time to wise up.

On April 29, 2013, at the National Institute of Mental Health (NIMH) website, Director Thomas Insel, the highest ranking federal mental health official in the US, published a blog commentary: "Transforming Diagnosis." Insel wrote (4/29/2013):

"In a few weeks, the American Psychiatric Association will release its new edition of the *Diagnostic and Statistical Manual of Mental Disorders* (DSM-5)...

"The strength of each of the editions of DSM has been 'reliability' - each edition has ensured that clinicians use the same terms in the same ways. The weakness is its lack of validity. Unlike our definitions of ischemic heart disease, lymphoma, or AIDS, the DSM diagnoses are based on a consensus about clusters of clinical symptoms, not any objective laboratory measure."

Not any objective laboratory measure.

Again: *Not any objective laboratory measure.*

This is on the order of the US Attorney General holding a press conference and admitting that every one of its criminal prosecutions, going back 70 years, was based on fraudulent cooked evidence.

If you or your child is ever in the presence of a psychiatrist who gets up on his high horse, makes a diagnosis, and tries to foist drugs on you, you might call attention to Thomas Insel's statement, tell the psychiatrist who Insel is, and read his statement out loud, in the sober and somber style of a mortician.

Ditto if you're dealing with a teacher, school counselor, psychologist, or principal who thinks he knows anything at all about "mental health."

Courtesy of Dr. Fred Baughman, Rappoport uncovered two more smoking guns.

The first is a letter, dated November 10, 2008, sent from Supriya Sharma, MD, a director general of Health Canada, to a private citizen (name withheld).

Health Canada is the equivalent of the FDA in America.

Dr. Sharma is "responding on the Minister's behalf"—the Health Minister of Canada, a post roughly comparable to the US Secretary of Health and Human Services.

Here is Dr. Sharma's key passage:

"For mental/psychiatric disorders in general, including depression, anxiety, schizophrenia, and ADHD, there are no confirmatory gross, microscopic or chemical abnormalities that have been validated for objective physical diagnosis."[24]

Dr. Sharma is readily admitting that the diagnosis of mental disorders has no basis in actual science.

Now I have to say I do recognize ADD and ADHD. They really do exist. I've seen parents with terrible problems, trying to raise children with these disorders to a normal life. But then I view both these conditions as entirely treatable and for four decades I have been able to resolve most cases that came to me with detox, diet and nutritional protocols. **I do not try to grab innocent, boisterous children, make this false diagnosis and use it as an excuse to put them on life-devastating drugs, such as ritalin, adderall and the like**.

Dr. Baughman's second smoking gun is an email sent from the FDA, he received dated March 12, 2009. It was written by Donald Dobbs, Consumer Safety Officer, Division of Drug Information, Center for Drug Evaluation and Research. It refers back to Health Canada and smoking gun #1:

"I consulted with the FDA new drug review division responsible for approving psychiatric drug products and they concurred with the response you [Dr. Baughman] enclosed from Health Canada.

"Psychiatric disorders (as Health Canada refers) are diagnosed based on a patient's presentation of symptoms that the larger psychiatric community has come to accept as real and responsive to treatment."

Could there be a better description of unscientific consensus?

Psychiatrists can tap dance all they want to about "remarkable progress," "new breakthroughs," "the need for more research money" and "chemical imbalances," but they're just blowing smoke, says Rappoport.

Perhaps psychiatry qualifies for status as a speculative hypothesis, on the level of "Jesus studied healing in Atlantis"—but in what universe does the profession deserve the unqualified backing of the federal government; the ability, under certain conditions, to have citizens placed in psych-ward lockdowns; and the indulgence of courts to hear testimony from "experts" about the mental state of defendants?

Yes, there are certainly people with severe problems. They show all sorts of signs of these problems. But the causes can stem from a variety of circumstances, and any health practitioner worthy of the name would approach each unique patient to find out what is relevant.

You will learn throughout this book that the vast majority of people who exhibit disturbances of mind are physically ill or deficient in some way; that's *physically ill*, not mentally ill.

But there's more... Oh yes!

Jon Rappoport cites two more pieces of information that attest to the unconscionable embarrassment to the medical profession that is known as psychiatry.

Here's a statement made by a prominent expert on an episode of PBS television's *Frontline* series. The episode title was: "Does ADHD Exist?"

PBS Frontline Interviewer: Skeptics say that there's no biological marker-that it [ADHD] is the one condition out there where there is no blood test, and that no one knows what causes it.

Barkley: (Dr. Russell Barkley, professor of psychiatry and neurology at the University of Massachusetts Medical Center): "That's tremendously naïve, and it shows a great deal of illiteracy about science and about the mental health professions. A disorder doesn't have to have a blood test to be valid. If that were the case, all mental disorders would be invalid...There is no lab test for any mental disorder right now in our science. That doesn't make them invalid." [*my underlining, K S-M*]

Rarely will you hear a scientist make as bold and definitive a statement against his own interests as that one. And Barkley was so egregiously ignorant about what science is that he spoke with blithe confidence.

Science, as opposed to a preferred special interest, demands confirmation of its assertions. That means physical tests. Definitive tests. You claim a disorder exists in the brain, you present a physical test that confirms it.

Again, you can search the entire DSM and try to find one such defining test for a diagnosis of any of the 300 so-called mental disorders, including the old standby, schizophrenia, and you'll go begging. You'll come up empty.

Think of the range and influence and power of psychiatry. Think about its partnership with central governments and pharmaceutical companies. Think about its ability to pronounce people insane or mentally ill, and what it can then coercively force on such hapless persons.

Think about all the politicians and pundits who blithely refer society's problems to the "need for more psychiatric treatment" and "earlier intervention" (with toxic drugs).

The entire profession of psychiatry, from top to bottom, is a staged event. It claims that millions and millions of people, including very young children, are suffering from disorders that have never been proven to exist.

Of course, many will respond with disbelief. "A total fraud? That couldn't be because there are professionals who know science and they say..."

I don't care what they say. I don't care what the consensus is. You want to play the game called science? You play by the rules of the scientific method. Otherwise, get out and play another game. Roll the bones, spatter chicken blood or buy a Ouija board.

Just don't pretend you are engaged in science.

It's All Just Opinion

OK, one more mind-boggling twist, then I'm done. One of the great psychiatric leaders, who has been out in front inventing mental disorders, went public. He blew the whistle on himself and his colleagues.

His name is Dr. Allen Frances, and he made very interesting statements to Gary Greenberg, author of a *Wired* article: "Inside the Battle to Define Mental Illness," (Dec.27, 2010).[25]

Dr. Allen Frances is the man who, in 1994, headed up the project to write the then-latest edition of the psychiatric bible, the DSM-IV.

In an April 19, 1994, *New York Times* piece, "Scientist At Work," Daniel Goleman called Frances "Perhaps the most powerful psychiatrist in America at the moment..."[26]

Well, of course he's "powerful". He's writing the fairy story, laying it out as a canon of diagnosable mental disorders for colleagues, for insurers, for the government, for Bih Pharma (who will sell the drugs matched up to the 297 DSM-IV diagnoses), you're right up there in the pantheon.

Powerful cannot be translated to mean competent, however. It's a joke.

Long after the DSM-IV had been put into print, Dr. Frances talked to *Wired's* Greenberg and said the following:

"There is no definition of a mental disorder. It's bullshit. I mean, you just can't define it."

As Jon Rappoport remarks, that's on the order of the designer of the Hindenburg, looking at the burned rubble on the ground, remarking, "Well, I knew there would be a problem."

1.3 What About The Drugs? You Want To Believe In Those?

Every new diagnosis that is sneaked into the *Diagnostic and Statistical Manual* (DSM) comes with the implication there is a drug which will fix it. Big Pharma wants more diagnoses, so they can sell more drugs.

They care little if the drugs work or cause devastating side effects. What this game is about is respectability. If it's in the Manual, it's "real", so we can cook up some chemistry and claim to treat it.

The sad thing is that psychiatric cases are often already tormented by life and so a few extra layers of misery, unpleasant side-effects, and troubled thinking are easily written off as part of the patients problems. "We don't really have to listen to all these complaints about symptoms being caused by the medication because these people are already judged below rational, medically speaking."

That's the typical doctor or psychiatrist speaking.

Antipsychotic' drugs such as Risperdal, Zyprexa, Seroquel and Geodon are used literally to chemically lobotomize millions of adults and children because the resulting apathy and indifference are seen as an improvement over their previously distressed and distressing state of mind or behavior.

Millions more adults take 'tranquilizers' like Xanax, Ativan, Klonopin and Valium, suppressing their overall brain function in order to reduce feelings of anxiety. A large percentage of our nation's children have their spontaneity reduced or even crushed by stimulant drugs such as Ritalin, Concerta, Adderall and Strattera, causing them to become more docile and more obsessively attentive to rote work (like robots, in other words).

Let me re-introduce Peter Breggin, a humane and brave psychiatrist, who stands out against the abuse of his colleagues (they ignore him). His book of *Brain-Disabling Treatments in Psychiatry* details much of what I'm talking about in this section.[27] According to Breggin, people misunderstand the nature of mind-altering pharmaceuticals. These substances do *not* "fix things"; they damage and shut down key brain pathways. They are designed to do that. "People commonly use alcohol, marijuana and other non-prescription drugs to dull their feelings but they do not fool themselves into believing they are somehow improving the function of their minds and brains. Yet when people take psychiatric drugs, they almost always do so without realizing that the drugs "work" by disrupting brain function, that the drugs cause withdrawal effects, and that they frequently result in dangerous and destructive mental reactions and behaviors.

In *Brain-Disabling Treatments in Psychiatry* Breggin introduces the concept of medication spellbinding—the capacity of psychoactive drugs to blunt the individual's appreciation of drug-induced mental dysfunction and, at times, to encourage a misperception that they are doing better than ever when they are, in fact, doing worse than ever. In the extreme, medication spellbinding drives individuals into bizarre, out-of-character destructive actions, including suicide and violence. Medication spellbinding is an aspect of the brain-disabling principle that explains why so many individuals take drugs of all kinds, from antidepressants to alcohol, when they are causing them great harm and even destroying their lives.

Here are some examples of officially-listed, commonly encountered side-effects of psychiatric drugs:

Adverse effects of Valproate (given for a Bipolar diagnosis) include:
- acute, life-threatening, and even fatal liver toxicity;

- life-threatening inflammation of the pancreas;
- brain damage.

Adverse effects of Lithium (also given for a Bipolar diagnosis) include:

- intercranial pressure leading to blindness;
- peripheral circulatory collapse;
- stupor and coma.

Adverse effects of Risperdal (given for "Bipolar" and "irritability stemming from autism") include:

- serious impairment of cognitive function;
- fainting;
- restless muscles in neck or face, tremors (may be indicative of motor brain damage).

In the 1950s a class of anti-depressant drugs was developed called the monoamine oxidase inhibitor (MAOIs), closely followed by the tri-cyclic anti-depressants (TCAs).

While sometimes effective, both these classes of drugs cause troublesome side effects and have complex, potentially fatal, drug and food interactions. Abnormal heart rhythm is another dangerous complication. Side effects of MAOIs can be quite severe. Their mode of action is to block the breakdown of neurotransmitters like serotonin and norepinephrine, which are known to enhance mood.

What about ADHD? What about Ritalin?

In 1986, *The International Journal of the Addictions* published a most important literature review by Richard Scarnati. It was called "An Outline of Hazardous Side Effects of Ritalin (Methylphenidate)."[28] Scarnati listed a large number of adverse effects of Ritalin. He cited published journal articles which reported each of these symptoms.

For every one of the following Ritalin effects (selected and quoted verbatim), there is at least one confirming source in the medical literature:

- Paranoid delusions
- Paranoid psychosis
- Hypomanic and manic symptoms, amphetamine-like psychosis
- Activation of psychotic symptoms
- Toxic psychosis
- Visual hallucinations
- Auditory hallucinations
- Can surpass LSD in producing bizarre experiences

- Effects pathological thought processes
- Extreme withdrawal
- Terrified affect
- Started screaming
- Aggressiveness
- Insomnia
- Since Ritalin is considered an amphetamine-type drug, expect amphetamine-like effects
- Psychic dependence
- High-abuse potential DEA Schedule II Drug
- Decreased REM sleep
- When used with antidepressants one may see dangerous reactions including hypertension, seizures and hypothermia
- Convulsions
- Brain damage may be seen with amphetamine abuse.

SSRIs (Prozac, Zoloft, etc.) Well-documented side-effects:

- Birth defects, including anencephaly (little or no head and brain)
- Suicide in children and young adults
- Bruising and bleeding
- Hallucinations
- Worsening of irritability
- Nervousness
- Agitation
- Unstable mood
- Sleeplessness
- Nausea and vomiting
- Dizziness
- Erectile dysfunction
- Drowsiness
- Insomnia
- Weight gain or loss
- Headache
- Dry mouth
- Diarrhea

In the US alone, there are at least 300,000 cases of motor brain damage incurred by people who have been prescribed so-called anti-psychotic drugs (aka "major tranquilizers"). Risperdal (mentioned above as a drug given to people diagnosed with Bipolar) is one of those major tranquilizers.[29] Motor brain damage, in case you are wondering, means dysfunction of movements. One of the worst outcomes for patients is tardive dyskinesia: relentless twitching and jerking, every minute of every waking hour, till the patient collapses exhausted in bed at night. This is a notorious side-effect, or should I say permanent damage, from taking tranquillizers of the class benzodiazepines (Valium, etc.), but also including the newer so-called atypical drugs like Risperdal, Zyprexa, Seroquel, Abilify, and Invega. Tardive akathisia is a relentless desire to wriggle and squirm that can be likened to a torture of the patient.

These disorders tend to become irreversible, especially if the drug is continued after the initial symptoms appear. There is no effective treatment.

Oh yes, the psychiatrists were concerned about this—not concerned for the patients, of course, but for themselves. They were worried about getting sued.

On October 7, 1983, the official American Psychiatric Association newspaper, *Psychiatric News*, declared in a headline: TD CASES UNDERSCORE IMPORTANCE OF APA REPORT. It told members that two major cases had set a precedent for settlement for damages, due to tardive dyskinesia, at $760,000 and $1 million (1983 values).

Psychiatrists were warned again in January 1984 by another professional rag *Clinical Psychiatry News* to expect: A FLOOD OF TARDIVE DYSKINESIA MALPRACTICE LAW SUITS.

How many? Well the APA's own task force, in July 1985, estimated that at least 10 – 20% of patients in mental hospitals and at least 40% of longer term patients would get more than minimal signs of tardive dyskinesia.

A Sad, Sad Story

This is from Peter Breggin's book, *Toxic Psychiatry*. I warn you, it's grim:

"Roberta was a college student, getting good grades, mostly A's, when she first became depressed and sought psychiatric help at the recommendation of her university health service. She was eighteen at the time, bright and well-motivated, and a very good candidate for psychotherapy. She was going through a sophomore-year identity crisis about dating men, succeeding in school, and planning a future. She could have thrived with the help of a sensitive therapist.

"Instead of moral support and insight, her doctor gave her Haldol. Over the next four years, six different physicians watched her deteriorate neurologically without warning her or her family about tardive dyskinesia and without making the [tardive dyskinesia] diagnosis, even when she was overtly twitching in her arms and legs. Instead they switched her from one neuroleptic to another, including Navane, Stelazine, and Thorazine. Eventually a rehabilitation therapist became concerned enough to send her to a general physician, who made the diagnosis [of medical drug damage]. By then she was permanently physically disabled, with a loss of 30 percent of her IQ.

"...my medical evaluation described her condition: Roberta is a grossly disfigured and severely disabled human being who can no longer control her body. She suffers from extreme writhing movements and spasms involving the face, head, neck, shoulders, limbs, extremities, torso, and back—nearly the entire body. She had difficulty standing, sitting, or lying down, and the difficulties worsen as she attempts to carry out voluntary actions. At one point, she could not prevent her head from banging against nearby furniture. She could hold a cup to her lip only with great difficulty. Even her respiratory movements are seriously afflicted so that her speech comes out in grunts and gasps amid spasms of her respiratory muscles...

"Roberta may improve somewhat after several months off the neuroleptic drugs, but she will never again have anything remotely resembling a normal life."[30]

"It is no exaggeration to call tardive dyskinesia a widespread epidemic and possibly the worst medically-induced catastrophe in history."[31]

Telephone Exchange Model

Not only do psychotropic drugs cause such extensive damage; they basically do not work. Let me share my telephone exchange model.

If you are receiving a lot of telephone complaints, unwanted and abusive calls, there is one way you could solve it all:

Bomb the telephone exchange! That would wipe out the wiring system and equipment, kill the operators and wreak havoc, preventing any more unwanted calls. Problem solved! But not the way you would want it solved. Remember, all the abusive of complaining callers are out there. Nobody is happy. Nothing is solved. You just interrupted the flow of bad news, that's all.

The brain is like a communication exchange system; a very subtle one. If you drop a bomb in the brain, it will malfunction and maybe the patient will no longer be able to complain. He or she will still feel bad. But they won't be talking to you; you have "cured" him or her.

We all know that's baloney (except that psychiatrists live by this model).

Despite all the propaganda, antidepressants such Prozac, Paxil, Zoloft and Cymbalta have no scientifically demonstrable effectiveness and are proven to cause suicidality, as well as violence and mania. They too 'work' by causing mental disabilities such as apathy and euphoria that are misinterpreted as improvements. They block spontaneous and coherent communication. This is the "bomb in the telephone exchange" model.

Meanwhile, their continued widespread use is determined in part by the fact that withdrawal produces severe psychiatric symptoms, including anxiety and depression. In short, it is too difficult and painful for people to stop taking them.

That's the trouble: All psychiatric drugs have the potential to cause withdrawal reactions, including the antidepressants, stimulants, tranquilizers, antipsychotic drugs and 'mood stabilizers' such as lithium.

When the individual's condition grows markedly worse within days or weeks of stopping the psychiatric drug, this is almost always due to a withdrawal reaction. However, misinformed doctors and misled parents, teachers and patients think that this is evidence that the individual 'needs' the drug even more, when in fact he or she needs time to recover from withdrawal effects.

It perpetuates the myth that drugs are "working".

This psychiatric drug plague is accelerating across the land. See the website: SSRIStories. org for accounts of people committing suicide and homicide while on (or dangerously withdrawing from) drugs like Prozac, Zoloft, and Paxil.

1.4 The Rise and Rise Of Biological Psychiatry

Biological psychiatry is a contradictory term (an oxymoron, actually) and I do not want you to confuse that concept with what are the majority of teachings in this book. My stand, backed by torrents of workable science, is that the vast majority of psychiatric and mental health issues are not mental at all but based on disordered metabolism, be that food allergies, nutritional deficiencies, hormonal imbalances, heavy metal poisoning, chemical sensitivity, Candida, parasites (weird feelings, hallucinations, pains) or a host of other *correctable* physical conditions that—unlike psychiatric diagnoses—can be identified with proper science-based testing and remedies by simply reversing the pathology process.

In other words, such individuals are NOT mentally ill. You might just as well say someone who popped LSD and had weird hallucinations was mentally ill. That's obviously not true; a physical substance caused the hallucinations, not mental or psychiatric disease.

No drug "treatment" of such ills is needed, only rectification of the physical problem found. In my example, all that would be required is for the individual to stop taking the LSD—no more hallucinations—problem solved! The proposition of a cure is that no further symptoms are encountered and no other treatment is required. The task is over. The patient is now satisfied.

That's my model: *physical organic disease creating psychological disturbance and distress.*

Now, despite the name, biological psychiatry is poles apart from what may be called the holistic psychiatry concept. It posits the idea that all mental illness is caused by some kind of chemical imbalance—too much dopamine, too little serotonin and so on. All we have to do is correct the imbalance and the patient will recover. Boom. Magic.

Unfortunately, there is a little too much magic. For one thing, all modern psychiatrists go straight to the prescription pad and never even investigate to see first if the patient has any correctable organic disease. But the most important failure of their model is they do not, and cannot, test for any such biological imbalance... *because these have been shown repeatedly not to exist.* It's a myth. A fairy story. Or a lie, if you want it unvarnished.

This will shock most readers who will naturally want to be reassured that I'm writing nonsense here. This must have all been proven by science, surely? Medicine has advanced steadily, through the application of sound science. You couldn't get 100,000 psychiatrists from all round the world to keep up this pretense, if indeed what I am saying is true.

But you'd be wrong. I'm going to advance abundant proof that psychiatry has nothing to offer that stands up to scrutiny. You also need to be aware that a growing number of psychiatrists themselves are disturbed by the status quo and completely reject the "chemical imbalance" model as the cause of mental ills.

How did all this nonsense take root then? To understand that, we need to look at some history.

History

It all started with the drug chlorpromazine (Thorazine, USA; Largactil elsewhere), launched in 1954. Up to that point it could be argued that psychiatry wasn't a medical science at all; it was just a system of controlling distressed patients and a pretty cruel and grim one at that. There are twentieth-century historical accounts of patients locked up, living in filth, often naked or with only rags to wear; women even being strapped to beds and trolleys while they were molested; demented individuals chanting, screaming and moaning; all rounded out with the stench of urine and feces.

Yes, it would have turned the reader's stomach. But in the day this monumental abuse was kept secret. Few ever saw the Belsen-like conditions in a psychiatric ward. It was just people farming, the souls of men and women were shorn from them, as they were processed like meat and churned out the other end dead or so incapacitated they could not reasonably complain.

Treatments varied from the ridiculous to the cruel: high pressure hoses, prolonged baths, injections of metallic salts, horse serum and even arsenic. Henry Cotton, superintendent at Trenton State Hospital in New Jersey, reported in 1916 that he cured insanity by removing the patients' teeth... one has little hope that the anesthesia was adequate.

The surroundings were equally disgusting: leaking roofs, moldy walls, damp and rotting floors, where grossly overcrowded patients were obliged to sprawl, for lack of seats or beds.[32] Eventually really desperate measures were introduced, like insulin coma therapy, electroconvulsion therapy and that abhorrence of all right-thinking doctors: lobotomy (permanently tearing up the patient's forebrain, so the patient could no longer protest, and yet calling that a remedy). This grotesque mutilation was nicknamed "surgery of the soul" by the *New York Times* in one of its more lyrical moments. Amputation of the soul, more like.

It wasn't until after the Second World War that matters began to significantly improve. The National Institute of Mental Health was formed in the USA to oversee reforms. But changes were slow and understanding of mental illness fell far behind the enthusiasm generated by post-war euphoria. It was not an exaggeration to state that, up until mid-twentieth century, treatment of hospitalized psychiatric patients was not in any real sense a medical science.

Moreover, psychiatry is a peculiar specialty in which the patient's interests are not necessarily paramount. Considerations for other family members entered into "treatments"; social issues were included, like "public safety"; and, of course, there was a legislative interest in what was done with mental health patients. The public had to be protected.

Now, suddenly in 1954, psychiatry had a drug! A real treatment! It was now a proper medical discipline. Troublesome patients could be whacked on the head with a chemical cosh, which would render them quiet and manageable.

Chlorpromazine was immediately billed as the "penicillin" of psychiatry or the equivalent of insulin for fighting diabetes. Unlike barbiturates and opiates, chlorpromazine did not cause generalized brain suppression (sleep and unconsciousness), which is potentially dangerous. This was the birth of what has become known as psychopharmacology. There were miracles in the making. Diseases such as depression, anxiety and psychosis were real and exact and the new treatment knocked out the pathological problem without harming the patient. It was a cure! (I'm being heavily ironic here).

French Navy surgeon Henri Laborit spoke of this advance at a conference in Brussels and described the tranquillizing effect of chlorpromazine as "a veritable medicinal lobotomy." How apt this expression really was you will come to realize before the end of this section.

Well, that was the public perception of the time, fueled by media frenzy and not a little dishonesty among scientists jostling for power, money and prestige. The latter half of the twentieth century was a time when the public was gulled into believing in the boundless wonders of science and its inevitable goodness. Certainly the idea of fake or fraudulent science had not surfaced.

Remember also at this time the use of insulin, vitamin B12, cortisol and above all antibiotics had exploded on the world stage and people were being kept alive by drugs who would surely have died in the past. It did seem that pharmacology was the answer to diseases. There was an expectation that a drug intervention could be developed for virtually every ill.

When *Time* magazine suggested chlorpromazine was a "wonder drug" and lavished praise on it, even stating that patients willingly took the pills and once they did, they fed themselves heartily and lapsed into deep and satisfying sleep, the public and the medical profession bought it, hook, line and sinker.[33] With the media spewing such praise, why would anyone bother with the science behind this? Now, with twenty-twenty hindsight, we can dispassionately examine the true history of antipsychotic drugs, tranquillizers and other neuroleptics (the latter means drugs which take hold of the nervous system and quell it).

The Treated Patient

French psychiatrists Jean Delay and Pierre Deniker, who introduced the use of chlorpromazine in psychiatry, described the "psychic syndrome" induced by chlorpromazine, in a series of articles published in 1952:

Seated or lying down, the patient is motionless on his bed, often pale and with lowered eyelids. He remains silent most of the time. If questioned, he responds after a delay, slowly, in an indifferent monotone, expressing himself with few words and quickly becoming mute. Without exception, the response is generally valid and pertinent, showing that the subject is capable of attention and of reflection. But he rarely takes the initiative of asking a question; he does not express his preoccupations, desires, or preference. He is usually conscious of the amelioration brought on by the treatment, but he does not express euphoria. The apparent indifference or the delay of the response to external stimuli, the emotional and affective neutrality, the decrease in both initiative and preoccupation without alteration in conscious awareness or in intellectual faculties constitute the psychic syndrome due to the treatment.[34]

This doesn't really sound like a happy state, does it? In fact, Delay and Deniker concluded that chlorpromazine induced deficits similar to *encephalitis lethargica*, a degenerative and often fatal illness thought to be due to a virus and which was the subject of Oliver Sacks book "Awakenings", (also made into a movie starring Robert de Niro and Robin Williams).[35]

Nearly five million people were affected by this famous "outbreak" of encephalitis, a third of whom died in the acute stages. Many of those who survived never returned to their pre-existing "aliveness". "They would be conscious and aware - yet not fully awake; they would sit motionless and speechless all day in their chairs, totally lacking energy, impetus, initiative, motive, appetite, affect or desire; they registered what went on about them without active attention, and with profound indifference. They neither conveyed nor felt the feeling of life; they were as insubstantial as ghosts, and as passive as zombies."[36]

It was worse than that because patients gradually deteriorated into a profound Parkinson's-like state. And guess what? That's what happens to patients on this type of drug (phenothiazines) long-term. It's a condition I described already, called tardive dyskinesia (section 1.3).

The "Next Big Thing"

In 1955 Wallace Laboratories brought Miltown to the market. It was an anxiolytic, meaning it dissolved anxiety. It was soon followed by me-too drugs and brands. Hoffman-La Roche developed chlordiazepoxide and started selling it in 1960, as Librium.

Its running-mate Valium (diazepam) was soon born and sales went stratospheric. The Age of Tranquillizers was born. This new class of drugs were known by their chemical name as the benzodiazepines. They were said to be safe and non-addictive, something we now know to be totally untrue. Yet for several decades they were handed out like candies at the least excuse. The whirlwind of pain that was to come was not recognized for a long time, except for a few cautious physicians.

Another group of compounds started with iproniazid, originally developed as an anti-tuberculosis drug. Respiratory physicians noticed that patients tended to become euphoric while being treated for TB using this compound or another very like it (imipramine). So it was sold as an antidepressant, Tofranil, from 1958. Soon afterwards came amitripyline (Elavil). This new class of drugs became known as the tri-cyclic antidepressants (TCAs). Very quickly it became clear they were toxic and dangerous. Serious side effects included seizures, an increased risk of suicide in those under 25 years of age, agranulocytosis, thrombocytopenia, eosinophilia, leukopenia, urinary retention, glaucoma, and a number of heart issues.[37] Nevertheless, amitriplyline has stayed. It is on the WHO Model List of Essential Medicines, even today.

The armory of psychiatric medications was growing apace. By 1967, one in three American adults was on some kind of "psychoactive" medication.[38] This "first generation" of antipsychotic drugs, as they were known, created a drug-induced brain pathology by blocking the neurotransmitter dopamine and essentially shutting down many higher brain functions. The search for something better was on!

Eventually, as we all know, Prozac was born and in 1986 the world changed!

Prozac Heaven

Fluoxetine (Prozac) is one of a class of drugs called selective serotonin re-uptake inhibitors, known more commonly by the abbreviation SSRIs. The "imbalance" theory argues that depression in caused by a significant lack of serotonin, the "happy" neurotransmitter. In fact this is scientific nonsense, as we shall see soon.

But that is the biological psychiatry explanation. It follows therefore that boosting serotonin levels will cheer up the depressed patient. As a result, we saw an explosion of this class of "anti-depressants": sertraline (Zoloft), citalopram (Celexa), citalopram (Lexapro), paroxetine (Paxil, Pexeva), fluvoxamine (Luvox) and trazodone (Oleptro), to name the main ones.

These are now considered second generation anti-depressants. But do they work any better, or are they any less toxic, than the first generation drugs they replace?

It emerged in time that Eli Lilly (Prozac's manufacturer) had covered up the severe complications and side-effects of fluoxetine. The drug caused mania, tendency to suicide and murderous violence in a significant number of the individuals who took it. *One FDA reviewer even warned that Prozac appeared to be a dangerous drug, but it was approved anyway*. How wicked is that?

Eli Lilly's shady tactic was simply to cover up the problems. This is they did in a number of ways. One trick was just to simply remove reports of psychosis from some of the data. They also went back and "recoded" some of the trial results. Let's say someone had a manic episode or a psychotic episode; instead of putting that down, they would just put down a return of depression, and that sort of thing.[39] Thus, within one decade, there were 39,000 adverse reports about Prozac that were sent to the USA Medwatch reporting system. There were more adverse event reports received about Prozac in its first two years on the market than had been reported on the leading toxic tricyclic antidepressant in 20 years. By the way, the FDA tries to keep these adverse reports from the public, so it's very hard to get the real data from their website. And now Google has joined the covert ops, hiding "inappropriate" data from the public.

Remember, Prozac is pitched to the American public as this wonderfully safe drug, so what are people complaining about: trivial headaches and mildly off-color? No! Mania, psychotic depression, nervousness, anxiety, agitation, hostility, hallucinations, memory loss, tremors, impotence, convulsions, insomnia, nausea, suicidal impulses. It's a wide range of serious symptoms.

And here's the kicker. It wasn't just Prozac. Once we got the other SSRIs on the market, like Zoloft and Paxil, by 1994 antidepressants were among the top 20 most complained about drugs on the FDA's Medwatch list. In other words, every one of these drugs brought to market started triggering mania, hallucinations, psychotic depression, and other serious adverse events.

People got murdered. Consider...

Did you know that mass shootings are almost all the acts of people crazed on psychiatric drugs, notably SSRIs?:

1. Myron May, November 2014, Tallahassee (Hydroxyzine, Wellbutrin, Seroquel)

2. Aaron Ybarra, June 2014, Seattle, (Prozac)

3. Jose Teyes, October 2013, Sparks, Nevada (Prozac)

4. Matti Saari, September 2008, Kauhajoki, Finland (SSRI and a benzodiazepine)

5. Richard Lopez, January 2001, Oxnard, California (Prozac and Paxil)

6. Eric Harris and Dylan Klebold, April 1999, Columbine, Colorado. Harris was on Luvox (Klebold's records remain sealed)

7. Toby Sincino, October 1995, Blackville, South Carolina (Zoloft)

8. Adam Lanza, 2014, Sandy Hook Elementary School, (Calexa, Lexapro)

The list of mass murders "goes on and on", as they say.

The cover-up attempt tries to argue that it's not the drugs that trigger the violence; it's the mental illness that is being treated. They say that there are many more that need treatment to prevent these tragedies.

Yet Dr. David Healy, an internationally known psychiatrist and expert on psychopharmacology, stated that pretty much any psychotropic drug can trigger violence up to and including homicide. According to Dr. Healy, if the depression caused the violence, then we should not find that ninety percent of school shootings are associated with psychotropic drugs.

Big Pharma Cover Up

Beware the science of someone who is trying to sell something has been my lifelong cynical maxim. Nothing exemplifies this more than the massive cover up attempts at showing their dollar-busting drugs are not just ineffective but outright dangerous.

Big Pharma insists it is unaware of drugs' true risks until a wide swath of the population uses them and "safety signals" emerge. Facts sometimes suggest this is disingenuous. In many cases, the Pharma companies "discover" the real problems only after their drug patent has finally expired.

Years before the label of the antipsychotic Seroquel was changed in 2011 to warn the drug "should be avoided" in combination with at least 12 other medications because of heart risks, at least 99 articles in the U.S. National Library of Medicine linked the drug to "sudden death", "QT prolongation" (a heart disturbance that can lead to death), "cardiac arrest" and "death."

Then there's Paxil. Paroxetine was a top selling SSRI antidepressant drug for GlaxoSmithKline during the "happy pill" craze when Big Pharma was telling everyone they had "depression." But in 2004, soon after its approval, the New York Attorney General charged that research about the drug published in the *Journal of the American Academy of Child and Adolescent Psychiatry* (known as "Study 329") buried the drug's true risks of suicide in adolescents.

There were also questions about where the research appeared. *The Journal of the American Academy of Child and Adolescent Psychiatry* is a publication of the American Academy of Child and Adolescent Psychiatry which lists the funders of its "treatment guidelines" for children and adolescents with bipolar disorder as Abbott, AstraZeneca, Eli Lilly, Forest, Janssen, Novartis and Pfizer.

There could not be a more outrageous conflict of interest. It's mind-boggling crime *and they get away with it*. Not one Big Pharma executive has ever been jailed for mass slaughter with lies.

And there were more questions about the Paxil research. Former Boston Globe reporter Alison Bass and others reported that the paper was not even written by the 22 doctors and researchers listed as "authors" but by a medical communication company hired by GSK.

In 2006, "author" Martin Keller, former Professor Emeritus of Psychiatry at Brown, acknowledged that GSK had given him tens of thousands of dollars during and after the time the study was conducted.

Then, in September 2015, when many reporters, psychiatrists, researchers and professors had given up the Paxil fight, the *British Medical Journal* (BMJ) published a reanalysis that amounted to a reversal of the original study. The new research demonstrated that Paxil indeed increases risks of suicide in young people and adolescents.

But many pill-pushing doctors continue to fight evidence of Paxil's suicide risks and similar SSRIs. "There is a very reasonable possibility that it has discouraged patients from taking antidepressants and physicians from prescribing these medications [and] the government should rescind the black-box warning on antidepressants altogether," Richard A. Friedman, a professor of clinical psychiatry at Weill Cornell Medical wrote in the New York Times a month before the Paxil reanalysis.[40]

The Science Doesn't Hold Up

OK, you argue; the psychotropic drugs you are writing about are maybe crap. But that doesn't mean the biochemical imbalance theory is faulty, does it? Yes it does.

"Chemical imbalance" has become the watchword for the new chemical psychiatry. Patients are told they have it virtually upon entering the clinic; this despite the fact there is no known test for such a condition, as I have said.

Let's look at the real science. Remember in the sections that follow, that this is psychiatry's own research I'm quoting, not the ranting of some AIDS-denialist type folks.

This isn't a lesson in psychobiology so let's just take a quick peek into the research to show serotonin lack (depression) and dopamine excess (psychosis). What's the evidence?

The staggeringly complex human brain, with its 100 billion neurons and 150 trillion synapses, was boiled down to just one little problem (don't laugh yet): not enough serotonin. That's it! This is the "cause" of depression. Not enough was being released at the synapses or too much was re-absorbed too fast. So, all we would have to do is block the re-uptake of serotonin and the patient would be magically cured. Hence: SSRIs, selective serotonin re-uptake inhibitors.

But is it true? Investigators couldn't study serotonin at the synapses; the reactions were too fast, almost instant. So, they elected to test for 5-hydroxyindole acetic acid (5HIAA). By testing for quantities in the cerebrospinal fluid (the fluid that bathes the brain, spinal cord and meninges), they could *it was claimed* have a measure of how deficient the depressed patient might be.

In 1969, Malcolm Bowers at Yale University was the first to report: 5HIAA levels were not "significantly" lower in depressives. Two years later, a team at McGill University said they too have failed to find any significant difference in levels.

Not sounding good for the theory! In fact Bowers was back in 1974 and found that *depressed patients who had not taken antidepressants had absolutely normal levels of serotonin.*

The serotonin theory was about to be declared dead, when in 1975 Marie Asberg and colleagues at the Karolinska Institute in Stockholm, Sweden, claimed to have found a "subgroup" of depressed patients (20 out of 68 eight patients) who did, on average, have lower serotonin levels. The next thing you know US psychiatrists were writing that one third of depressed patients (20/68, remember) had low serotonin levels.

But this is a story of complete wishful thinking. Re-examining Asberg's data, it was obvious that the "normal" controls also had variable levels of cerebrospinal 5HIAA. There was no difference in this distribution between the controls and the patients. What we call the bell curve was the same in both groups. In fact half the depressed patients had serotonin levels *above* the median level! She had DISPROVEN the serotonin hypothesis, not found a significant sub-group.[41]

The theory had one more shot at life in 1984, when NIMH investigators under James Maas looked at whether amitriptyline responders had low serotonin levels, as the theory would predict. They did not. In Maas's words, "Contrary to expectations, no relationships between cerebrospinal fluid 5-HIAA and response to amitriptyline were found".[42]

Maybe the dopamine excess theory of schizophrenia and psychosis would have more luck?

Antipsychotic drugs were claimed to lower dopamine levels and thus benefit psychosis. So the first order of business was to see if that was correct.

It wasn't. True, they found two dopamine receptors, called D1 and D2. Antipsychotics blocked 70-90% of the D2 receptors. So far so good.

But the same Malcolm Bowers almost immediately blew that out of the water, by announcing he could find no levels of dopamine metabolites in unmedicated schizophrenics. The key word is *unmedicated* (untreated) patients. Dopamine is metabolized to homovanillic acid (HVA) and it should therefore appear in excess quantity in the cerebrospinal fluid. None was found.

"Our findings," Bowers wrote, "do not furnish neurochemical evidence for over-arousal in these patients, emanating from a midbrain dopamine system."[43]

Others soon published similar findings. In 1975, Robert Post at the NIMH reported that HVA in 20 unmedicated schizophrenics were not significantly different from normals.[44]

Autopsies looking at schizophrenic brains also failed to find abnormal levels of dopamine.

So, since dopamine levels were entirely normal in schizophrenics, the next step in trying to nail this twisted theory in place was to turn attention on the dopamine receptors. Maybe they had too many receptors? If so, they might be hypersensitive to dopamine.

Bingo! In 1978 Philip Seeman at the University of Toronto announced in *Nature* that this was so. At autopsy, the brains of 20 schizophrenics had 70 percent more D2 receptors. But Seeman was no fool and realized that the increased number of D2 receptors might have resulted from the long-term administration of neuroleptic drugs.[45] A number of studies eventually confirmed that this was indeed the case. When rats were fed neuroleptics, their D2 receptors quickly increased in number.[46]

If rats were given a drug that blocked D receptors, that receptor subtype increased in density.[47] That's quite logical: if the D2 receptors are interfered with, the body reacts by trying to impose more receptors.

Finally, investigators in France, Sweden, and Finland used positron emission tomography to study D2-receptor densities in living patients who had never been exposed to neuroleptics, and all reported "no significant differences" between the schizophrenics and "normal controls."[48] [49] [50] [51]

It comes down to this:

"The low-serotonin hypothesis of depression and the high-dopamine hypothesis of schizophrenia had always been the twin pillars of the chemical-imbalance theory of mental disorders, and by the late 1980s, both had been found wanting. Other mental disorders have also been touted to the public as diseases caused by chemical imbalances, but there was never any evidence to support those claims."[52] The Drugs Don't Work!

The truth is that biological psychiatry is washed out; it's a fraud. Its perpetrators are guilty of abuse, dishonesty and outright professional negligence. The psychiatric associations, government regulators, the World Health Organization, individual doctors and the trillion-dollar might of the pharmaceutical industry are backing a criminal scam.

That's the only way that continued prescription of drugs that are based on a discredited theory, are proven not to work and have ample evidence of being dangerous could be explained. These people don't even believe their own story.

Dr. Ronald Pies, the editor-in-chief emeritus of the *Psychiatric Times*, made this startling admission in the July 11, 2011, issue; "Psychiatry's New Brain-Mind and the Legend of the 'Chemical Imbalance'"

"In truth, the 'chemical imbalance' notion was always a kind of urban legend - never a theory seriously propounded by well-informed psychiatrists."

For decades, the whole basis of psychiatric drug research, drug prescription, and drug sales has been: "we're correcting a chemical imbalance in the brain." Now the editor-in-chief of a major professional journal says it's basically a hoax; an urban legend, for goodness' sake!

Dr. Pies continues with this fatuous remark:

"In the past 30 years, I don't believe I have ever heard a knowledgeable, well-trained psychiatrist make such a preposterous claim [about chemical imbalance in the brain], except perhaps to mock it...the 'chemical imbalance' image has been vigorously promoted by some pharmaceutical companies, often to the detriment of our patients' understanding."

His claim is a total falsehood. First of all, many psychiatrists have explained and continue to explain to their patients that the drugs are there to correct a chemical imbalance. They must know this is not true. Therefore they are liars and fraudsters.

And second, if all well-trained psychiatrists have known, all along, that the chemical-imbalance theory is a fraud, then why on earth have they been prescribing tons of drugs to their patients, since those drugs are developed on the false premise that they correct an imbalance?

Wild Off-Label Prescribing Of Antipsychotics

Don't think the problem is confined to legal, supposedly scientific prescribing. There are tens of millions of prescriptions filled every year which bear no relation to what the powerful psychotropic drugs are supposed to do. Or prescriptions which violate scientific integrity, even given the scanty science backing of Big Pharma's peddled drugs.

This is called off-label prescribing, meaning using the drug for a purpose it is not designed to fulfill.

One study of primary care records published by the *British Medical Journal* has revealed that more than half of the prescriptions for antipsychotics in the United Kingdom are prescribed to individuals with no diagnosis of a serious mental illness at all. [53]

This is shocking in itself.

Investigators at University College London also found that off-label antipsychotic prescribing is more likely to occur in women, older people, and socially and economically disadvantaged individuals (to shut them up, of course).

"In this study of antipsychotic prescribing in a large primary care database representative of the UK, approximately half of the prescriptions for first-generation and second-generation antipsychotics are issued to people who have no record of serious mental illness...in their clinical notes," the researchers, led by Louise Marston, PhD, write.

International and national guidelines urge caution concerning the use of antipsychotics; for patients who do not have a diagnosis of psychosis, their use is recommended only in a limited number of cases.

"Furthermore, they are more likely to be prescribed to older people, who may be more sensitive to adverse effects, such as movement disorders and cardiometabolic risk," they add.

The drugs are associated with serious adverse effects, including extrapyramidal symptoms (read: tardive dyskinesia) with first-generation antipsychotics and weight gain and lipid/glucose dysregulation with second- generation agents. Moreover, antipsychotics may be linked to increased rates of stroke and all-cause mortality in patients with dementia.

This makes them wholly inappropriate and even dangerous, yet doctors and health care staff go on prescribing these wretched drugs to that most vulnerable population: the elderly.

Of course when there is trouble—the patient gets very sick, distressed or wild—it's great. All the attendants have to do is blame the patient's age. "He/she was senile. What do you expect?" which nicely diverts from the harm these drugs are capable of.

Speculating on the possible explanations for the high rate of antipsychotic prescribing to people without a psychotic diagnosis, the team dismisses the notion that it is due to psychotic disorders going unrecorded in the notes, either because of patient preference or to avoid stigma.

"It may be that clinicians and/or mental health professionals quite frequently add antipsychotics to the treatment plan for people with non-psychotic disorders, either for agitation, poor sleep or anxiety or due to their general reputation as tranquilizing medications," the authors note.

In truth, the elderly in care are often subject to what I would call chemical coshing: hitting them over the head with a drug to knock them out, so the patient is no further trouble; in fact quite easy to manage for criminally lazy and inattentive attendants.

It's shabby and frightening. Don't get old! Or if you do, make sure you are taken care of at home, with people who love you and care.

Sadly, for hundreds of millions of elderly individuals, they are sold into care management in a system which is not unlike slavery and exploitation.

1.5 Do You Trust The Prescribers and Care Attendants?

It's healthy to berate the pharmaceutical industry for its crimes and dishonesty; to attack the ruthless incompetence of academic science that claims to understand the mind's working and (even more dishonestly) claims to understand the process when it's broken.

But that doesn't cover all the difficulties. There is the matter of who is administering the pills: literally, giving out the pills? This layer is a source of constant danger to the supposed mentally ill patient.

It's not just Big Pharma lies and fake science that dirty the waters here: it's phoneys and incompetents in the mental health profession, who abound everywhere, it seems.

Take the Adam Lanza case (the Sandy Hook Elementary School shooting in Newtown, CT). It emerged that Lanza was being supervised by a dangerous incompetent by the name of Kathleen Koenig, a nurse specialist in psychiatry at Yale. While seeing her, Adam tried Lexapro, which psychiatrist Dr. Paul Fox had prescribed.

Lanza's mother, Nancy Lanza, reported to Koenig, "On the third morning he complained of dizziness. By that afternoon he was disoriented, his speech was disjointed, he couldn't even figure out how to open his cereal box. He was sweating profusely…it was actually dripping off his hands. He said he couldn't think…He was practically vegetative." This stuff is supposed to help? It's a joke.

Later the same day, Nancy Lanza wrote, "He did nothing but sit in his dark room staring at nothing." Arrogant Kathleen Koenig wasn't listening and apparently pooh-poohed these concerns stating, "He had a biological disorder and needed medication," she claimed. Ultimately, it seems that Koenig labeled Nancy Lanza "non-compliant," when in reality this mother was acting responsibly.

But now it gets interesting: according to the State Police Report, Koenig acknowledges that she had prescribed Adam Lanza the mind-altering drug, Celexa, and that Nancy Lanza had "immediately" reported what she believed to be serious adverse reactions to the drug. Yet the Lexapro incident apparently was not reported to investigators by Koenig, subsequent to the shooting. What was she hiding? Just her own dangerous incompetence?

Koenig was clearly in over her head and had far too much freedom and power: she apparently prescribed a "small dose" of Calexa, which had disastrous effects and then concealed the fact.

Immediately after the Calexa, Koenig received a phone call from Nancy Lanza which reported her son was "unable to raise his arm." Nancy Lanza was reporting her son was attributing this symptom to the medication. Koenig attempted to convince Nancy Lanza that the medication was not causing any purported symptoms which Adam Lanza might be experiencing. That's the kind of scary ignorance and incompetence I am seeking to highlight here.

Adam Lanza stopped attending and Koenig contacted Dr. Paul Fox, who agreed that his behavioral-based therapy would remain the primary course of treatment for Adam Lanza. But Lanza never showed for any further treatments.

So did Kathleen Koenig's massive "fail" lead to the deaths of twenty children and six adults at the Sandy Hook school that fateful day? I think probably, yes. But it cannot be proven.

As an aside, on the theme of general trustworthiness and competence, in 2012 Lanza's primary psychiatrist Dr. Paul Fox was accused of having sexual relations with his patients, surrendered his license to practice medicine in New York and Connecticut, destroyed his records and moved to New Zealand.[54]

How Bad Can It Get?

In a 2014 case, a psychiatrist settled out of court for $700,000 damages, after an expert witness (Dr. Peter Breggin, no less) found within a reasonable degree of medical certainty that the psychiatrist in question had committed the following negligent acts:

(a) Prescribing antipsychotic drugs for five years when they were not indicated or needed. The drugs included Risperdal, Seroquel and Zyprexa.

(b) Failing to taper and discontinue from Risperdal during years of exposure.

(c) Failing to warn the patient about the side effects of Risperdal, Seroquel and Zyprexa, including the dangers of tardive dyskinesia/tardive akathisia, and failing to educate the patient and family so that they could properly recognize the earliest signs of tardive dyskinesia/tardive akathisia.

(d) Failing to obtain informed consent.

(e) Continuing to prescribe the offending drugs after the patient began to show signs of tardive dyskinesia.

(f) Failing to properly re-evaluate, examine and assess the need for Risperdal periodically; and failing to record in the medical record these procedures and a plan for evaluating and discontinuing the medication.

(g) Failing to have or to display sufficient knowledge about the use of a neuroleptic such as Risperdal.

(h) Failing to conduct routine, periodic examinations for tardive dyskinesia and failing to record them in the record.

(i) Resuming neuroleptic treatment for a full year with Seroquel and Zyprexa after he recorded the diagnosis of tardive dyskinesia in the medical record.

That's a catalogue of criminal negligence and incompetence. Are we supposed to believe this doctor was a one-off case? That's what the profession would like us to think. But why should we believe that?

Mark well the words of British psychiatrist R D Laing (pronounced lane):

I am still more frightened by the fearless power in the eyes of my fellow psychiatrists than by the powerless fear in the eyes of their patients.

R D Laing (much loved by the 60s "freedom generation") was an old-fashioned sort of psychiatrist. "Old school" meant showing love and care and supporting the patient's self-determinism. We believed that hurt people needed care, comfort, understanding and leading out of the desperate trap they had fallen into.

But by the time I went to med school in 1963, the revolution was under way. The patient's feelings and dignity were no longer a concern. They were defective, damaged, inferior, broken people. Psychiatry was being converted to wholesale mechanistic and biochemical "control". New technologies were emerging, not just violent and crude lobotomy, or shock treatment, which had been around, but drugs which literally took away any sense of self or being.

Psychotherapy and counseling were soon deliberately purged from the training curriculum. Psychiatrists would not be taught—or more explicitly would be taught not to—talk at length with the patients and try to understand their plight.

By 1987, at a symposium *Training Psychiatrists for the 90s: Issues and Recommendations*, one of the presentations was entitled "Psychotherapy Will Not Be Central In Psychiatric Education" and the speaker, an influential psychiatrist, came out flatly against teaching psychiatrists to be skilled at delving the patient's problems.

Children Now Targeted Too

This is very worrying. Children being tended by psychiatrists is all wrong, in my view. They are being deliberately targeted for dosing with medications which are notoriously difficult to discontinue (very reminiscent of the way that tobacco companies got kids addicted early on in life). Children with problems that were once handled by remedial education or improved parenting and now being diagnosed as having mental disorders, that need "treating" with drugs, medical staff and even hospitals.

It's the latest thing, investigative journalist Jon Rappaport tells us. "Psychiatrists are giving children in poor neighborhoods Adderall, a dangerous stimulant, by making false diagnoses of ADHD, or no diagnoses at all. Their aim? To "promote social justice," to improve academic performance in school.

"The rationale is, the drugged kids will now be able to compete with children from wealthier families who attend better schools.

"Leading the way is Dr. Michael Anderson, a pediatrician in the Atlanta area. Incredibly, Anderson told the New York Times ("Attention Disorder or Not, Pills to Help in School") his diagnoses of ADHD are "made up," "an excuse" to hand out the drugs.

"We've decided as a society that it's too expensive to modify the kid's environment. So we have to modify the kid," Anderson said.

It would be hard to find a clearer mission statement from a psychiatrist: mind control.

But the whole program is based on a lie, says Rappoport, to wit: that ADHD drugs can enhance school performance.[55]

The following pronouncement makes a number of things clear: The 1994 *Textbook of Psychiatry*, published by the American Psychiatric Press, contains this review (Popper and Steingard): "Stimulants [given for ADHD] do not produce lasting improvements in aggressivity, conduct disorder, criminality, *education achievement*, job functioning, marital relationships, or long-term adjustment."

So this is the industry's own publication, admitting that their drugs don't do what their mischievous and dishonest psychiatrists claim.

Beware this evil profession is what I say. It's the new targeting of children that troubles me most. Children, as we all know, are fanciful, imaginative and not troubled by adult views of "reality" (whatever that is). But that's not madness; that's the joy of being young and exploring.

"Take a child who wants to invent something out of thin air, and instead of saying no, tell him he has a problem with his brain, and then stand back and watch what happens. In particular, watch what happens when you give him a toxic drug to fix his brain. You

have to be a certain kind of person to do that to a child. You have to be, for various reasons, crazy and a career criminal." (The Underground, Jon Rappoport)

Here are a few facts that should give you pause:

According to NAMI (National Alliance on Mental Illness), "More than 25 percent of college students have been diagnosed or treated by a professional for a mental health condition within the past year."

NAMI: "One in four young adults between the ages of 18 and 24 have a diagnosable mental illness." [so they claim]

According to healthline.com, 6.4 million American children between the ages of 4 and 17 have been diagnosed with ADHD. The average age for the child's diagnosis is 7.

The British Medical Journal: "The number of UK children and adolescents treated with antidepressants rose by over 50% from 2005 to 2012, a study of five Western countries published in European Neuropsychopharmacology has found."[56]

In a 2014 article from the National Center for Health Statistics, entitled "Are Children Being Overmedicated?", it was estimated that 7.5 percent of U.S. children between ages 6 and 17 were taking medication for "emotional or behavioral difficulties". The CDC reports a five-fold increase in the number of children under 18 on psychostimulants in the years from 1988-2010. This is awful. The rate of antipsychotic prescriptions for children increased six-fold over this same period.[57]

So why hasn't psychiatry been discredited and disowned? Because there is money in it. Big money. Pharmaceutical money. And because the public is in a trance. Mothers and fathers are quite willing to take their children to these brain poisoners...lambs to the slaughter.

The silence of the lambs.

It's happening everywhere Big Pharma has inserted its sticky tentacles (which is EVERYwhere). Given that safety studies are very poor and the children more likely to be at risk, this is a major worry.

For instance, a 2016 US study found that the use of so-called atypical antipsychotics (or 2nd generation antipsychotics) in 4 to 18-year-old patients significantly increased between 1993 and 2010 in the United States. Yet over 65% of those visits did not have any US FDA-approved diagnosis. During 2007 to 2010, the most common mental disorder was ADHD, accounting for 24% of total pediatric prescriptions.[58]

Again, more than half.

Integrated Drug-Free Treatment

Do not fear, reading this book of natural therapies, that a psychiatrically-distressed patient *must have* drug treatment; "it's for their own good"; they are a danger to themselves and others if they don't get the "right treatment". That is simply an industry hoax, perpetuated by underperforming psychiatrists and industry shills.

Why prescribe drugs at all, when modern drug-free experimental programs are producing better outcomes? Consider these studies:

1. The Pilot Project Soteria Berne Ciompi, L. Swedish researchers who opened a Soteria-style house in Berne reported that this approach produced good results. They noted that "patients who received no or very low-dosage medication demonstrated significantly better results." (Page 148.)

Soteria houses are often seen as gentler alternatives to a psychiatric hospital system perceived as authoritarian, hostile or violent and based on routine use of psychiatric (particularly antipsychotic) drugs.[59]

2. Two-Year Outcome in First Episode Psychosis Treated According to an Integrated Model. Is Immediate Neuroleptisation Always Needed? Lehtinen, V. *European Psychiatry* 15 (2000):312-320.

In this study by Finnish investigators, 43% of the patients in the experimental group didn't receive any antipsychotic medication, and overall, the outcomes for the experimental group "was equal or even somewhat better" than those treated conventionally with drugs.

3. Integrating Intensive Psychosocial Therapy and Low-Dose Medical Treatment in a Total Material of First Episode Psychotic Patients Compared to "Treatment as Usual.[60] Swedish physicians sought to replicate the Finnish approach involving selective use of antipsychotic drugs. Only 45% of the patients in their experimental group were on antipsychotics at the end of three years, and those on the drugs were taking a very low dose of Thorazine. This experimental group had much lower hospital use than those treated conventionally with drugs during the three-year study.

4. Five-Year Experience of First-Episode Nonaffective Psychosis in Open-Dialogue Approach. Finland's Jaako Seikkula reports on his "open-dialogue" program in Western Lapland that involves minimizing the use of neuroleptics in patients diagnosed with schizophrenia and other psychotic disorders. At the end of five years, 82% of his patients did not have psychotic symptoms, 86% had returned to their studies or were working, and only 14% were on a disability allowance. Only 29% of his patients had ever been exposed to an antipsychotic drug during the five years, and only 17% were on antipsychotics at the end of five years.[61]

All Scandinavian studies, please note. You won't find US dollar-based medicine even willing to consider looking at drug-free approaches, so rapacious is the grip of the pharmaceutical industry on psychiatry.

I find the Jaako Seikkula paper especially admirable, in that without the use of drugs *82% of patients were symptom free and 86% were back at work or at study.*

As I said, the "chemical imbalance" theory is totally washed up. It's for frauds and pseuds only.

It's even arguable that administering drugs will block any successful recovery. New research reveals that mindfulness-based cognitive therapy (MBCT) may be most helpful when drugs are not used. The study, published in the current issue of *Psychotherapy and Psychosomatics*, found that the participants in a randomized control trial for MBCT who showed the greatest improvement were those who had not taken antidepressants.[62]

Drug-free is the way to go. Be assured, be confident, be knowledgeable in this!

There may be one possible exception...

1.6 Do Psychedelic Drugs Have Anything To Offer?

Maybe so. Trouble is, use and study of this class of drugs has been illegal since the hysterical moral and political backlash of the 1960s. Thanks to the verbal ravings of Timothy Leary and Richard Alpert (later known as Baba Ram Dass) the establishment of the day was convinced that psychedelic tripping was no different to insurrection and social disorder. No good could come of it. It had to be stopped.

By the late 60s, these substances had been banned in the US, Canada and Europe. Research ground to a halt. But that was fifty years ago. Maybe it's time to get things back in proportion.

First of all, let me separate myself from the mass of mainstream writers and investigators in this field. They uphold the mind-is-matter theory of "brain as Being" model as a given; a point of unchallengeable faith.

Why, they say, we do drugs and that changes the brain and that changes thought, as if it is an irrevocable sequence. Messing around with thoughts and chemicals PROVES that we are just brain.

But I say different. What happens with psychedelic drugs is not that the brain is stimulated but that the brain is knocked out, put out of the equation altogether. We revert to being natural non-material mind, beyond the reaches of neurotransmitters, chemicals and physiology. We become just pure mind. Pure consciousness.

Which is why we are able to create any reality we want: fantastic images, changing landscapes of the mind, reaching out into the great regions of the Cosmos, interconnecting with other people, new worlds and other beings... It's what natural consciousness wants to do. It's primed to do. Consciousness creates our experience, as quantum science has been telling us for decades. The whole of reality is just an invention of consciousness. No other model explains what is happening to us, or our world.

Therefore if we unfetter our conscious minds, which psychedelics have the special capacity to do, we experience first-hand the wonders of limitless Being and fun plastic reality.

Personal Experience

For the sake of transparency, let me state clearly I have NO experience of taking psychedelic substances. In my teens I was too scared to mess with my mind (I have never regretted the decision) and by the 1970s, these substances were illegal.

For a few hours I was once given morphine post-operatively and it was a grim experience. I had a chemical anesthetic once (I have no idea what it was), while the surgeon went back in via the esophagus, to retrieve a stuck gallstone. It was the most terrifying nightmare of my life, flying through mental hyperspace at horrendous (but of course hallucinatory) speed, absolutely without any control of what was happening to my mind and unable to stop it or blank out the overwhelming sensations.

It was an experience I would never again allow myself to undergo.

But I have made my life a study and practice of the adventures of non-material mind and Being. So I speak from a great deal of experience gathered, I might say, under controlled conditions, rather than the random effects of hallucinatory drugs.

Therefore I speak with some insight and personal knowledge.

Psychedelics Arise Again

A psychedelic renaissance has been announced many times, without ever delivering on the high hopes. But this time it feels different. There is a growing band of respected scientists whose work is finally bearing fruit – not only in terms of benefits for patients, but also unprecedented insights into the workings of a healthy mind.

That's right. I like this work because it is often based on the responses of healthy and "normal" people (whatever that means), not just those in distress.

We may have a whole new class of drugs to transform mental illness into a less harrowing experience. Not only that but to teach patients that their "troubles" are not even a disease or malfunction—just something unfamiliar and which has lacked a grounded explanation that is comforting.

The idea that psychedelics might be used to treat mental illness emerged in the 1950s, a decade or so after Swiss chemist Albert Hofmann first described his experiences of taking LSD. By the mid-1960s, roughly 40,000 people had been given LSD as part of treatments for all manner of mental illnesses, from obsessive compulsive disorder to addiction, depression and schizophrenia.

The results were extremely good.

One might say, if psychedelics had not been banned, the history of psychiatry would have been very different.

Instead, we got antidepressants. Big Pharma launched selective serotonin reuptake inhibitors (SSRIs). Their loose "interpretations" of success in early trial results fueled the idea that depression is caused by a deficiency in serotonin. But recently, this idea has been called into question, as more and more studies suggest SSRIs are not at all as effective as we have been led to believe.

SSRIs probably have an effect for just 1 in 5 people. Even when they do work, there are problems, not least that coming off the drugs brings severe side effects.

The picture is no less grim for other mental illnesses: there is a chronic shortage of new treatments, NO effective drugs and precious few ideas about what else might be done.

The Multidisciplinary Association for Psychedelic Studies (MAPS)

Then, in the late 1990s, a US non-profit called the Multidisciplinary Association for Psychedelic Studies (MAPS), started promoting the revival of psychedelics for the treatment of PTSD. After a few individuals were determined enough to go through the arduous process of getting approval to work with psychedelics, the US Food and Drug Administration (FDA) decided to treat psychedelics like other drugs, meaning researchers were not banned from working with them.

Two decades later, those efforts are finally paying off. The psychedelic rebirth is entering a new stage, with a series of startling new insights appearing in the pages of scientific leading journals. Clinical trials of psychedelics or psychedelic-assisted therapy as it's called, have started making significant progress.

Take MDMA, better known as the party drug ecstasy. MDMA is not a classic psychedelic in that it doesn't induce hallucinations, but instead works by flooding the brain with serotonin, which makes users feel euphoric. These mood-altering effects are the reason researchers became interested in using it as a tool to assist psychotherapy for people with post-traumatic stress disorder (PTSD).

PTSD is claimed to affect roughly 7 percent of people in the US at some point in their lives. The most effective treatment involves memory reconsolidation, the method we use in Supernoetics® piloting (section 3.12). People are asked to recall traumatic events so that their memories of them can be stripped of fearful associations by processing them in a new way.

The problem is that recall can sometimes be so terrifying that they have to stop receiving this form of therapy. MDMA appears to help, not only because it extinguishes anxiety and stress, but also because it triggers the release of oxytocin, a pro-social hormone that strengthens feelings of trust towards therapists.

Last year, at the Psychedelic Science 2017 conference in Oakland, California, a group led by Michael Mithoefer at the Medical University of South Carolina presented results from trials in which 107 people with PTSD underwent a psychotherapy while under the influence of MDMA. A year or so after having the therapy, roughly 67 percent of them no longer had PTSD, according to a measure based on symptoms such as anxiety levels and frequency of nightmares. About 23 percent of the control group, which had psychotherapy and a placebo drug, got the same benefit.

So, with MDMA the results for this very tough condition were almost triple!

Psychotropic drugs (anti-psychotics) are worthless, measured against this scale of success.

In fact, the FDA was so impressed that it granted MDMA "breakthrough therapy" status, which will accelerate the path towards approval. If all goes well, it could be in use as soon as 2021.

The Real Deal

If recent research is anything to go by, however, true psychedelics—those that induce the characteristic changes in perception that scientists insist are just hallucinations—might end up having the biggest impact on mental health. That's because psilocybin, the active ingredient in magic mushrooms, is beginning to look like the real deal: a genuinely effective, long-lasting treatment for depression.

The change started in 2006, when Roland Griffiths, a psychiatrist and neuroscientist at Johns Hopkins University in Baltimore, replicated the results of a notorious study from 1962. He showed that a large dose of psilocybin can induce mystical experiences in volunteers without any mental health problems, including feelings of ego dissolution, a sense of revelation, ineffability and transcendence of time and space. *Readers will recognize this description as the very powerful and positive state that Abram Maslow dubbed "peak experiences" and they are to be desired and envied.*

What's more the feel good factor persisted. 14 months after taking the drug, 22 of the 36 participants said the experience improved their well-being or life satisfaction, and rated it as one of the top five most meaningful experiences of their lives.

Researchers are now writing about "psilocybin-assisted therapy". Psilocybin seems to work in exactly the opposite way to SSRIs; instead of causing emotional blunting, it makes the patients feel more alive, more connected, more available emotionally.

The good point is that these drugs are not difficult to handle; in fact far safer than most conventional drug trials. As Solomon Snyder, also at Johns Hopkins, wrote at the time: "The ability of these researchers to conduct a double-blind, well-controlled study tells us that clinical research with psychedelic drugs need not be so risky as to be off-limits to most investigators."

Figuring that psychedelic experiences would be particularly valuable to people confronting a terminal illness, Griffiths and others began trials designed to assess the safety and efficacy of psilocybin to treat anxiety in people with advanced cancer. In the largest of those, Griffiths recruited 51 volunteers. Half of them were given a small placebo-like dose during one session, then a high dose five weeks later. For the other half, the sequence was reversed.

The results were published last year. There was a marked reduction in depression and anxiety symptoms compared with placebo after the high-dose session, and for 80 percent of them those benefits continued to be felt six months later. An associated study at New York University reported similar results.

Meanwhile, Robin Carhart-Harris, a neuroscientist at Imperial College London, has been working with people with depression that has resisted all available treatments. In a trial involving 20 people, participants had two sessions – one on a single low dose of psilocybin (10 milligrams), one on a single high dose (25 mg) – during which they each separately lay listening to specially chosen music, accompanied by therapists.

The findings, also reported last year, were impressive. Those two doses, combined with the psychological support, were sufficient to lift depression in all 20 participants for three weeks, and to keep it at bay for five of them for three months.

This is majorly different from conventional therapy and, of course, the pharmaceutical companies won't like it. The more frequent the doses, the more medicines sold. It's kind of brutal. The very BEST therapy means as little treatment as possible and long-lasting benefits.

PART 2

THE SUFFERING SEVEN

There are thousands of varied psychological states that could be called pathological. The DSM-V gives 300 conditions that all lack for any objective proof, as I said. But there are detailed descriptions there, purporting to separate out these states of mind. Some are nonsensical "about to feel bad" states (I'm not kidding).

How are we to proceed, in the face of overwhelming possibilities?

I have decided to narrow the next stage of our enquiry down to seven key conditions; what we may call, if you like, the "Big Seven" of psychiatry and mental health.

These are:

1. Depression

2. Bipolar Disorder

3. Schizophrenia

4. Alzheimer's and Dementia

5. Anxiety States, including Phobias

6. Attention and Behavioral Deficit Disorders (ADD, ADHD etc.)

7. Addictions

I could add an 8th: crime, violence and delinquency. In fact, I intend to append a section on it here. But I have excluded it from what I am calling "The Big Seven".

Let's start with depression.

2.1 Depression

We all feel depressed from time to time. Almost everyone has experienced upset and used the expression "I am depressed". However, this is usually a transient state of affairs.

Real depression is a clinical condition and more protracted and severe than everyday feelings of "the blues". The patient's deep gloom and sense of helplessness can be so crippling at times that he or she may consider the possibility of ending it all. In the WHO promotion for their 2007 World Suicide Prevention Day we were told that, on average, almost 3000 people commit suicide every day. Every 30 seconds, the loss of a person who killed themselves shatters the lives of family and friends. For every person who completes a suicide, 20 or more may attempt suicide. For family and friends affected by suicide or attempted suicide, the emotional impact may last for many years.

This appalling toll tells us all too clearly that conventional treatment for depression has a long way to go. On the larger social scale there have been a number of spectacular incidents in which a clinically depressed patient ran amok and committed multiple murders, before ending their own life. Here we seem to have a remarkable modern development of "suicide with multiple mortality".

In virtually every case, we find that the perpetrator was taking powerful psychotropic drugs and since murderous violence is a documented side-effect of these drugs, it seems right to blame the medication and not some underlying deep distress within the perpetrator.

In other words, the drug caused the murders, not the depression.

Classification

It is important to remember that there can be many subdivisions of a mental disorder. Depression, for example, is not generally categorized by severity but by presentation.

- major depressive disorder (MDD)

- persistent depressive disorder

- seasonal affective disorder (SAD)

- psychotic depression

- peripartum (postpartum) depression

- premenstrual dysphoric disorder (PMDD)

- and 'situational' depression.

I have kept bipolar disorder separate to depression, since the manic component too is often very striking.

There are also types of depression you may not have heard of: dysthymia and "atypical depression".

It's pointless trying to separate out these types. These are just labels, which add nothing to our understanding. It is merely a pretense of knowledge, which the psychiatric profession loves. The holistic approach has a great deal to offer, even a complete resolution, to all types of depression, so it is doubtful that breaking it into different symptom groupings serves any real purpose.

How Depressed Are You?

It is useful to have some objective scoring method, to assess just how depressed a person is. One of the simplest and most often used in the Zung Self-Rating Depression Scale, designed by Duke University psychiatrist William W.K. Zung MD (1929-1992). It is a 20-item self-report questionnaire that is widely used as a screening tool, covering affective, psychological and somatic symptoms associated with depression. The questionnaire takes about 10 minutes to complete, and items are framed in terms of positive and negative statements.[63]

Each item is scored on a scale ranging from 1 to 4. A total score is derived by summing the individual item scores, and ranges from 20 to 80. Most people with depression score between 50 and 69, while a score of 70 and above indicates severe depression.

Try it!

For each item below, please check the column which best describes how often you felt or behaved this way during the past several days.

	A little of the time	Some of the time	Good part of the time	Most of the time
	(1)	(2)	(3)	(4)
I feel down hearted and blue.	○	○	○	○
Morning is when I feel the best.	○	○	○	○
I have crying spells or feel like it.	○	○	○	○
I have trouble sleeping at night.	○	○	○	○
I eat as much as I used to.	○	○	○	○
I still enjoy sex.	○	○	○	○
I notice that I am losing weight.	○	○	○	○
I have trouble with constipation.	○	○	○	○
My heart beats faster than usual.	○	○	○	○
I get tired for no reason.	○	○	○	○
My mind is as clear as it used to be.	○	○	○	○
I find it easy to do the things I used to.	○	○	○	○
I am restless and can't keep still.	○	○	○	○
I feel hopeful about the future.	○	○	○	○
I am more irritable than usual.	○	○	○	○
I find it easy to make decisions.	○	○	○	○
I feel that I am useful and needed.	○	○	○	○
My life is pretty full.	○	○	○	○
I feel that others would be better off if I were dead.	○	○	○	○
I still enjoy the things I used to do.	○	○	○	○

Conventional Therapy And Its Shortcomings

Did you know that among those who seek professional help for depression, less than half of patients will be correctly diagnosed as depressive?[64]

Of those who are diagnosed with depression, only one half will receive any form of therapy for their illness.[65]

Finally, among those who do receive treatment, only 25% will receive an adequate antidepressant dose and duration of treatment.[66]

These figures are bound to be conservative, since many depressed people do not admit to their problem openly.

For decades the main treatment was electro-convulsive therapy (ECT). Some crazed psychiatrists still justify it, mainly among hospitalized patients for severe depression. Unwanted outcomes include personality changes and memory loss. Moreover patients sometimes injure themselves during the seizures.

In the 1950s a whole class of anti-depressant drugs was developed called the monoamineoxidase inhibitor (MAOIs for short), closely followed by the tri-cyclic anti-depressants (TCAs). While sometimes effective, both these classes of drugs cause troublesome side effects and have complex, potentially fatal, drug interactions. Their mode of action is to block the breakdown of neurotransmitters like serotonin and norepinephrine, which are known to enhance mood.

The latest major class of drugs—the selective serotonin re-uptake inhibitors (SSRIs)— all act similarly, by preventing the natural re-absorption of serotonin by the nerve endings. The justification for this is that depression is some kind of serotonin lack. But that is not only unproved, it is proven NOT to be the case (see section 1.4).

It's just more flimflam from the pharmaceutical companies and slow-witted, lazy or dishonest psychiatrists.

Fluoxetine (Prozac) was the first SSRI. It has been joined by paroxetine (Paxil®), sertraline (Zoloft®) and numerous others, several of which have become virtual household names.

Holistic Mechanisms of Depression

Depression is the best paradigm model for all mental disorders, so I will spend some time going in depth with this condition. You can apply all you read here to virtually any state of mental illness. The general holistic principles and the universal causes that can be remedied will appear later, so I don't propose to work through them for each and every one of my "Big Seven".

Depression is a good place to start, because it exemplifies the fact that many pathways can lead to the same symptomatology. There is no scientific justification for saying depression is all one disease process. Is a sore throat and accompanying fever all one disease process? Of course not. It could be strep, Epstein-Barr, tonsillitis, quinsy, cancer, leukemia, an allergy (yes, even with a fever), and—most likely—any one of numerous viruses.

What interests us in this book is causes. What are the many causes of depression and what can we do about them?

First, there is reactive depression. If there is something to be depressed *about*, is that really a disease? Many of us have felt depressed and unworthy, when we flunk an exam, lose a bunch on the gambling table, or even worse, a beloved person dies or walks out. The response to these many setbacks can be severe. We may characterize it as grief. But is that an illness? (see section 3.1 Is Grieving an Illness?)

Or maybe the depression is coming from another persona from within. You will read about the Complex of Self model later. It means there are different thinking entities within our psychic domain. Maybe the sadness is coming from one of these? That would be especially likely if you are normally a vibrant joyous person and find yourself inexplicably plunged into gloom from time to time. It isn't you! Not the real you... (see section 3.15 for The Complex of Self explanation).

The Role Of Inflammation

One of the great surprises has been the discovery that depression has a pronounced inflammatory component. Increased levels of inflammatory proteins, such as interleukin one-beta (IL-1b) and tumor necrosis factor- alpha (TNF-a), suggest that low-grade, body-wide inflammation accompanies depression. Moreover, levels of these inflammatory markers correlate well with the severity of depression.[67]

Even if inflammation didn't cause your depression, if you lie around on the sofa, moping, not moving, eating comfort foods and watching garbage on TV, you will pretty soon PUT yourself into an inflammatory state!

A recent study carried out at Tel Aviv University in Israel is the first published report of deliberately induced inflammation causing signs of experimental depression in mice. Significantly, this effect was blocked by the administration of the SSRI fluoxetine (Prozac®), which may suggest an entirely different pathway for the mode of action of SSRIs than what is being hyped. Maybe they are just anti-inflammatories (like aspirin!).[68]

Omega-3 fatty acids are an essential dietary factor in combating inflammation. Patients with the lowest levels of essential omega-3 fatty acids tend to be the most severely depressed, while healthy control subjects are more likely to have normal levels of omega-3s, as measured in red blood cell membranes.[69]

So right away, we have an important holistic suggestion for reducing the severity of depression: omega-3s, in the form of EPA and DHA (eicosapentanoic acid and docosohe-aenoic acid), are well-known anti-inflammatory nutrients. Indeed, lack of essential fatty acids make far more sense as a cause of mental illness than supposed serotonin deficiency, or dopamine excess.

In 2006, researchers analyzed results from six published studies on depression and omega-3 fatty acids. They found that omega-3 fatty acids can significantly reduce symptoms of depression among adults.[70] Note the negative role that omega-6 fatty acids play... although "essential" by name, they are far too prevalent in modern diets and considerably outweigh omega-3s. This creates a relative omega-3 deficiency.

According to a recent study, depressed people have lower levels of omega-3 fatty acids in relation to pro-inflammatory omega-6 fatty acids, and the severity of symptoms correlated with the ratio of omega-6 to omega-3 fatty acids. Moreover inflammatory markers — interleukin 6 (IL-6) and tumor necrosis factor α (TNF-α) — showed a direct correlation with the omega-6:omega-3 ratio.[71]

Here's a gem: studies among prison inmates by Bernard Gesch in the UK report that aggression and violence is reduced, as well as mood improved, by supplementation with omega-3 fatty acids. Apparently, the chance of being murdered is 30 times greater in countries with a low fish consumption, according to Joseph Hibbeln MD, working at the US National Institutes of Health (NIH).[72]

Omega-3s are best obtained from marine sources and true grass-fed beef. Vegetarians will need plant sources, such as flaxseed. Dose: 1000- 2000 mgms daily.

To lower your omega-6 intake, cease eating manufactured food and rely instead on healthy wholefoods, such as fruit, vegetables, salads and fish.

Curcumin As Good As Prozac?

Interestingly, I found one important study that suggested curcumin (derived from Turmeric) may have similar anti-depressant effects to SSRIs. That would undoubtedly be due to the inflammation-quenching effect of curcumin, one of the best anti-inflammatories known! I already referred to the Tel Aviv University study above, which highly suggested that SSRIs may work via an anti-inflammatory effect. So, the two may have an identical action.

Omega-3s and curcumin, of course, are far safer than SSRIs and there is no known case of someone going on a mass shooting rampage after downing a curry!

"This study provides first clinical evidence that curcumin may be used as an effective and safe modality for treatment in patients with MDD without concurrent suicidal ideation or other psychotic disorders."[73]

You can find other ways to lower inflammation in a later section (5.1).

Finally Up To Date

2017 has been exceptional for nutritional psychiatry. Drew Ramsey, MD, assistant clinical professor of psychiatry from Columbia University in New York City and a practicing nutritional psychiatrist, said, "2017 has been an exciting year for nutritional psychiatry. We now have two randomized controlled trials showing significant efficacy for the treatment of clinical depression with dietary and nutritional interventions."[74]

Ramsey was talking about two notable studies: When people with severe depression followed the Mediterranean diet, they experienced a significant reduction in symptom severity that lasted up to 6 months.

In one of the first randomized controlled trials to examine the effect of the Mediterranean diet supplemented with fish oil in people with severe depression, researchers found the diet to be associated with a marked reduction in depression symptoms.

While both the intervention and control groups experienced significant mental health improvements, participants eating the Mediterranean diet experienced a greater reduction (45%) in the severity of their depression compared with the control group (27%).

This is only the second randomized controlled trial to use a Mediterranean dietary intervention in people with severe depression. The first trial, published earlier in 2017 in BMC Medicine, was also conducted in patients with moderate to severe depression.

In that study, following the Mediterranean diet was found to be associated with significant improvements in depression scores. But they did not test the efficacy of supplementing fish oil omega-3s. The most recent study wanted to boost those levels because previous research showed that people with depression had very low levels of omega 3s compared with the national average.[75]

Depression and The Microbiome

When thinking of inflammation, one should immediately think of the microbiome: organisms within the gut that are capable of creating a great deal of systemic (body-wide) inflammation. Indeed, I wrote an entire book, speaking to that theme: *Fire In The Belly* (Mother Whale Inc. Las Vegas, 2012, 2017).

Some patients are becoming tired of problems associated with small intestinal bacteria overgrowth (SIBO) and "Candida" (see section 5.5) and resorting to what is jokingly known as "fecal transplants" or eating shit, to you and me (www.thepowerofpoop.com). It's a desperate solution and not really necessary. We know from modern research that the microbiome will change quite quickly, often within hours, if the patient modifies what he or she is eating.

This is now proven science. Gut microbiomes may have a significant impact on mood and cognition, which is leading experts towards a new frontier in neuroscience (I've been there for decades... yawn). Studies have shown that an increase in the amount of good bacteria in the gut can curb inflammation and cortisol level, reduces symptoms of depression and anxiety, lowers stress reactivity, improves memory and even lessens neuroticism and social anxiety. This shows that, probably the beneficial gut bacteria or probiotics function mechanistically as delivery vehicles for neuroactive compounds.

Thus, we have a new science specialty called "psychobiotics". A psychobiotic is a live organism, when ingested in adequate amounts, produces a health benefit in patients suffering from psychiatric illness. Study of these novel class of probiotics may open up the possibility of rearrangement of intestinal microbiota for effective management of various psychiatric disorders.[76]

The important thing is to get off the damaging Western standard diet, with its excess of sugar, food additives and vitiated nutrients. Any natural wholefood diet will improve matters almost right away. Perhaps the "Stone Age Diet" which made me famous—today known as paleo eating—is the optimum way to restore a natural bowel flora (BBC television christened me the "Stone Age Doctor" in 1995).

Swallowing cartloads of probiotics is of doubtful benefit, even though yoghurt, etc. contains what we value in replacement organisms. The whole method falters unless the patient takes what are called pre-biotics at the same time (fiber, etc. to support the growth of probiotics).

Be aware that parasites too and heavy metals being excreted by the liver, via bile, can greatly inflame the intestinal tract. More of that later.

Your Heart Speaks Your Mind

C-reactive protein is another inflammatory protein found at higher levels in depressed persons. It is also commonly found in patients with cardiovascular disease, pointing to some as-yet-unfathomed connection between depression and the heart.[77, 78]

An even more explicit association with cardiovascular disease was revealed by a recent study showing that depressive states can actually lead to thickening of the arterial linings and hence reduced blood flow. Moreover, this study specifically ruled out other negative emotions, anxiety, hostility and anger as having the same effect on cardiovascular health. Only depression.[79]

Another new report reveals that heart failure patients with highest levels of the cytokine TNF-1 have an almost 5-fold risk for depression.[80]

So maybe there is something to the old-fashioned idea that our heart holds our emotions! It's a two-way traffic, of course. Emotions influence our heart and vascular system. One of the sure-fire ways to drop dead of a heart attack or stroke is to be continually unhappy or stressed.

Depression can indeed be a killer, beyond suicide. Cardiovascular disease and cancer are major pathways to this outcome.

You need to work on your emotions, as surely as you work on your inflammation markers. There are many approaches, from emotional freedom technique to meditation, with all stations in between.

Highly recommended (in this work) is my own development of Supernoetics® piloting. More about that in section 3.12 and online. You can see more details in the **Valuable Resources** section in the back of the book.

Homocysteine

Homocysteine, a general marker for inflammation, is also indicative of heart disease. It basically denotes a failure of the healthy re-methylation process, known to repair DNA and prevent aging.

Up to 50% of depressed people have homocysteine levels that are *significantly* above normal, considered to be greater than 10 millimoles per liter (mmol/L) of blood.[81], [82]

Levels above 10 mmol/L are considered unsafe and indicate a risk of serious cardio-vascular and neurological damage. It is recommended to aim for a level of 8 mmol/L or less. 6 mmol/L is even better. One study found each 3-unit increase in homocysteine caused a 35% increase in heart attack risk.[83]

My recommendations are as follows:

Homocysteine levels can be lowered by a number of nutrients, some of which (especially S-adenosyl-L-methionine, or SAMe) have been found to improve depression independently. In Europe, SAMe is sold as an antidepressant and is available on prescription.

A recent Canadian review elaborated extensive evidence for the fact that SAMe provides a mechanism for removing toxic homocysteine.[84]

Take 400 to 1200 mg of SAMe daily without food.

SAMe should not be taken along with drugs, especially antidepressants, because there is a risk of serious interactions.

People who have bipolar disorder should not use SAMe, because it increases the risk of manic episodes.[85]

What remains unclear to date is whether lowering homocysteine levels has any benefit in reducing depression scores. Nevertheless, I consider it prudent to keep homocysteine levels as low as possible, certainly less than 8 mmol/L.

See also *Life Extension Magazine* October 2006: Homocysteine as a Risk Factor for Disease, for a comprehensive overview.

The Cortisol Connection

Hormones too can influence mood and behavior. Cortisol levels are consistently elevated in depressed subjects, due to over-stimulation of the hypothalamic-pituitary-adrenal axis (HPA axis, section 5.9), which regulates cortisol secretions. Concomitant secretions of vasopressin increases this effect.[86]

Vasopressin thus reinforces depression negatively and is felt to be the probable trigger for suicide. Oxytocin (the "love or bonding hormone"), on the other hand, lowers cortisol levels.[87]

It is better not to consider depression as simply a response to stress but also as some fundamental dysfunction of the HPA axis. In depressed patients cortisol levels peak in the afternoon, whereas they peak around 8.00 am in a normal individual.

A 2007 study reported that patients diagnosed with unipolar depressive disorder, some recovered, some were still depressed.

Cortisol and ACTH levels were measured and clearly abnormal in the both groups, compared to controls. What is revealing is that the recovered group also scored badly, showing their HPA axis had remained abnormal, even while mood was restored. This points to some underlying malfunction of the HPA axis that has yet to be clarified.[88]

While it is not established that cortisol levels are causative in depression, it makes sense to attempt to reduce the stress response. Meditation, because of its deeply introvertive action, may not be appropriate for depression cases. But therapeutic massage, aromatherapy with essential oils, moderate exercise, hobbies, laughter and social support are all tried and proven methods of lowering stress levels.

A study, which was reported by Valencia Porter, MD, of the Scripps Center for Integrative Medicine (SCIM) in La Jolla, California, and colleagues involved a review of the charts of 569 patients who had been enrolled in the "Healing Hearts" program—a 6-month, integrated rehabilitation program incorporating yoga, exercise, stress management, and nutrition counseling. The improvements were surprisingly robust, according to Dr Porter.[89]

It should be obvious that similar interventions could help patients with many other disorders and imbalances.

Feel-Good Supplements

A number of recognized supplements could be helpful in reducing overall stress and creating a "feel good" sensation:

Phenylethylamine (PEA). This compound is an endogenous neuroamine and has been called the "love molecule" (don't mix it up with oxytocin, sometimes called the love hormone). PEA unquestionably increases mood and leads to sustained relief of depression in a significant number of patients. PEA works as rapidly as amphetamine but does not produce tolerance.[90]

PEA is found in chocolate but the highest concentrations are found in the blue-green algae *Aphanizomenon flos-aquae* (AFA). Phycocyanin, the blue pigment in AFA, is a natural selective COX-2 inhibitor with strong anti-inflammatory properties, which suggests it may also act directly against the inflammatory component of depression.

Recommended dose: aim for about 800 mgms of AFA.

Phenylalanine. This is a related compound and a number of studies have shown it to be effective against depression. It leads to an increase in the body's natural PEA levels (measured by urinary excretion). Side effects are few and include mild headache, low blood pressure, and agitation. Phenylalanine may also help regulate disordered glucose metabolism, another aspect of depression (see next).[91]

Take 200- 500 mg daily of phenylalanine.

Tryptophan and 5-hydroxytryptophan (5HT). Available as dietary supplements, these two substances are immediate precursors to serotonin (which is actually 5-hydroxytryptamine). In some countries, tryptophan is licensed as an antidepressant. More study is needed on the use of these supplements in depression, to establish efficacy. If depression and other mental disorders are not a result of serotonin imbalance, as all the evidence suggests, then it is difficult to see why tryptophan should have much effect, other than as a sleep remedy. Up to you!

Take 500 to 1000 mg of tryptophan once or twice daily on an empty stomach

Disordered Glucose Metabolism

The link between obesity and depression has been long known. "Comfort eating" is a laymen's concept that has all but crept into the medical canon.

A 2007 study indicated women with high levels of depressive symptoms have an increased risk of developing metabolic syndrome (obesity and insulin resistance, among other factors).[92]

Now a recently published 10-year study has shown that older adults who show a high level of depressive symptoms, or experience a significant deterioration in mood, are more likely to develop type 2 diabetes.[93]

It may not work the other way round though. An almost contemporaneous study implied that successful lowering of depression scores had no beneficial effect on glycemic control.[94]

However, this is contradicted by a somewhat earlier study, which showed that depression improvement can produce better glycemic control, independent of favorable changes in weight and diabetes self care.[95]

Recommendations:

Keeping glucose levels under control is one of the most important health interventions that any of us can undertake. For many years, resting insulin levels have been taken as the number one marker for aging and early death.

The simplest corrective intervention is with knife and fork. Patients should limit their carbohydrate intake to a maximum of 120 grams daily and this to be taken in the form of complex carbs (whole grain, pulses etc). The rest of the diet should consist of vegetables, fruits (2 pieces), salads, fish, fowl and lean meat—the Mediterranean diet.

Chromium has long been known to be outstanding for regulating glucose levels. The recommended adult dose is 400 mcg daily. Other supplements to consider are:

- DHEA: 10-50 mg per day to start (men), 10-30 mg per day to start (women); assess effect via repeat blood test

- Lipoic acid: 150 mg once or twice daily

- Mixed tocopherols (vitamin E): 400 IU twice daily with mixed tocotrienols (75 mg twice daily)

- Vitamin A: 5000 IU per day, with mixed carotenoids (for example, lutein 5000 mcg, lycopene 3000 mcg, and zeaxanthin 360 mcg) daily

- Pycnogenol: 200 mg daily

See also section 5.8 Hypoglycemia.

Hormonal Factors Contributing To Depression.

Thyroid. Without doubt the main hormonal imbalance missed in depressed patients is thyroid insufficiency. It has been estimated that at least 10- 15% of people suffering from depression are undiagnosed hypothyroid.[96]

The real figure must arguably be far higher, since few depressed patients are investigated for hormonal dysfunction. Low T3 (the most active thyroid hormone) is associated with resistant depression and a tendency to relapse quickly.[97], [98] Conversely a series of open studies seemed to suggest that (T3) has a beneficial effect in a majority of patients with depression refractory to tricyclic therapy.[99]

However, according to a 2005 study, T3 did not enhance SSRI efficacy (paroxetine).[100]

Right now you should get yourself over to Janie Bowthorpe's website: www.StopTheThyroidMadness.com! There's a link in the **Valuable Resources** section in the back of the book!

Meanwhile, there is a whole section on hormone imbalances later in the book. You are referred to that.

In men, for example, the male menopause or andropause is just as significant an event for men as for women and symptoms are remarkably similar.

Testosterone levels should be checked in depressed men of any age. Studies repeatedly show low levels of testosterone in depressed men and this was re-inforced yet again by a 2006 Canadian study which found middle-aged men with depression have reduced levels of bioavailable testosterone.[101]

Carnitine is a supplement that may be equal to testosterone in its ability to improve sexual function, boost low moods, increase energy, and promote weight loss through its effect on fat and glucose metabolism. A dose of 2000 mg per day of acetyl-L-carnitine has been found effective in most studies.[102]

Low estrogen too is linked to depression in women. Patients using estrogen replacement therapy to alleviate menopause symptoms appear to experience reduced depression. In some older women being treated for depression, estrogen replacement therapy may actually improve the effects of conventional antidepressants.

Progesterone. This normally very positive and helpful hormone has a paradoxical reverse effect in depression and should be administered as a supplement only with extreme caution. Progesterone, and even more so synthetic progestogens, increase monoamine oxidase activity.[103]

Nutrient Deficiencies

Nutrient deficiencies have long known to provoke or exacerbate depression. Any vitamin deficiency will impact general health but the B complex group (including folate) are particularly important for healthy brain function by regulating energy metabolism, assisting in the production of chemicals that affect mood, and contributing to the myelin sheath surrounding and protecting nerves. B-vitamin deficiencies may therefore impair memory and increase anxiety, confusion, irritability, and depression.[104]

B1 (Thiamine) is vital for the functioning of healthy nerve tissue. The recommended daily allowance is 1.5 mg. This is pathetically low, as we shall see later. For one thing, infections, large volumes of urine, alcohol, antacids and HRT all increase B1 requirements.

B3 Niacin. This vitamin has long been known to be helpful in depression but citations are remarkably lacking. A 2003 study showed that niacin was a potent inhibitor of proinflammatory cytokines, which may indicate a possible mode of action.[105] Vitamin B6 (pyridoxine). In 2005, a team of researchers from Yale University examined all the published studies on vitamin B6 and depression. Although the researchers lost all evidence of the benefits from vitamin B6 treatment by combining the results of all the studies, they did find that premenopausal women suffering from depression benefited from vitamin B6.

B6 is known to help lower homocysteine levels.

Vitamin B12 (cobalamin). Deficiency in vitamin B12 has been cited as a risk factor for developing depression. People with high vitamin B12 levels have better treatment outcomes for major depression.[106]

Vitamin B12 supplementation is important for depressed individuals, particularly older patients, in whom low vitamin B12 levels are common.[107]

Folic acid. Treatment resistant depression has been linked to low blood levels of folic acid. Folic acid deficiency causes high homocysteine blood levels. Folate-deficient people are also more likely to be deeply depressed and for longer periods.[108]

This variety of depression responds poorly to antidepressant medication (hence treatment resistant), but naturally does respond to folic acid. Because relapse is associated with low serum folate, it is important to maintain folate supplementation for at least a year following a depressive episode.

Magnesium. This mineral is a vital cofactor in over 300 enzyme functions in the body, many concerned with detoxification pathways and many are found in the brain. The consequences of magnesium deficiency vary from heart arrhythmias to seizures, diabetes to hypothyroidism.

Magnesium deficiency has long been known to be a causal factor in depression.[109]

One study noted that magnesium levels in cerebro-spinal fluid were low in patients who had attempted suicide and moreover correlated with levels of 5- hydroxyindoleacetic acid, a metabolite of serotonin.[110]

Another study showed that the calcium/magnesium ratio is abnormally high in depression sufferers.[111]

Magnesium deficiency is associated with increase in C-reactive protein, one of the main markers for chronic inflammation.[112]

This may be yet another pathway in which magnesium helps depression scores.

Unfortunately, magnesium is very depleted in the typical Western diet. Few people reach the RDA of 400 mg for an adult male. Magnesium is mainly found in unprocessed nuts, grains, beans, seeds and green leafy vegetables.

Zinc. Decreased blood levels of zinc are associated with depression and maintaining a healthy zinc level in the brain is essential to normal brain function.[113] [114] Animal studies show that antidepressants and electroconvulsive shock treatments change zinc concentrations in areas of the brain associated with depression. [115] In an animal study, zinc was also shown to enhance antidepressant effects of imipramine, the original MAOI.[116]

Toxic Burdens

Heavy Metal Toxins. As well as testing for deficiencies, the alert physician will investigate possible toxic burdens. Heavy metal poisoning is a well-recognized health problem in today's industrialized world. Toxic metal poisoning can interfere with healthy enzyme systems and this may lead to a multitude of symptoms, including depression.

The treatment is chelation. This may require an office procedure. But many available sulfur-containing food substances have chelation properties (that is, will help take out the unwanted metals), especially garlic, kelp (seaweed) and cilantro. Chlorella, an algae, is known as a magnet for heavy metals: take 2- 6 tablets daily. Lipoic acid is also a chelator and has fantastic all-round health benefits. Take 200 mg daily of lipoic acid, in divided doses.

Zinc is a pre-cursor of metallothianein, a protein capable of chelating lead and arsenic.[117]

An Integrated Plan Works Best

Here's a highly instructive case of the value of measures recommended all through this book. It's a wise and witty saying that the symptoms are not the disease; the person's lifestyle is the disease!

A 45-y-old, married, Caucasian female with a history of diagnosed bipolar disorder with psychotic features, premenstrual dysphoric disorder, panic disorder, and repeated occurrence of suicide attempts and self-mutilating behavior presented for outpatient management. She reported limited gains through conventional treatment consisting of medication. The patient was prescribed a dietary, detox, and meditation regimen for one month, after which supplementation was added to support detoxification, digestion, hormonal balance, and nervous system structure and function. Additional lifestyle management therapeutics included daily meditation, dry-skin brushing, and coffee enemas.

Conclusion • This case exemplifies dramatic clinical remission after cessation of medication treatment and engagement of lifestyle interventions, which included dietary change, meditation, and detoxification. When medication demonstrates limited results, tapering combined with dietary interventions as the first-line therapy should be considered.[118]

Food Allergies

In his *Anatomy of Melanchology* (1621) Robert Burton, an English cleric, noted: "Milk, and all that comes of milk, as butter and cheese, curds etc., increase melancholy." It is the first recorded recognition that food intolerance could cause depression. Since then it has become abundantly clear that many foods can and do have this selective adverse effect in intolerant individuals

It is essential that patients suffering from depression and other symptoms of mental dysfunction be investigated competently for the possibility of food reactions. The bench mark is elimination and challenge eating but there are many pitfalls in this seemingly simple procedure, which will confuse the unwary.[119]

Multiple Chemical Sensitivity (MCH). Patients with multiple chemical sensitivity (section 5.3) are known to suffer depression. They have long had to endure the scorn of the medical profession and the presumption that their sensitivities are illusory and that depression is actually the cause of their syndrome, not the other way round.

All antioxidants, especially vitamin C, are useful detoxers. One of the most powerful antioxidants of all is glutathione. It also plays a vital role in the cytochrome P-450 oxidation pathway. Any sulfur donor will help too, such as cysteine and sulfur-containing foods: garlic and brassicas.

Take Vitamin C, 2-10 grams daily, glutathione 250 mgm daily (only the liposomal form will work orally) and L-cysteine 50 mgms. These may be available as combination capsules, depending on the supplier.

It makes sense to protect the liver and kidneys, our main detox and excretion organs, against the present chemical blizzard we are all experiencing. Milk thistle (Sylimarin) is a highly effective herbal remedy known to support the liver.

Finally, The Homeopathic Connection.

Let's not forget the gentle healing of homeopathy. The full treatment of psychiatric symptoms can be complex and require full training as a homeopath. But there are simple options for the lay person. HEEL makes a number of useful compounds:

Ignatia-homaccord is good for the depression of grieving (Ignatia amara).

Nervo-Heel is suggested for reactive depression (exogenous) and *Psorino-Heel*, supported by *Nervo-Heel* and *Ignatia-Homaccord*, for endogenous depression.

Possibly the best thought-out depression remedy is Deprex by Vaxa.

Deprex contains remedies which help the body to naturally regulate hypothalmic activity and balance the natural production of serotonin and norepinephrine. Deprex also contains Ignatia, as well as Avina sativa extract (oats).

The latter is excellent for nervous exhaustion, and sleeplessness. Deprex also contain homeopathic lithium carbonate; lithium is the main orthodox treatment for bipolar depression.

You can find the relevant websites in the **Valuable Resources** section at the back of the book.

There are several homeopathic ingredients that aid in the reduction of Depression symptoms such as: insomnia, headaches, restlessness, fatigue, changes in appetite, uncontrollable weeping, etc.

Mild exercize is good for all types of depression but, please, just light exercize. Obsessively overdoing it (like the Crossfit cult) will almost certainly misfire; it's the beginning of obsession and mania. If some light exercize makes you feel good, that does NOT mean that more will make you feel better.

But what we call "small dose" exercise, yes.

A large study of healthy adults conducted in London suggests that an hour a week of low-intensity exercise may be all it takes to prevent depression.

"Being active is good for you — even in small doses. Taken regularly, exercise is good for you, and it probably prevents mental ill health," senior author Matthew Hotopf, PhD, director of the South London and Maudsley NHS Foundation Trust National Institute of Health Research Biomedical Research Center at Kings College London, the United Kingdom, told Medscape Medical News.

"So, if physicians have a patient with a history of depression, this advice is probably particularly important: do regular, small amounts of enjoyable exercise. Patients don't have to run a marathon," Dr Hotopf added.

Dr. Mats Hallgren, PhD, a researcher at the Karolinska Institute in Stockholm, Sweden, was lead researcher in a similar study involving 946 patients with mild to moderate depression who were assigned to undergo either yoga or stretching, moderate aerobic exercise, or vigorous aerobic experience.

Hallgren confirmed the benefits of exercise on depression were maintained 12 months after baseline assessment, even if the patient didn't stick to the recommendations fully.

"I think the recommendation should not be to exercise only once a week, because people need to exercise more than once a week for general health, so for that reason alone, we should recommend that people exercise three times a week," Dr Hallgren said.

Apparently there was no added benefit to exercizing more than an hour at a time.

The study was published online October 3, 2017, in the *American Journal of Psychiatry*.[120]

2.2 Schizophrenia: Is There Such A Thing?

We should probably avoid the term schizophrenia, not because I don't believe in it, but because it seems to be a whole range of behaviors and thought dysfunction, from hearing voices and hallucinating, to psychotic unreality and detachment, with many stages between.

In other words, schizophrenia is not a disease, it's a symptom—or more exactly a whole battery of click-to-fit symptoms.

At its worst, this tendency is characterized by fantasy and delusion, and a frightening sense of mental fragmentation. At its least, the patient could fairly be described as "out of touch with reality".

There is no meaningful hierarchy of mental illness, but if there was, the schizoid range would definitely follow on from depression. Maybe it is not so common but it is definitely a most severe disability, indeed possibly the worst.

In his book *Schizophrenia - The Sacred Symbol of Psychiatry*, professor Thomas S. Szasz, MD, says "There is, in short, no such thing as schizophrenia".[121]

In the Epilogue of their book *Schizophrenia - Medical Diagnosis or Moral Verdict?*, Theodore R. Sarbin, Ph.D., a psychology professor at the University of California at Santa Cruz who spent three years working in mental hospitals, and James C. Mancuso, Ph.D., a psychology professor at the State University of New York at Albany, have this to say: "We have come to the end of our journey. Among other things, we have tried to establish that the schizophrenia model of unwanted conduct lacks credibility. The analysis directs us ineluctably to the conclusion that schizophrenia is a myth".[122]

In his book *Against Therapy*, published in 1988, Jeffrey Masson, Ph.D., a psychoanalyst, says "There is a heightened awareness of the dangers inherent in labeling somebody with a disease category like schizophrenia, and many people are beginning to realize that there is no such entity".[123]

Rather than being a bona-fide disease, so-called schizophrenia is a nonspecific category which includes almost everything a human being can do, think, or feel that is greatly disliked by other people (or by the so-called schizophrenics themselves). There are few so-called mental illnesses that have not at one time or another been called schizophrenia.

Because of this, schizophrenia is hard to define objectively. Typically, definitions of schizophrenia are vague or inconsistent with each other, even contradictory. Most doctors and even most psychiatrists would point to the symptom of a "split personality"; that's certainly the most popular definition.

But a pamphlet published by the National Alliance for the Mentally Ill titled "What Is Schizophrenia?" says "Schizophrenia is not a split personality".

In her book *Schiz-o-phre-nia: Straight Talk for Family and Friends*, published in 1985, Maryellen Walsh says, "Schizophrenia is one of the most misunderstood diseases on the planet. Most people think that it means having a split personality. Most people are wrong. Schizophrenia is not a splitting of the personality into multiple parts".[124]

(Please be sure to carefully read my multiple self model, section 3.15. It may contain all the answers you are looking for!)

The American Psychiatric Association's (APA's) *Diagnostic and Statistical Manual of Mental Disorders* (Second Edition), published in 1968, defined schizophrenia as "characteristic disturbances of thinking, mood, or behavior" (p. 33). That means precisely nothing. Characteristic of what? ...of schizophrenia, of course.

In the 1980 edition, the DSM-III was still saying: "The limits of the concept of schizophrenia are unclear" (p. 181).

I need not go on. Uncertainty and confusion about what schizophrenia actually IS confounds the profession (however, that doesn't stop them labeling it as an excess of dopamine, requiring urgent medication!)

Perhaps this is a case like the late US Supreme Court Justice Potter Stewart, who famously declared in a celebrated obscenity case that, although he could not define pornography, 'I know it when I see it'.

The fact that schizophrenia is a complex of different disease processes is surely why the confusion exists. Until mainstream medicine starts to look at causes, instead of symptoms, that will persist indefinitely.

Instead there is an obsession to make schizophrenia into a single disease and give it a single cause: some kind of chemical imbalance, which can be treated with suitable drugs.

However, the official definition of schizophrenia maintained and published by the American Psychiatric Association in its Diagnostic and Statistical Manual of Mental Disorders (DSM) for many years specifically excluded organically caused conditions from the definition of schizophrenia.

Contrast this with a statement by psychiatrist E. Fuller Torrey, MD, in his book *Surviving Schizophrenia: A Family Manual*, published in 1988. He says boldly that "Schizophrenia is a brain disease, now definitely known to be such".[125] Of course, if schizophrenia is a brain disease, then it is organic. There is no evidence to back up this statement. The science points to the opposite. But by now we have to get used to psychiatrists simply lying through their teeth, to justify the expensive and tragically-destructive treatments they hand out as a "cure".

It was not until the publication of the revised DSM-IV in 1994 that the APA position was rescinded in regard to schizophrenia.

From then on, all bets were off. We are allowed to say it is an organically based disorder so that's the line the industry uses! No evidence for it, as we saw in section 1.3, but if they can make this theory stick, then they are cleared to sell a lot of unnecessary and unworkable drugs as the "proper" treatment!

Characteristics

There are certain consistent symptoms that presumptive schizophrenic patients report, any one of which may be present in any combination with the others, in any given patient. This alone means there is little correlation between thoughts, emotions and behavior.

Common are hearing external voices, paranoia (jumpy and suspicious), ideas of reference (the patient has a fixation that people are watching him, or beaming energies or thoughts into his mind), there may be delusions, hallucinations, depersonalization, agitation (restless, pointless movements and gestures), or inertia (sitting around in a motionless, nonreactive state). There may be excitation of emotions, so that someone ecstatically happy could be labeled schizoid, according to the DSM-II (1968); or showing lack of any real feelings, which the 1987 edition, DSM-III-R, allows a person can be "diagnosed" as schizophrenic because he displays neither happiness nor sadness! (p. 189),

As attorney Bruce Ennis says in his book *Prisoners of Psychiatry*: "schizophrenia is such an all-inclusive term and covers such a large range of behavior that there are few people who could not, at one time or another, be considered schizophrenic".[126]

For example, people who are obsessed with certain thoughts or who feel compelled to perform certain behaviors, such as washing their hands repeatedly, are usually considered to be suffering from a separate psychiatric disease called "obsessive-compulsive disorder" (OCD). However, people with such obsessive thoughts or compulsive behaviors have also been called schizophrenic (e.g., by Dr. Torrey in his book *Surviving Schizophrenia*, pp. 115-116).

Psychiatrist Dr. Torrey, cited above, admits: "The definitions of most diseases of mankind has been accomplished. ... In almost all diseases there is something which can be seen or measured, and this can be used to define the disease and separate it from non-disease states. Not so with schizophrenia! To date we have no single thing which can be measured and from which we can then say: Yes, that is schizophrenia."

Psychiatrist William Glasser, M.D., says in his book *Positive Addiction*, published in 1976: "Schizophrenia sounds so much like a disease that prominent scientists delude themselves into searching for its cure" (Harper & Row, p. 18). This is a silly endeavor, because these supposedly prominent scientists can't define "schizophrenia" and accordingly don't know what they are looking for.

Lawrence Stevens JD, a lawyer who represents psychiatric "patients", argues that schizophrenia is really just based on disapproval. Labels like pornography or mental illness indicate disapproval of that to which the label is applied and nothing more.

The term schizophrenia, according to Stevens, is a reflection of the speaker's or "diagnostician's" values or ideas about how a person "should" be, often coupled with the false (or at least unproven) assumption that the disapproved thinking, emotions, or behavior results from a biological abnormality.

Clearly there is SOMETHING going on. I myself have met babbling individuals, who are totally out of touch with reality (mad, if you like) talking to people who are not present. I recall a very strong and aggressive young man who had grabbed a nurse's breast and gripped it really tightly, apparently unaware that what he was doing was wrong. He seemed in a daze. I had to prize his hand off the frightened girl, leaving her breast blue with savage bruises, before subduing the man (this was on the open wards, by the way).

But is that schizophrenia? It certainly fits Lawrence Stevens's dictum that it is something we would all disapprove of.

Back to the claim it is a brain disease...

The Only Thing We DO Know Is That It's NOT Metabolic

According to three Stanford University psychiatry professors, "two hypotheses have dominated the search for a biological substrate of schizophrenia." They say these two theories are the transmethylation hypothesis of schizophrenia and the dopamine hypothesis of schizophrenia.[127]

The transmethylation hypothesis was based on the idea that schizophrenia might be caused by "aberrant formation of methylated amines", similar to the hallucinogenic pleasure drug mescaline in the metabolism of so-called schizophrenics. After reviewing various attempts to verify this theory, the authors concluded: "More than two decades after the introduction of the transmethylation hypothesis, no conclusions can be drawn about its relevance to or involvement in schizophrenia" (p. 107).

Columbia University psychiatry professor Jerrold S. Maxmen, M.D., succinctly describes the second major biological theory of schizophrenia, the so-called dopamine hypothesis, in his book *The New Psychiatry*, published in 1985: "...many psychiatrists believe that schizophrenia involves excessive activity in the dopamine-receptor system...the schizophrenic's symptoms result partially from receptors being overwhelmed by dopamine".[128]

But in the article by three Stanford University psychiatry professors referred to above they say "direct confirmation that dopamine is involved in schizophrenia continues to elude investigators" (p. 112). In 1987 in his book *Molecules of the Mind* Professor Jon Franklin says "The dopamine hypothesis, in short, was wrong".[129]

I wrote extensively about the failure of this hypothesis in section 1.3. It not only lacks evidence to support it; there is direct evidence it is WRONG.

Other efforts to prove a biological basis for so-called schizophrenia have involved brain-scans of pairs of identical twins, when only one is a supposed schizophrenic. They do indeed show the so-called schizophrenic has brain damage not present in the identical twin. The flaw in these studies is the so-called schizophrenic has inevitably been given brain-damaging drugs as a supposed treatment and it is these drugs that have caused the damage, not so-called schizophrenia. Anyone "treated" with these drugs will have such brain damage, a fact side-stepped by investigators.

These brain scans actually prove that current drug medications are hurting patients and damaging their brains, not a demonstration of the causes of any disease.

In *The New Harvard Guide to Psychiatry*, published in 1988, Seymour S. Kety, M.D., Professor Emeritus of Neuroscience in Psychiatry, and Steven Matthysse, Ph.D., Associate Professor of Psychobiology, both of Harvard Medical School, say "an impartial reading of the recent literature does not provide the hoped-for clarification of the catecholamine hypotheses, nor does compelling evidence emerge for other biological differences that may characterize the brains of patients with mental disease."[130]

Belief in biological causes of so-called mental illness, including schizophrenia, comes not from science but from wishful thinking or from desire to avoid coming to terms with the experiential/environmental causes of people's misbehavior or distress. The repeated failure of efforts to find biological causes of so-called schizophrenia suggests it really belongs in the category of socially/culturally unacceptable thinking or behavior, rather than in the category of biology or "disease" (like the man who viciously grasped a nurse's breast, above).

Even the proponents of the biological model of schizophrenia stumble and are confounded; they admit it.

In his book *Schizophrenia Revealed - From Neurons to Social Interaction* (W.W.Norton, New York, 2001), Michael Foster Green, Ph.D., a professor in the UCLA Department of Psychiatry and Behavioral Sciences, and chief of the treatment unit of the Department of Veterans Affairs Mental Illness Research, Education and Clinical Center, does his best to promote the idea that so-called schizophrenia is biological. He nevertheless makes the following admissions: "...we do not yet have an adequate understanding of schizophrenia... a specific brain abnormality in schizophrenia has remained elusive ...schizophrenia cannot be diagnosed by a brain scan".[131]

Nor diagnosed by any other objective test. It's all just opinions. But opinions wickedly manipulated by a crazy, dishonest pharmaceutical industry, with a whale of a profit return on its evil mind!

Here's a better story...

Carl Pfeiffer

Carl C. Pfeiffer, M.D., Ph.D. (1908–1988) was a US physician and biochemist who researched schizophrenia, allergies and other diseases. He was Chair of the Pharmacology Department at Emory University and considered himself a founder of orthomolecular psychiatry and published in the Journal Science.

Of all the disorders he studied, Pfeiffer was focused most intently on Schizophrenia. He used the terms: "the waste basket diagnosis", "the plague of mental disease", "demon possession" and insanity. He felt the word schizophrenia was an inadequate and misleading diagnosis. He believed that "disperceptions of unknown cause" was a more appropriate definition.

He made major contributions to the understanding of trace element and mineral metabolism in the schizophrenias; made a rational division of the schizophrenias into three biochemical groups, and discussed amino acids in medicine. Carl Pfeiffer was one of the original members of the Committee on Therapy of the American Schizophrenia Association.

In his book, 'Twenty-Nine Medical Causes of Schizophrenia', he gives a comprehensive list of medical causes of schizophrenia broken down into three categories: well-known, less-known, and almost unknown. Here are the first two categories. Practitioners will satisfy themselves as to the third group of obscure causes.

Well-known

- Heavy metal toxicity
- Sleep deprivation
- Folic acid/B12 deficiency
- Homocysteinuria
- Drug intoxications
- Hypothyroidism
- Porphyria (George III's disease)
- Pellagra
- Dementia paralytica

Less Well-known

- Psychomotor epilepsy
- Hypoglycemia
- Cerebral allergy
- Wheat-gluten sensitivity
- Histapenia – copper excess
- Histadelia
- Pyrroluria
- Wilson's disease
- Chronic Candida infection
- Huntington's chorea

Note that Pfeiffer lists hypoglycemia as one of the potent hidden causes of schizophrenia. He estimates the frequency of the less well-known causes as:

- histapenia with excess copper: 50% of schizophrenias
- histadelia with low copper: 20% of all schizophrenias
- pyrroluria, a familial double deficiency of B6 and zinc: 30%
- cerebral allergies: 10%
- hypoglycemia: 20%

These latter 5 causes and treatments are dealt with in more detail later, in Part 5.

Switching To The Holistic View

Searching for physical causes has been very rewarding for some but there is no consistent pattern, to indicate we are on the trail of "real" cause. I have personally had great results with using the food allergy approach. Frank Dohan MD has also had some success in this regard, particularly eliminating grains and gluten.[132]

In a later study from the Danish population registers, persons whose parents had celiac disease (gluten allergy) were three times as likely to later be diagnosed with schizophrenia.[133]

In the end, this is all about brain allergies, which will be discussed in the exploration and treatment section. Food allergy is clearly one of the common causes of brain inflammation and dysfunction.

It is interesting to note that there is a clear association between autoimmune diseases and what is commonly diagnosed as schizophrenia: rheumatoid arthritis, thyroid disorders, type 1 diabetes and celiac disease. Currently the evidence is strongest for thyroid disorders (see section 5.9) and celiac disease.[134]

I know from decades of experience that food allergies largely underpin autoimmune diseases. Also chemical sensitivity and heavy metal poisoning (lead, mercury, etc.)

It seems to me that what we are calling schizophrenia, is really an autoimmune disease of the brain. In other words: encephalitis, or inflammation of the brain.

I'll need to persuade some heavy guns to investigate it meaningfully. But if you step back and think about it, what could be a more likely cause of the endless kaleidoscope of bizarre and disturbing symptoms?

A researcher at the University of Oxford, Belinda Lennox, agrees. She and her team found a proportion of the cases with antibodies attacking NMDA receptors. These receptors are widespread throughout the brain and pivotal in action. Among other things, this receptor is involved in the formation of new memories. When the immune system attacks the NMDA receptor, it becomes inflamed, and one of the possible symptoms is psychosis.[135]

In my own texts, I have described food and chemical allergy symptoms as bizarre, protean and highly subjective. Proteus was a Greek sea god, son of Poseidon (Neptune), who kept changing his form whenever he appeared.

Symptoms can be very bizarre, such as headache every Monday but no other day (onions with Sunday dinner), epilepsy after eating carrots, drunk after eating potatoes or orange, hallucinating after cheese, strange body image with excess wheat intake, and sexual arousal after eating chicken – these are all true cases from my files.

Subjective symptoms seem to create even more hostility with physicians, yet patients sometimes have difficulty describing what they feel: I have heard complaints such as "hot water running down the inside of my skin" and "seeing myself down at the end of a long tunnel"; the feeling of "derealization", that everything has become unreal, unfamiliar and strange; and so-called "Alice In Wonderland" syndrome, where the patient experiences a distortion of time, space or body image.

Well, isn't that all a bit like schizophrenia?

Treatments

The mainstream treatment of schizophrenia is with prescription antipsychotic drugs, many of which produce severe adverse effects; are linked to an incentive for monetary profit, benefiting pharmaceutical corporations; lack sufficient evidence for safety and efficacy; and have been grossly misused.[136]

That schizophrenia may be caused or aggravated by a deficiency of essential nutrients appears to be unknown or marginalized by the majority of health care providers under the sway of Big Pharma propaganda.

Because of that bias, the claim that "antipsychotic medications represent the cornerstone of pharmacological treatment for patients with schizophrenia," is meaningless. They never look outside their model for something better.[137]

Waves of different antipsychotic drugs have been developed throughout the last 60 years, yet these have done nothing to decrease the prevalence of schizophrenia; in fact it has increased dramatically.[138]

Of course that could be due to an increase in enthusiastic diagnosis of schizophrenia, citing ever more and more tenuous complaints. *Remember there are no criteria for diagnosis schizophrenia, other than pure opinion.*

So the bar for success is very low.

"For schizophrenia, the recovery rate with drug therapy is under 15%. With nutritional therapy, the recovery rate is 80%." - Abram Hoffer, MD, PhD

The orthomolecular approach may be, at least, an integral part of a treatment program that optimizes general health and leads to a life free from schizophrenic symptoms, with few or no negatives. Compared to the savage side-effects of psychotropic drugs, merely to switch from a drug approach to a natural one would be an enormous advance.

But considering the outcomes are far better, the orthomolecular approach could be taken as the standard.

Food Allergies and Schizophrenia

Young Jacob was a Jewish boy, aged 19. His mother contacted me in desperation; he was severely out of touch with the real world, hallucinated strange realities, talked at length with his "voices" and seemed to be getting worse. At times he would walk around, in full and open discussion with Jesus, Bob Dylan, Abraham Lincoln and several other very public figures I cannot now remember.

I very quickly established that Jacob had food allergies. Several were quite severe. Eventually, it emerged that cheese was the main trigger for his schizoid symptoms. When he stayed off this food, he was as normal as you and me.

But if he should eat cheese, all his symptoms came back, full force, and he was diagnosably insane for about four days—until the cheese left his bowel, at which point he reverted to normal.

I mention this case particularly because Frank Dohan MD (1907-1991) became a noted expert in the correlation between wheat allergy and schizophrenia. The association was strong and significant; moreover, the trait appeared to run in families. He spent the latter part of his busy and varied life trying to persuade colleagues of this important inter-relation.[139]

But Dohan missed the key point I learned over the years: any food allergy can cause any bracket of symptoms.

Since his pioneering, David Perlmutter has now taken up the story and is promoting it in his book *Grain Brain*.[140] It turns out that schizophrenics have 50 to 100 times the incidence of celiac disease (gluten sensitivity) compared to the general population.

Put the other way round, celiac doctors also noticed their patients were schizophrenic about 10X as often as the general population. That's a lot! In addition, epidemiological studies of Pacific Islanders and other populations showed a strong, dose-dependent relationship between grains intake and schizophrenia. The native gluten-free populations had an extremely rare occurrence of schizophrenia - just 2 per 65,000 versus about 1 per 100 as we have in the grain-eating West.

When native populations turned to Western grain-based diets (flour, bread, pizza, sugar, and beer), schizophrenia became common. In some clinical trials, gluten made new-onset acutely ill schizophrenics much worse, but unfortunately gluten-free restrictions only occasionally helped with long-term patients.

The link is there but there is clearly more to this than just gluten, as I have been saying and writing for nearly 40 years! It turns out that schizophrenics tended to have a lot of anti-wheat antibodies floating around in their systems, but these antibodies were entirely different from the ones that people with celiac disease have. That means that the usual test for gluten issues, the tests for celiac, wouldn't come up positive in schizophrenics, even though they have unusual immune reactions to wheat. I know David Perlmutter and admire his work. But he needs to look beyond the limited model of just grains. My view is that any food can potentially do it.

A food allergy reaction is highly inflammatory. It doesn't take much systemic inflammation to cause cerebral dysfunction. Therefore it is important for the health practitioner to be alert to any and all food allergies as a contributory or causal phenomenon for mental symptoms. Some of the reactions I have seen are quite bizarre.

The important point is that every patient with problematic psychological dysfunction should, as a matter of course, be investigated for food allergies and intolerance. And I do mean *investigated*. There is a current fad or trend, ignorant in the extreme, which seems to think that gluten and casein are the only significant food allergies of note. My experience is that any person can react to any food. We are all, as Roger J. Williams said, unique in our biochemistry.

I have given pretty detailed instructions in this book explaining how to uncover food allergies, by elimination and challenge dieting. But it can become complex and therefore I refer the reader to two further resources:

My book Diet Wise and it's accompanying teaching system **Diet Wise Academy** are linked in the **Valuable Resources** section in the back of the book.

Remember not to overlook related topics, such as chemical sensitivity, molds, yeasts, Candida, and heavy metal overload.

Niacin and Schizophrenia

Research into possible genetic causes of schizophrenia has not found any obvious candidate. Apparently, many gene mutations are associated with schizophrenia, but none yet found have an influence strong enough to be considered THE cause. This isn't surprising, since schizophrenia is so clearly not just one disease but a whole family of interrelated conditions, implying many different causes.

Orthodox treatment is unsuccessful in the main and only "controls" the condition, by shutting down mind and Being. But time and again nutritional strategies have been shown to be highly effective, even fully restorative (providing the regimen is maintained).

Many schizophrenic patients have severe nutrient dependencies that can be treated with niacin and other vitamins and nutrients. A dependency isn't quite the same as a deficiency state: it means the individual's needs for that nutrient are higher than normal, so he or she is dependent on getting plenty (well above average, anyway).

Interest in the use of niacin therapy for testing and treatment of schizophrenia and many other conditions appears to be rapidly expanding. For a therapeutic effect, pioneer psychiatrist Abram Hoffer recommended gradually increasing doses up to 3,000 mg/day of niacin in divided doses, along with 2,000 mg/day or more of vitamin C and other essential nutrients. For some people, high doses can cause temporary side effects, so many people take niacin for its health benefit at lower doses (500 - 1,000 mg/day). Niacinamide does not cause the skin flush but may not be quite so effective.[141]

The trouble is that Hoffer and Osmond's theories about how niacin could treat schizophrenia were never proven sufficiently to convince orthodox psychiatrists. However, many professionals did acknowledge that they were getting surprisingly good results, with or without the correct explanation.[142]

Niacin Skin Test

The "problem" with using high-dose niacin as a treatment is the alarming skin flush reaction. The new patient can find it quite unnerving.

The skin turns bright red and feels literally on fire for several minutes, before the reaction subsides. This is a normal consequence of niacin activating prostaglandin pathways that cause vasodilation in the skin and is not harmful. To avoid the skin flush, one starts with small doses [typically 25 mg/day] and gradually increases the dose over several days to achieve a therapeutic effect.[143]

However, some schizophrenics don't get this niacin flush, which suggests they may have a different metabolic pathway for the nutrient. Or that they have a severe degree of B3 deficiency (and likely other essential nutrients too). For this reason it has been suggested that niacin applied to the skin or taken orally could be used as a test for latent schizophrenia. Interestingly, Hoffer noted that in some cases, where schizophrenics recovered, they reverted to a normal skin flush. So this could be important.[144]

A number of recent studies show that about one third of schizophrenics have a blunted niacin skin flush, suggesting that this test can be used as a diagnostic tool.

Several of these recent studies attempt to determine what metabolic disturbance might cause problems for the brain. Although most of these studies don't explicitly discuss the use of niacin as a treatment, the underlying theme is that niacin treatment can help many schizophrenics.

This is such an important holistic psychiatry issue I have given several in the Valuable Resources section at the back of the book. It was compiled by Robert G. Smith of Orthomolecular News (you can find his link in the same area).

Smoking And Schizophrenia

Finally, a surprise topic in the management of schizophrenia.

Scientists have found that smoking and schizophrenia are tightly linked, but are not sure why. Could nicotine actually be helping the disorder?

People with schizophrenia smoke up to three times more than the general population and more than most psychiatric populations. Schizophrenia patients who smoke also have higher levels of nicotine in their bodies because they tend to extract more nicotine per cigarette than other smokers.

Nicotine and its brain receptors—proteins on the surface of cells that receive chemical messages—are keys to understanding the links between smoking and schizophrenia. Already, research has revealed that:

- Nicotine and its receptors are involved in functions such as cognition or thinking ability, reward, movement, and pain relief.

- Schizophrenia patients have fewer and more poorly functioning nicotinic receptors, especially in the hippocampus, cortex, and cells that wrap the thalamus—brain areas involved in several cognitive and sensory deficits of schizophrenia.

- Increased nicotine intake—from smoking cigarettes or sometimes from a skin patch, gum, or nasal spray—may temporarily normalize sensory disruptions of schizophrenia.

Here's where addled scientific thinking comes in. Because schizophrenics have few nicotine receptors, it is lame to assume that smoking benefits such patients by giving them "rewards". It's just as logical to think that smoking has a much more damaging impact on their thinking because of lack of suitable receptors.

Thus there are two schools of logic. One group which thinks schizophrenics smoke more because it helps them; in other words patients who smoke are self-medicating. The other group thinks that smoking it particularly harmful to certain individuals and is causing, or increasing the risk of, schizophrenia.

I am firmly of the latter group. If you stop mental health patients smoking, many diseases—not just schizophrenia—dramatically improve. It's only logical, since nicotine and its combustion products are chemical pollution and overload (most science investigations of nicotine simply didn't examine the question of tar and burn products from cigarettes).

Now a large meta-analysis study from King's College has really put the seal on it, finding that smoking actually increases the odds of schizophrenia.

The team looked at 61 past studies of almost 290,000 participants, and ran statistical analyses to determine any connections between smoking and the likelihood of having or developing schizophrenia. They found that daily smokers were at least two times more likely to develop schizophrenia than non-smokers. It is said that correlation does not mean causation. That's true. But the team also found that daily smokers tended to develop psychosis about a year earlier than non-smokers. That makes the theory that smoking is merely a consequence of the illness seem very unlikely.[145]

I visit the smoking relationship to schizophrenia again, in more detail, in section 5.8.

Avatar Therapy

Finally, something completely out of left field... talking to a computer avatar! Devized by Prof Julian Leff, from University College London, so-called avatar therapy has helped patients hearing voices to cope better with hallucinations, a 2017 UK trial has found.

This could be a major step forward. It is the premise of this book and the opinion of this author that "voices" are quite real; just a manifestation of other non-material thinking presences (entities) within a patient's psychic space.

Meantime, psychiatrists go on labeling this phenomenon "auditory hallucinations." The voices can be rude and threatening. But isn't this what any thinking human being would resort to, if completely ignored or derided as not real? We would whine and complain, yes? Possibly become aggressive.

Talking to the voices in a calm, rational and polite way, as if they were "real" and entitled to express themselves (provide they do so respectfully and not threateningly) is the best—and only really successful way—to calm the voices. Once listened to, they settle down, instead of yelling and screaming for attention!

Substituting an avatar is about as near to the truth that mainstream psychiatrists can go at this time. Not surprisingly, it works because it is a kind of dummy conversation with the voices.

The present study, looking at 150 people, was published in *The Lancet Psychiatry* journal 23 Nov 2017). It follows a much smaller pilot study in 2013. Run by King's College London and University College London, 75 patients who had continued to hear voices for more than a year, were given six sessions of avatar therapy while another 75 received the same amount of counseling.

In the avatar sessions, patients created a computer simulation to represent the voice they heard and wanted to control, including how it sounded and how it might look.

The therapist then "voiced" the avatar while also speaking as themselves in a three-way conversation to help the patient gain the upper hand.

Prof Tom Craig, study author from King's College London, said getting patients to learn to stand up to the avatar was found to be safe, easy to deliver and twice as effective as counseling at reducing how often voices were heard.

"After 12 weeks there was dramatic improvement compared to the other therapy," he said. "With a talking head, patients are learning to confront and get replies from it.

"This shifts the idea that the voice is all-controlling," Craig said.

Patients are encouraged to talk to the avatar and take control of the conversation, saying things such as, "I'm not going to listen to you any more."

Seven patients who had had the avatar therapy and two from the counseling group said their hallucinations had completely disappeared after 12 weeks. It would be trivial to claim that avatar therapy had more than triple the success of CBT (2:7). But there is a clear difference.

Sir Robin Murray, professor of psychiatric research at King's College London's Institute of Psychiatry, said "If a wholly psychological intervention such as avatar therapy can produce such an improvement, then it should make us rethink the way we conceptualize auditory hallucinations."[146]

Well, I hope so Murray!

Researchers are now evaluating whether repeated "booster" sessions of avatar therapy would be beneficial.

2.3 Bipolar Disorder

Originally known as manic-depressive psychosis, because the person gets both disorders, in spades!

Bipolar disorder is a condition in which the sufferer cycles through bouts of mania or hyper-agitation, followed by inertia and deep depression. The switches can be very dramatic and unpredictable, making this condition very difficult to live with for both patients and family. In its lesser form, the patient may only be aware of racing thoughts, fatigue and insomnia, loss of appetite and sexual dysfunction, rather than depression *per se*.

Bipolar is usually classified as a severe variant of depressive illness. However, as you will see, ecstatic (but unhealthy) highs are just as much a part of the picture.

From happiness highs (mania) to deep lows (depression), bipolar disorder is a chronic mental illness characterized by extreme swings in mood. These drastic mood changes can happen a few times a year or multiple times in a single day.

Bipolar disorder is responsible for the loss of more disability-adjusted life years (DALYs) than all forms of cancer or than major neurologic conditions such as epilepsy and Alzheimer's disease[1], primarily because of its early onset and chronicity across the life span.

Aggregate estimates of the prevalence of bipolar disorder indicate that approximately 1.0% of the general population meet lifetime criteria for bipolar disorder. In the USA, this figure may be higher: approximately 5.7 million adult Americans, or about 2.6% of the U.S. population age 18 and older.[147] Understanding Bipolar in One

The best way to get a grasp of the bipolar (two-part) nature of this disorder is to consider the effects of alcohol. Suppose somebody is getting steadily drunk. He or she will start by being lively and loquacious (talkative); he or she is larger than life; wants to save the world; he or she is the best lover in town, etc. etc. We've all been there, or at least seen these dudes in action during happy hour.

They are grand. They are happ-y!

But as the person keeps drinking, the drunkenness and excitement rises to a crescendo; he or she gets noisy, irrational and out of control. Then, inevitably, he or she starts coming down the other side. They slow down, mumble their words, stagger around and finally (if no-one takes them home), they will crash out under the table, in a stupor.

Next day he or she feels awful; like death warmed up; heavily hung over; apologetic, morose and very depressed!

This is the nature of bipolar disease: over-revved or excited, followed by slowed down and depressed. Up and down; up and down. Hence the term bipolar.

The downs are just depression. That's bad. But the UPs can be quite spectacular! I met one at med school who wanted to shoot the rapids on the Irwell river in Manchester, UK; buy a million dollar hotel with a bouncy check; molested countless women as if he were irresistible; and he finally tried to gatecrash the BBC television studios and announce himself on air, before the police were finally summoned to take him off the streets!

Usually, the mania phase, or hypomania (just a bit less than mania), is less dramatic than this case: can't sleep, talking all the time, rapidly swirling moods, mind tumbling with ideas, driving faster than is safe and spending money like there is no tomorrow.

This is close to the way a lot of people behave; just a bit too much. Normal but just too much! Which is why many bipolar people go undiagnosed and untreated. It can affect close personal relationships, job performance, and ability to function consistently in daily life. The patient may not recognize how their behavior impacts those around them.

50% of all bipolar disorder diagnosed occurs between 15-25 years old.

During periods of mania, bipolar disorder can increase productivity, creativity, and energy levels. So he or she looks good! Hesitant to give up these "highs," some patients are reluctant to undergo treatment.

The most common symptoms can be summed up as follows:

- Unexpected and dramatic changes in mood from euphoria to deep sadness.

- Energy that ebbs and flows without apparent cause.

- Inflated self-esteem and grandiose plans.

- Inability to concentrate, racing thoughts, or rapid speech.

- Feelings of extreme irritability or aggressiveness.

- Engaging in high-risk behavior: fighting, reckless driving, shopping sprees, or unprotected sex.

- Fluctuations in eating and sleeping patterns.

- During the depressive lows, those who suffer with bipolar disorder may focus on self-harm, thoughts of death, or may attempt suicide.

In the high phase, physical energy levels can seem limitless. The body moves smoothly, there is little or no fatigue. But it doesn't last. The elevated phases are short, mild and generally manageable, but the shift into severe depression or a mixed mood state occurs sometimes within minutes or hours, certainly within days and will last weeks, often without any periods of normality. Indeed, the patient often loses track of what normality is.

He or she becomes unable to concentrate to read a novel or watch TV. His or her brain slows right down. The patient seems to drop out of touch with other people and the world around them.

Risk Factors for Bipolar Disorder:

Most cases of bipolar disorder occur in teens and adults, as I said, but children as young as six years old have been diagnosed bipolar, something that many mental health experts would disagree with. In a sense, all kids are bipolar!

Bipolar disorder has been linked to other serious conditions such as attention-deficit/ hyperactivity disorder (ADHD), substance abuse, post-traumatic stress disorder (PTSD), and physical ailments such as obesity, heart disease, and thyroid dysfunction.

Other aspects of the condition include:

- Immediate family member that is a blood relation with a history of mental disorder, alcoholism, or suicide.

- Stress in daily life.

- Alcohol or drug abuse.

- Unexpected trauma such as the death of a loved one.

- A history of physical, emotional, or sexual abuse.

At some stage or other, every bipolar patient will consider ending it all.

Bipolar disease has one of the highest risks of suicide. Legal troubles, relationship problems, substance abuse, and poor work performance are just a few of the regular issues that bipolar disorder—diagnosed or undiagnosed—can trigger. The safety of the patient and other people is paramount.

Dealing With Bipolar Disorder

Treatment for this form of depression is ongoing and involves the patient taking responsibility for their recovery.

Everything that was written in section 2.1 about depression applies to bipolar disorder, which is after all only a type of depression. All treatable physical disorders must be corrected: blood sugar (especially important), toxic overload, nutritional deficiency, hormonal imbalances and particularly food allergies.

Think again of the person getting drunk, being uninhibited, and then crashing. Something is removing the blocks and then poisoning out the brain. In this example we know it is the alcohol.

But what else can do this? Drugs, obviously. Dope, amphetamine (especially), ecstasy and narcotics.

What most doctors and psychiatrists miss is that it can be something simple, like a food allergy (wheat, corn, egg, caffeine, etc.), sugar overload, mold allergy, stealth pathogens, or heavy metal poisoning.

It's all covered later in this book. The point is that bipolar people are NOT mentally ill, no matter how strangely he or she behaves; however outrageous, antisocial and even dangerously he or she lives, while in the grip of the syndrome.

Something is driving the brain fire and that something is the real culprit. Once found and dealt with, the whole issue of bipolar—or depression altogether—simply vanishes!

I repeat: this is not a mental sickness, this is brain inflammation.

The Inflammation Factor

Brain inflammation has many causes. But it will not be diagnosed, unless doctors and practitioners think of it.

As proof of the concept, I put it to you that bipolar disorder is strongly associated with immune dysfunction. Replicated epidemiological studies have demonstrated that bipolar disorder has high rates of inflammatory medical comorbidities, including autoimmune disorders, chronic infections, cardiovascular disease and metabolic disorders.

Inflammatory markers called cytokines have been shown to be a part of the presentation (how it looks) of bipolar disorder. Overall, it gives the impression of a chronic low-grade inflammation, with further increases in pro-inflammatory cytokine levels during mood episodes.

Several mechanisms have been identified to explain the bidirectional relationship between bipolar disorder and immune dysfunction. Key mechanisms include cytokine-induced neurotransmitter changes (especially monoamines), increased oxidative stress, pathological microglial over-activation, hypothalamic-pituitary-adrenal (HPA) axis over-activation, alterations of the microbiome-gut-brain axis and sleep-related immune changes.

Note that all of these factors play a part in any neurological or so-called mental disorder. Fixing these conditions individually is part of the very tenets of holistic psychiatry.

Several proof-of-concept clinical trials have shown a positive effect of anti-inflammatory agents in the treatment of bipolar disorder.[148]

We can do better in this present work, which is to find and eliminate the causes of systemic and neurological inflammation in the body, not just tune out the symptoms of inflammation. Why mop up the spillage when it makes more sense to turn off the overflowing faucet?

The Ups and Downs Of Addicted Life

By far the most interesting discovery in psychiatric medicine, though most psychiatrists are unaware of its existence, is in the realm of 'brain allergy', whether due to real allergy, intolerance, low–grade poisoning, etc., the effects can be subtle, amusing, bi-

Normal writing

1 2 3 4 5 6 7 8 9 10
11 12 13 14 15 16 17 18 19

and after challenge testing

zarre, dangerous or disastrous, in varying combinations. I have seen an allergy lead to heightened sexual feelings, murderous assault, schizophrenic psychosis, woolly thinking, hallucination, hyperactivity, depression, anxiety, learning difficulties, dyslexia and autism, with many intermediate types and mixtures of symptoms.

One of the tests we used at my office, for minimal brain dysfunction during an acute allergic response, was to have the patient write his or her name and the numbers 1 to 10. Some of the results were outlandish, to say the least. All my UK records are gone but my good friend Dr. Doris Rapp made a practice of collecting such records and an example is included here, so show clearly what brain allergy can do to normal intellectual function.

Minimal brain dysfunction in children is probably one of the commonest allergic effects. It may lead to antisocial acts, poor concentration, learning difficulties and emotional unhappiness. Dyslexia is an interesting and unusual condition which may respond dramatically to the clinical ecology approach. I had an extraordinary case in my Dublin office, of a young boy Eamonn, who wrote his name backwards (mirror-image style) while under the influence of wheat and apple. I have often pondered what extraordinary complexity of brain processing took place, in order to write a word in reverse!

Some youngsters afflicted with these problems have a very hard time in life; everyone thinks they are naughty, stupid or lazy and they get no help and may even be scolded or punished for things they have no control over.

Naturally, if undetected these difficulties may roll on into adult life. There the condition shifts emphasis often, causing more inner neurosis and unhappiness. Patients may brood and feel melancholy; life doesn't seem worth living and many patients have said they would like to end it all, if only they had the courage.

In this context it is worth quoting in full from my food allergy writings, relating the seminal work of the late Dr. Theron Randolph. I published it in my book *Diet Wise*. It is too important to not repeat here.

Chicago pioneer doctor Theron "Ted" Randolph, who began to notice unusual cerebral manifestations in his patients, went to the trouble of cataloguing these and drawing up a table (see below). It is one of the most rewarding studies of human behavior I know. Randolph realized that there were varying stages of excitation and depression during allergic and hypersensitivity reactions, passing through gradually deepening levels, as the brain became more and more overcharged or somnolent. Moreover, people would "roller-coaster ride" between different stages. These ups and downs, he pointed out, were exactly like the manifestations of addiction.

Two points need making clear. Firstly, there are no hard–and–fast gradations: these symptoms blend subtly one into another and indeed it is possible to have 'minus' reactions present at the same instant as 'plus' reactions. Secondly, each individual, though he or she may move around on the ladder, tends to gravitate towards a permanent level appropriate to him or her. Even this 'chronic' level may move in time, usually ultimately tending towards the extreme minus end of the scale, which represents a total inability of all body resources to oppose stress. So-called "allergic" reactions are thus, in reality, short-term departures from this chronic level.

Minus reactions are easy to equate with illness but the over–stimulatory phase is not, except in its extreme. Rather it is sometimes looked on as a good thing to be 'energetic', charging around all the time, 'getting things done'. Moreover, inappropriate laughter and enthusiasm tend to be viewed as evidence of a cheerful disposition when in fact they are merely the result of a minor degree of intoxication, corresponding to a plus 1 or 2 reaction. This only becomes clear when working daily with people being allergically challenged and using provocation techniques, such as Miller's method (serial end-point skin titration); the difference between genuine emotion and a pathological state then becomes easy to discern.

Stimulatory and Withdrawal Levels of Manifestations

Directions :Start at zero (0). Read up for predominantly Stimulatory Levels. Read down for predominantly Withdrawal Levels

LEVEL	SYMPTOM MANIFESTATIONS
PLUS ++++ MANIC WITH OR WITHOUT CONVULSIONS	Distraught, excited, agitated, enraged and panicky. Circuitous or one-track thought, muscle twitching and jerking of extremities, convulsive seizures, and altered consciousness may develop.
PLUS +++ HYPOMANIC, TOXIC, ANXIOUS AND EGOCENTRIC	Aggressive, loquacious, clumsy (ataxic), anxious, fearful and apprehensive; alternating chills and flushing, ravenous hunger, excessive thirst. Gigging or pathological laughter may occur.
PLUS ++ HYPERACTIVE, IRRITABLE, HUNGRY, AND THIRSTY	Tense, jittery, hopped up, talkative, argumentative, sensitive, overly responsive, self-centred, hungry and thirsty, flushing, sweating and chilling may occur as well as insomnia, alcoholism, and obesity.
PLUS + STIMULATED BUT RELATIVELY SYMPTOM FREE	Active, alert, lively, responsive and enthusiastic with unimpaired ambition, energy, initiative and wit. Considerate of the views and actions of others. This usually comes to be regarded as 'normal' behaviour.
LEVEL 0 BEHAVIOUR ON AN EVEN KEEL, AS IN HOMOEOSTASIS	Children expect this from their parents and teachers. Parents expect this from their children. We all expect this from our associates.
MINUS – LOCALIZED ALLERGIC MANIFESTATIONS	Running or stuffy nose, clearing throat, coughing, wheezing, (asthma), itching, eczema and hives, gas, diarrhoea, constipation, colitis, urgency and frequency of urination, and various eye and ear syndromes.
MINUS - - SYSTEMIC ALLERGIC REACTIONS	Tired, dopey, somnolent, mildly depressed, oedematous with painful syndromes (headache, neckache, backache, neuralgia, myalgia, myositis, arthralgia, arthritis, arteritis, chest pain), and cardiovascular effects.*
MINUS - - - DEPRESSIONS AND DISTURBED MENTATION	Confused, indecisive, moody, sad sullen, withdrawn, or apathetic, Emotional instability and impaired attention, concentration, comprehension, and thought processes (aphasia, mental lapse, and blackouts).
MINUS - - - - SEVERE DEPRESSION WITH OR WITHOUT ALTERED CONSCIOUSNESS	Nonresponsive, lethargic, stuporous, disoriented, melancholic, incontinent, regressive thinking, paranoid orientations, delusions, hallucinations, sometimes amnesia, and finally comatose.

* Marked pulse changes or skipped beats may occur at any level.

The speed with which people can move from one phase to another is on occasion quite astonishing. I have witnessed patients, challenged with a food or chemical, appear excited, giggling and intoxicated yet within minutes be slumbering soundly, difficult to rouse. It is well known that for every 'high' there tends to be a corresponding low. The transition can be sharp and the effect very unpleasant indeed. So much so that patients who have never touched alcohol can suffer alarming hangover symptoms. Indeed the inebriation effect caused by foods has often been taken for drunkenness, leading on occasion to unfortunate encounters with the police, who have needed a great deal of convincing.

Not all psychiatric manifestations are food allergies, of course. But all psychiatric illness, I believe, is complicated by organic food-related inflammatory processes and these aspects of an individual's illness, even assuming there are genuine psychogenic (coming from the psyche, caused by the mind) components, will only respond to the ecological approach. Drugs (more chemical pollution) are the last thing that these individuals require; yet that is usually their fate.

Incidentally, sexual excitation and destimulation follow patterns that are similar, and Randolph produced a table to this effect too:

Changes in Sexuality at Various Levels of Reaction

++++   Performance commonly impossible

+++   Excessive desire: poorly co-ordinated performance

++   Hypersexuality in both desire and performance

+   Normal to slightly heightened sexuality

Normal

-   Normal to slightly reduced sexuality

--   Debility and diminished desire and performance

---   Female frigidity and male impotence occur

----   Frigidity and impotence the rule

Physical Causes

You need to clean up your act. Not easy to do when you are feeling down. So get ready and get started when you are on the way UP!

You need to establish which foods are brain-inflammatory in nature. That means following a whole elimination and challenge dieting regimen. Full details on how to do this are given in a later section of this book.

No parties and events at this time. Stop smoking (tobacco is a pronounced brain allergen)

Sleep is very crucial. See section 3.4 for data on that.

I mentioned the benefits of "small dose" exercize in the previous chapter. There is also more information on brain-friendly exercize in section 5.1 (inflammation)

Then you need to fill up on supplements, meaning don't go silly with quantities, but make sure you are not deficient. A good multi-formula is a great start. Beware of the source supplies; for example vitamin C is often manufactured from corn; vitamin E starting from wheatgerm; B vitamins are usually made from yeast. These could be allergy issues.

Lithium Is King

I'm sure you have heard of the important reputation of lithium for bipolar disorder. Indeed, it is crucial. You cannot afford to be deficient.

The prestigious medical journal the *Lancet* reports that "Lithium increases human brain gray matter." As you may know, gray matter is the tissue found in the outer layer of your brain known as the cortex.

Neuroscience adds, "Lithium may help generate entirely new cells in your brain."

Further proof? Researchers treated mice with lithium in dosages equivalent to human therapeutic range. Then they performed autopsies and examined their brains.

The scientists found a 25% increase in the number of dividing cells in the brain's hippocampus—a clear indication of the growth of new brain neurons (neurotrophic effect).[149]

We now know this is important to bipolar patients: this new growth of brain tissue is helpful to cycling mood disorders. There is a growing body of evidence suggesting that mood stabilizers and antidepressants exert neurotrophic effects and may therefore be of use in the long-term treatment of other neuropsychiatric disorders.

Put another way, lithium grows new brain tissue and so do antidepressants. Which would you rather take?

Self Medication

Big Pharma likes to pretend lithium is a drug and charges a bunch. In fact it's just a natural mineral, readily available, cheap and does the job just as well as the proprietaries, such as Eskalith, Lithobid, Lisconium and Priadel. Ironically, the drug companies are really into orthomolecular medicine—they just don't admit it!

They will try to tell you that it is not safe to self-dose with lithium. That's just to scare you off and make you go for the prescription version. You must have repeated blood tests, they will tell you. But that's only if you are using a high-dose regimen, such as doctors prescribe.

You can take care of your own lithium, in much the same way as you would supplement zinc, magnesium and calcium!

According to Jonathan Wright, M.D., America's top authority on lithium orotate, a total daily intake of 30 milligrams of elemental lithium will have unnoticeable effects on serum lithium levels, with levels usually residing in a non-detectable range. Even 40 mg per day appears to be completely safe, presenting no negative side effects or signs of toxicity.

According to Wright there is no need for routine blood lithium measurements.

Note: lithium carbonate, the "drug" form is very different from the orotate or chloride forms. Lithium carbonate is not recommended for self-medication.

At the least sign of the return of restlessness, high mood and overactivity, go back to your prescribed dose of lithium carbonate. It is only a mineral supplement after all. But I am surprised by the number of muddle-headed doctors who think that patient should be taken off lithium when they are doing fine.

If you don't get the lithium you need, take it by yourself. It's basically a medication for life, unless you do find your serious food, chemical and mold triggers.

Arachidonic Acid

Another discovery is that people with bipolar have disordered essential fatty acid regulation in the brain, which results in damaging inflammation and interferes with brain function. Specifically bipolar brains release an excessive amount of the omega-6 fat called arachidonic acid which promotes inflammation and a relative deficiency of the omega-3 fats docosahexaenoic acid (DHA) and eicosapentaenoic acid (EPA), which are anti-inflammatory.

Our bodies make some arachidonic acid from the omega-6 oil (linoleic acid) found in nuts and most seed oils but we can also consume a lot of arachidonic acid directly in manufactured foods (like donuts and cookies), with some also found in red meats and pork. Our body makes some DHA from the oil found in a few plant sources but very inefficiently. To obtain the sort of therapeutic levels needed by the bipolar brain we need to consume EPA and DHA directly by eating oily fish or taking fish oil.

Lithium supplementation counteracts the inflammation caused by the excessive arachidonic acid seen in bipolar cases, which is at least one of the reasons it is beneficial. You can help the lithium work better by attending to your omega-3 intake, at least 3 grams daily (6 capsules typically).[150]

Thyroid and Iodine

Note that lithium antagonizes iodine. If you are talking lithium, whether on a holistic regimen, or as prescribed by your doctor, you need to take iodine. We should all take iodine anyway. No one can afford to be short of this vital mineral. Without it the immune system doesn't function properly. Moreover the thyroid needs iodine and poor thyroid function is one of the risk factors for depression. It all adds up.

Accumulating evidence suggests that hypothalamo-pituitary-thyroid (HPT) axis dysfunction is strongly related to bipolar disorder. Hypothyroidism, either overt or more commonly subclinical, appears to the commonest abnormality found in bipolar disorder. Lithium-treatment has potent antithyroid effects and can induce hypothyroidism or exacerbate a preexisting hypothyroid state.[151]

There is a great deal in later section of this book that would benefit bipolar disorder. You are referred to these sections.

Things to avoid: do NOT use St John's wort or S-adenosyl methionine (SAMe). These are excitants and can trigger a manic episode. In fact avoid any "energizer" formula, such as those containing dimethyl glycine (DMG). That includes my own formulation: **Mito-Cell Rejuvenator**. It's great for extending youthful energies and is good overall for the nervous system. But because it greatly boosts energy, it should NOT be taken by patients diagnosed as bipolar.

Transcranial Magnetic Stimulation For Bipolar Depression

It is a moot point whether transcranial magnetic stimulation (TMS) is really "natural". But in the sense of meaning not orthodox drug therapy, then it certainly has a place.

The official line on TMS is as follows:

Some research showed that transcranial magnetic stimulation improved depression symptoms, while in other studies it didn't seem to help. If transcranial magnetic stimulation works for you, your depression symptoms may improve or go away completely. Symptom relief may take a few weeks of treatment.

However, in 2008 the FDA did reluctantly approve one TMS device, the NeuroStar TMS brain-stimulating device. Please understand this was a clearance, as opposed to a formal approval. It does not mean (in my view) that the NeuroStar TMS is the best available device.

The FDA's claimed clinical trials have not conclusively proven the efficacy of TMS, yet recognized studies showing that TMS-treated individuals were twice as likely as those who received a sham treatment to show clinical benefit.

However, some of the FDA reviewers expressed concerns that TMS for depression benefits appeared "small," "borderline," "marginal," and "of questionable clinical significance."

But that statistical pronouncement obscures the fact that some individuals did wonderfully well; for others, not much benefit. Your concern is not whether the FDA is impressed or not but whether you are among those individuals who will benefit greatly.

And the only way to find out is to try it!

TMS uses a magnetic field to stimulate specific areas of the brain that are associated with bipolar disorder. Treating bipolar disorder usually requires daily treatment sessions during the acute phase of treatment, which typically lasts between 4-8 weeks. So you will need your own device.

A review on PubMed reports that TMS could be effective in bipolar depression by stimulating the left prefrontal cortex or inhibiting the right prefrontal cortex. It has been proposed that in bipolar mania there is decreased cortical activity in the right side, with a relative increase in left-sided activity. Therefore TMS might have therapeutic effects in mania when the right prefrontal cortex is stimulated.

TMS appears to be relatively safe and well tolerated. There is no post-procedure recovery period and no risk from anesthesia, as with ECT. The most common side effects are headaches and pain at the site of the stimulation.[152]

Although TMS is not nearly so brutal and violent as ECT (which is an extreme kind of "TMS", if you think about it), it is not without side effects and is not recommended for patients with epilepsy or seizure disorders, and does not always deliver measurable results.

Also, it is most likely to NOT work in some of the circumstances where folks may need it most – those who have experienced psychotic breaks and seek to be less heavily medicated, and those who have suffered extended depression (over 4 years in duration) and show a pattern of treatment resistance.

On the up side, it is offered by the Mayo Clinic and some other highly reputable treatment centers. They wouldn't offer a treatment they knew didn't work, just to make money, would they?

Good Read: *Madness: A Bipolar Life* By Marya Hornbacher.

Ms. Hornbacher's life makes for an amazing read, and this memoir won't disappoint. The numerous setbacks she experiences only makes you appreciate every time she finds a moment of happiness or peace. Shortly into the book, you begin rooting for her, as though she were some fictional character in a novel. And that's the clincher — she's not fictional, she's real.

2.4 Anxiety States and Phobias

The labeling of our times has run the gamut from the 'Space Age' to the 'Age of Aquarius' to the age of 'Sexual Revolution'. However, the one epithet that probably fits more accurately than all the rest is the 'Age of Anxiety'.

Anxiety is the one negative force that cuts through all levels of society, affecting the rich and poor, young and old alike. Anxieties and tensions are insidious forces which exist below the surface of your awareness, smoldering and building up, until you reach a 'breaking point' and explode in a fit of anger or a violent argument, or some other unreasoned behavior.

Conscious worry and fear also enter the picture to compound the feeling of frustration already being experienced because you are not able to identify the source of the unconscious anxiety and thus eliminate it.

Anxiety may also manifest as over-indulgence in food, alcohol, cigarettes, sex or work, "pumping up" (gym), but also in headaches, fatigue, impotence, clumsiness, sleepless nights, or any number of physical ailments.

Consequently, if you are like most people, you will gulp down a handful of pills to alleviate that dull aching feeling, or your 'escape' will be in the form of the after-work booze-up. Or you'll change your job, or get a divorce, or move to another town, or some psychologist will tell you to 'adjust' to your problems.

Or you will grin and bear it because your religious leader piously proclaims that sorrow is this life's just reward, and so on.

But you find that you receive nothing but temporary relief and that you carry your problems with you wherever you go and whatever you do.

To add to this state of tension, is the sense of 'alienation' that modern society produces: a feeling of isolation, separation, loneliness, powerlessness, apathy, non-involvement, pessimism, meaninglessness, rootlessness, and lack of authentic values.

Alienation may be described as that state in which the individual feels dislocated from himself, from others, from the world in general. With mechanization, specialization and automation increasing every day, Man has become lost in the giant machinery he once controlled and created, and thereupon he has become a mere 'cog in the machine' - mechanized, reutilized, depersonalized, apathetic, insignificant, an object to be manipulated.

With the threat of nuclear annihilation on the one side, and on the other promises of a super-abundant age of leisure from the resources of high technology, man has become confused, uncertain, almost schizoid because he cannot relate to or solve problems of such magnitude.

Millions of people use reality TV, YouTube, movies and popular music to effect their "escape".

But perhaps most outstandingly these days: people find their escape in Facebook and social media. The figures have become staggering: As of the third quarter of 2016, Facebook had 1.79 billion active users, generating 4.5 billion likes. If Facebook was a country, it would now be the most populous in the world—even bigger than China.

Twitter comes a poor second, with 320 million users, but is still an international powerhouse, with 79 percent of its users living outside the US. Twitter is supported by 35 languages around the world,

True, social media engagement is safer than the chemical solutions listed above but does not make up for the paucity of good emotions in a person's life. The observable downside is that social media promulgate concerns and worries.

With the instant communications systems of mass media, informing Western man of the struggles for freedom of men throughout the world, he feels helpless in his inability to do anything about the situation. It means more anxiety, not less.

Learning about constant crime, the world seems a dangerous place. And stuck in urban dwellings, he becomes increasingly isolated from Nature with all of its beauty, peace and refreshing naturalness.

How Common Is Anxiety?

Anxiety disorders, which include panic disorder, generalized anxiety disorder, post-traumatic stress disorder, phobias, and separation anxiety disorder, are the most common class of mental disorders present in the general population.

Perhaps strangely, estimates of anxiety disorders are generally higher in developed countries than in developing countries.[153]

We are all familiar with the symptoms of intense anxiety:

- Feelings of dread, panic, fear, or uneasiness
- A sense of impending doom or disaster
- Tension
- Problems sleeping
- Cold or sweaty hands or feet
- Shortness of breath
- Heart palpitations
- Not being able to be still and calm
- Dry mouth
- Shaking

It is a very unpleasant state of mind. How much worse, then, when it is an almost continuous day-to-day experience.

Phobias too may trigger these unpleasant symptoms, if the object of fear cannot be avoided.

To understand anxiety states better, think of brain excitation. Caffeine, as we know, is a strong brain stimulant; it keeps you awake. Just be aware that any food or chemical reaction you can't tolerate is capable of doing the same thing.

Refer to the Ups and Downs table in section 2.3 for a clear picture of what happens as the brain is more and more agitated, leading, in the extreme, to outright mania. Remember also that what goes up must come down. Sooner or later the exhaustion phase sets in and the person becomes more and more depressed and lethargic. Really, anxiety and depression are just two aspects of the same spectrum of over-stimulation.

See also the section on Crime, Violence and Delinquency (section 2.8)

Neurotransmitters

The dominant neurotransmitters in anxiety are GABA (gamma amino butyric acid), serotonin and glutamate. Basically we want more GABA and serotonin, less glutamate. We can make chemical tweaks, with herbs and supplements, but there is still an onus on the sufferer to do some brain training. It's important to reprogram the amygdala and strengthen the frontal cortex to stop anxious thoughts and panic attacks hijacking our mind.

So meditation, yoga, any kind of gentle exercise, like Pilates, and multi-media sensory stimulation (section 3.10 MMSS) are the order of the day.

So how do we lower glutamate levels?

DON'T take glutamate or anything like it (aspartate, glutamine, MSG, etc.) It acts as an excitotoxin, but the actual agent is calcium influx. Go easy on the calcium supplements. Magnesium is the one you really want. 500 mg a day, minimum. 1,000 mg is better, at least till your nutritional balance is restored.

Magnesium has been nicknamed "Nature's tranquillizer".

You need more GABA, which is the natural opposite of glutamate: it calms the nervous system. Interestingly, GABA is very prominently involved with the neuronal connections of language. It actually puts the gaps between words. Decreased GABA leads to increased anxiety, increased aggressive behavior, decreased social behavior, decreased eye contact, and decreased bowel function.

GABA is widely distributed in the brain. Its natural function is to reduce the activity of the neurons to which it binds. Some researchers believe that one of the purposes that GABA serves is to control the fear or anxiety experienced when neurons are overexcited.

GABA receptors are probably the most common kind in the mammalian nervous system. It is estimated that close to 40% of the synapses in the human brain work with GABA and therefore have GABA receptors.

Research is indicating that a major factor in people who suffer from anxiety disorders or panic attacks and in people who have become addicted or dependent to street drugs, prescription drugs and alcohol is that they are likely to be suffering from low GABA activity.

Consider an amazing herb, which could be good for both relaxation and calming, also a memory helper (for dementias). It raises levels of GABA in the brain. You can grow it for free in your own garden or a pot!

Lemon Balm (Melissa officianalis)

This is a calming and soothing herb, with good effect on memory and cognition. So it's worth considering for both anxiety states and dementia.

It has a long history. Lemon balm is mentioned by Homer in *The Odyssey*. Beloved Swiss physician Paracelsus (aka. Philippus Aureolus Theophrastus Bombastus von Hohenheim, 1493-1541), thought it should be used for "all complaints supposed to proceed from a disordered state of the nervous system". Lemon balm is also given a mention in John Gerarde's massive (1700 pages) tome: *Herball, or Generall Historie of Plantes* (1597), where it is said to "quicken the senses."

Nearly a century later, the most famous English herbalist of all, Nicholas Culpeper (1616-1654) writes about it in his *Complete Herbal*.

But there is more than tradition today. A number of scientific trials give it the green light as therapy. Lemon balm has remarkable healing and regenerative effects on the brain. It's an antioxidant that can stimulate memory and reduce anxiety, too!

The principal active ingredient seems to be a compound called rosmarinic acid (RA). Researchers in India discovered RA reduces free radicals and protects the brain's nerve cells from deterioration.

Their results suggest RA might help prevent several neurodegenerative diseases caused by oxidative stress, such as Alzheimer's and Parkinson's disease (see section 2.5).[154]

In Finland, scientists assessed lemon balm extract for its effectiveness in mild to moderate Alzheimer's patients. They found the extract restricted the enzyme acetylcholinesterase, which reduces the neurotransmitter acetylcholine. Low acetylcholine levels inhibit the brain's signaling ability, which is common in Alzheimer's cases.[155]

Note that the much-touted Alzheimer's drug Aricept does only that: restricts the breakdown of acetylcholine.

A Relaxing "Chill" Herb

A study from Canada links the traditional relaxing effects of lemon balm to boosting levels GABA (Gamma-Aminobutyric Acid). The herb suppresses an enzyme, GABA-transaminase, which downgrades GABA in the brain. This enzyme is a main target in current anxiety and neurological disorder therapies.[156]

Researchers at the University of Northumbria in Newcastle, UK performed a randomized, placebo-controlled, double-blind study on 20 young participants. After receiving single doses of varying amounts of lemon balm extract, cognition as well as calmness improved in everyone who took part.[157]

A 2003 study published by the American College of Neuropsychopharmacology evaluated cognition and mood using active dried leaves of lemon balm. The scientists also found that memory performance improved and calmness increased in all participants.[158]

Yet another study, published in *Current Pharmaceutical Design*, showed lemon balm possesses cognition-enhancing properties and reduces reduces agitation. A good candidate then, for anxiety states, panic attacks and other states of tension or agitation.[159]

Note that lemon balm alters thyroid metabolism. If you have any thyroid-related condition, try this only under the supervision of your doctor.

L-Theanine

A good "antidote" to anxiety is L-theanine, a free amino acid found, among other places, in tea leaves (*Camellia sinensis* bush).

L-theanine, otherwise know as gamma-ethylamino-L-glutamic acid, is thought to be the key to tea's subtle but calming effects.

L-theanine is believed to counter the stimulating effects of caffeine by increasing the production of alpha and theta brain waves. Alpha waves are associated with a state of deep relaxation while being mentally alert. Theta waves are a sign of dreaming and deep trance. These effects are similar to the state achieved by those during meditation.

L-theanine increases GABA activity. It probably interacts with dopamine and serotonin as well, resulting in increased focus, improved memory and learning ability.

Dose: 100- 200 mg at night, before sleeping.

Excitotoxins

You have probably heard of excitotoxins. Neurosurgeon Russell Blaylock MD has been writing trenchantly for many years about this health hazard. Excitotoxin is his term for recognized toxic brain stimulant, such as aspartame, glutamate (MSG etc.) and cysteine. But it is vital to understand that any food or chemical can do this to any susceptible individual. Unfortunately, large amounts of these three particular amino acids are routinely added to our food, solely for the commercial benefit of the food manufacturers and despite concerns of the scientific community.

Glutamate, as monosodium glutamate (MSG), is added to many foods. It excites our taste buds and can make bland food taste good. In 1908 a Japanese scientist discovered that glutamate is the active chemical in the ancient drink *kombu*. By 1933 their annual consumption of monosodium glutamate in Japan was over ten million pounds.

Inevitably, the American food industry was soon following the Japanese lead and introduced MSG. Today MSG is added to most soups, chips, fast foods, frozen foods, ready-made dinners, and canned goods. And it has been a boon for the diet food industry, since so many low-fat foods are to all intents and purposes tasteless.

Often MSG and related toxins are added to foods in disguise. For example, among the food manufacturers favorite misleading names are 'hydrolyzed vegetable protein,' 'vegetable protein,' 'natural flavorings,' and 'spices'. Each of these may contain from 12 percent to 40 percent MSG.

Glutamate may surprise you; after all, isn't glutamate found naturally in our brains? It's a neurotransmitter. Why would it be toxic? Too much of anything is toxic, if you can't get rid of it. Unfortunately, sometimes our natural detox protection mechanisms break down.

If we lack sufficient necessary nutrients—specifically magnesium and antioxidants like vitamin C—we can get into a vicious cycle in which excitotoxins stimulate free radical formation and these free radicals in turn stimulate further excitotoxin accumulation. That's one of the reasons these nutrients are so vital.

Secondly, we have the so-called "blood-brain barrier" to protect our nervous system from toxins. But this barrier is not well developed in the very young and it may even be still under-functioning in adolescents. Some parts of the brain never develop a barrier system at all, for example, the hypothalamus, which is the key regulator of endocrine function (hormones).

If that wasn't enough danger, it has also been found that glutamate passes across the barrier of the placenta and enters the fetal bloodstream. Pregnant mothers are not being adequately warned about dangers to the fetus from junk chemicals in food and drink. Due to the pioneering work of John Olney, MD, pure MSG has been removed from baby food. However, the criminal profit-crazed food manufacturers continue to add an even more dangerous product, "hydrolyzed vegetable protein", which contains three known excitotoxins and has added MSG.

As noted by Richard C. Henneberry, PhD, "I consider it ironic that the pharmaceutical industry is investing vast resources in the development of glutamate receptor blockers to protect neurons against glutamate neurotoxicity in common neurological disorders, while at the same time, the food industry, with the blessing of the FDA, continues to add great quantities of glutamate to the food supply."[160] Sugar Is A Neuro-Excitant

Don't forget sugar fires up your brain. Some people cannot sleep if they consume sugar, especially deadly fructose. A 2012 study on rats, conducted by researchers at UCLA, found that a diet high in fructose hinders learning and memory by literally slowing down the brain. The researchers found that rats who over-consumed fructose had damaged synaptic activity in the brain, meaning that communication among brain cells was impaired.

Heavy sugar intake caused the rats to develop a resistance to insulin, a hormone that indirectly regulates the function of brain cells, by controlling blood sugar levels. Insulin strengthens the synaptic connections between brain cells, helping them to communicate better and thereby form stronger memories. So when insulin levels in the brain are lowered as the result of excess sugar consumption, cognition can be impaired.

"Insulin is important in the body for controlling blood sugar, but it may play a different role in the brain," Dr. Fernando Gomez-Pinilla, the study's lead author, said in a statement. "Our study shows that a high-fructose diet harms the brain as well as the body. This is something new."

It's also the last thing you want, if you are battling mental dysfunction!

This story was published by UCLA and the food industry immediately reacted, forcing them to alter the wording from high-fructose corn syrup to just fructose, to avoid the implication that the study focused solely on high-fructose corn syrup. Also, there were a couple of mistakes: high-fructose corn syrup is *not necessarily "six times sweeter" than cane sugar* they were told to say; and that Americans consume approximately 35 pounds of high-fructose corn syrup per capita annually, not "more than 40 pounds" as the original news release said. 35 pounds a year? Oh that's OK then, 5 pounds less than the original concern level![161]

There was more, incidentally: Gomez-Pinilla and study co-author Rahul Agrawal, a UCLA visiting postdoctoral fellow from India, studied two groups of rats that each consumed a fructose solution as drinking water for six weeks. The second group also received omega-3 fatty acids in the form of flaxseed oil and docosahexaenoic acid (DHA), which protects against damage to the synapses.

DHA is an important "essential fatty acid" containing omega-3s. This group of fats are "essential" because our body cannot make them. Yet they are vital for health.

"This is the mechanism that makes learning and memory possible, Gomez-Pinilla said. "Our bodies can't produce enough DHA, so it must be supplemented through our diet." Weight Gain

Consistently, the animals exposed to MSG were found to be short, grossly obese, and had difficulty with sexual reproduction. One can only wonder if the large number of people having difficulty with obesity today is related to early exposure to food additive excitotoxins since this obesity is one of the most consistent features of the MSG exposure.

One characteristic of the obesity induced by excitotoxins is that is doesn't appear to depend on food intake. This could explain why some people cannot diet away their obesity. No matter how hard the patient struggles, the pounds just do not come off. It is ironic that so many people drink "diet" sodas sweetened with NutraSweet® (aspartate)!

There is no chance of losing weight on such products. Anyone sensible discovers that sooner or later, but the industry propaganda lies continue to be rolled out.

For example, consider the claim that double-blind studies show that aspartame, glutamate and L-cysteine are quite safe:

These "studies" were faked. By using NutraSweet® (aspartame) as the "placebo" when testing glutamate, there would obviously be no difference between the "placebo" and the "active" chemical. It was cynical and deliberate.

Aspartate is a known excitotoxin. It would seem obvious even to the layman that you would not use a control substance to compare to a known toxin if the control contained the same class of chemical toxin. But that is exactly what was done.[162] Draw your own conclusions about this "science".

Neurodegenerative Diseases

Dr. Russell Blaylock, in his book *Excitoxins: The Taste that Kills*, Health Press, P.O. Box 1388, Santa Fe, NM 87504, 1994, explains in detail exactly which areas of the brain are involved in the neurodegenerative diseases: amyotrophic lateral sclerosis (ALS, Lou Gehrig's or Guam disease), Parkinson's, and Alzheimer's. All three diseases can develop gradually. "The symptoms of Parkinson's disease do not manifest themselves until over 80 to 90 percent of the neurons in the involved nuclei (called the substantia nigra) have died. The neurons didn't all suddenly die at the same time, rather they slowly and silently deteriorated over many years.

The same is true of Alzheimer's disease, he says. This is why prevention is so important.

At times, all three diseases, ALS, Parkinson's, and Alzheimer's, have developed one after the other in the same patients. For example, in Guam following World War II the natives developed exceedingly high levels of ALS and some of them later developed Parkinson's and Alzheimer's. The cause was in their diet of flour made from the seed of the false sago palm (cycad), which has poisonous aspartate constituents.

They had eaten this flour for centuries but only after soaking the sliced seeds in water for several hours. This was repeated several times, each time using fresh water. After the last soaking, a chicken was fed some of the wash water. If it lived, the seed was deemed safe to eat!

However, because of famine during the war, cycad flour became a much larger part of their diet. Also, fresh water was scarce so the precautionary washing measures were often abandoned or at least abbreviated. Adding to the problem, the famine could result in the natives having chronically low blood sugar—such low energy levels can block the detoxification of neurotoxins. Thus the people would be more vulnerable to the devastating neurodegenerative diseases.

Avoiding Excitotoxins

First we need to understand where these excitotoxins come to us. The answer is in manufactured foods. Fresh, raw foods are mainly OK but (true to form) Agribusiness wants L-cysteine to be used as a fake way of preserving the color of fresh fruits.

Here Is A Summary Of Food Sources For MSG:

Additives that always contain MSG:

- Monosodium Glutamate
- Hydrolyzed Vegetable Protein

- Hydrolyzed Protein
- Hydrolyzed Plant Protein
- Plant Protein Extract
- Sodium Caseinate
- Calcium Caseinate
- Yeast Extract
- Textured Protein
- Autolyzed Yeast
- Hydrolyzed Oat Flour

Additives that frequently contain MSG:

- Malt extract
- Malt Flavoring
- Bouillon Broth
- Stock Flavoring
- Natural Flavoring
- Natural Beef or Chicken Flavoring
- Seasoning Spices

Additives that *may* contain MSG and/or other excitotoxins:

- Carrageeenan Enzymes (Protease enzymes from various sources can release excitotoxin amino acids from food proteins.)
- Soy Protein Concentrate
- Soy Protein Isolate Whey
- Protein Concentrate.[163]

Phobias

Phobias, meaning unreasonable and panicky fear caused by certain circumstances, is really a kind of anxiety mode. Agoraphobia is well-known (fear of open places and crowds); claustrophobia is the opposite (fear of being shut in), herpetophobia is a fear of snakes; arachnophobia, fear of spiders and bugs.

Fancy Latin names like this are endless and add nothing to our understanding of the basic condition.

It is a waste of time to tell the person their fear is unreasonable (what I call the "pull yourself together treatment"). It has a very fierce grip on them. It is ineffective and even unkind to just suppose the sufferer is somehow weak-willed or inadequate. What is needed is some means of disconnecting the event or circumstance from the fear reaction it engenders.

See also Supernoetics® 3.12.

Stop or reduce consumption of products that contain caffeine, such as coffee, tea, cola, energy drinks, and chocolate.

Ask your doctor or pharmacist before taking any over-the-counter medicines or herbal remedies. Many contain chemicals, such as ephedrine, that can increase anxiety symptoms.

Cognitive Behavioral Therapy (CBT)

CBT is possibly the most widely-used therapy for anxiety disorders. Research has shown it to be more effective than medication in the treatment of panic disorder, phobias, social anxiety disorder, and generalized anxiety disorder.

CBT takes time and the person has to be led to a new psychic place, in which he or she has enough understanding about their condition to modify it.

The basic premise of cognitive behavioral therapy is that our thoughts—not external events—affect the way we feel. In other words, it's not the situation you're in that determines how you feel, but your perception of the situation.

Desensitization therapy is a technique in which the person is gradually exposed to their worst fears and (hopefully) learns to accept this exposure, without it triggering unpleasant fear reactions. If all goes well, the person builds up to possibly normal contact or exposure.

For example, fear of flying programs will start on the ground, with a stationary craft. The first few sessions will simply get the person used to the smell of the cushions, the cabin crew announcements and the engine noises, without ever leaving the ground. Gradually, more and more elements are added until, finally, the passenger agrees to a real flight.

"We're not saying you have to like to fly, but at least you have the tools to fly, and of course, practice makes perfect. Over time and repeated flights, your anxiety and phobias diminish dramatically," says Tony Martinez, who serves on the board of the San Mateo, California-based Fear of Flying Clinic.

Addressing Past Events

You will sometimes read remarks from various under-performing "experts" that addressing anxieties and miseries from the past is a waste of time. I assure you, it is not.

Our history makes us what we are. And sometimes the past can haunt us in a very forceful way. There are people who can't *think about* snakes, without breaking into a cold sweat. There is always something in their memory banks that leads them to fear snakes. Oddly, it might not even be because of an experience with snakes. It could be someone else's unpleasant encounter which, then described to the patient, was sufficient to make them scared.

TV these days is pretty bad at portraying graphic events that are likely to create second-hand fear, nausea and panic.

EFT (emotional freedom technique), NLP (neuro-linguistic programming) and similar pretend-it's-gone-away therapies have much to offer in an acute situation. But having dealt with many people who were vulnerable to terror, despite having "tapped" it away, or "moved it out of their mind space", supposedly, I can state firmly that it is my view this approach has not much to offer long-term.

We need to locate and flatten or defuse the emotional content of whatever experience is underpinning the fear or anxiety, to see it finally go away for good. Eliminating the negative emotional "charge" means the memory becomes clean and useful. In other words the memory does not disappear but becomes available without the distressing emotional content. My own specialty, which I light-heartedly called Punk Psychology®, is the best I know at locating and eradicating past unpleasant and charged events, which we call memonemes.

Assuming you have eliminated food allergies, hyperventilation and hypoglycemia attacks as a probable cause of these unpleasant anxiety or panic episodes, then a competent workout with someone who knows Punk Psychology®, should be able to trace and defuse the events or experience from your past that leads to these attacks being triggered. There is ALWAYS a hidden lever that can be pulled unconsciously, that causes a detonation of feelings.

Well, the trick is to explode the landmine, so at any future time when you step on the detonator, it can no longer blow up and cause hurt! (OK, crude metaphor, but you get the idea, I hope: all possibility of future return to the panic syndrome is exhausted; gone; impossible.

Interestingly, I hear that the founder of EFT, Gary Craig, has realized the importance of finding and blowing up the landmines, not just walking a path around them!

We call this approach "piloting" in Supernoetics® because we are skillfully leading the individual towards the source of the problem (ignoring later re-runs of this same phenomenon).

You can learn more about Punk Psychology® later in the book, in the section called Supernoetics® (section 3.12).

Panic attacks

Answer the following questions, if you think you may be experiencing panic attacks:

1. Do you experience sudden episodes of intense and overwhelming fear that seem to come on for no apparent reason?

2. During these episodes, do you experience symptoms similar to the following: racing heart, chest pain, difficulty breathing, choking sensation, lightheadedness, tingling or numbness?

3. During the episodes do you worry about something terrible happening to you, such as embarrassing yourself in front of others, having a heart attack or even dying suddenly?

4. Do you worry about having additional episodes like this?

One positive answer is suggestive of panic attacks. Two or more is conclusive.

A panic attack is a sudden rush of fear or anxiety that is very intense in character. Usually, one or more uncomfortable physical symptoms will be present, such as increased heart rate, dizziness or lightheadedness, shortness of breath, inability to concentrate, and confusion.

After a number of panic episodes, the individual can become afraid of being suddenly gripped by an attack. In other words, the fear becomes self-reinforcing. He or she may hesitate to be alone, to venture far from home, or to be in public places. Even when not experiencing an anxiety attack, the person with panic attacks often becomes increasingly nervous and apprehensive that one will occur. He or she attempts to remain physically and psychologically tense in preparation for the next attack.

Panic attacks are often treated with medication (anxiolytics). This is a poor solution, since the cause is not addressed and the patient left helpless against repeat episodes. Moreover, the main component of the disorder is fear and therefore the patient may be afraid to ever stop the medication. This leads to a life of toxic chemical burden.

Better remedies are relaxation techniques: autogenic training (see over), meditation, Chi'gung, yoga, etc.

You need to search out possible food and chemicals reactions, which are notorious for producing panic attacks yet easily dealt with (sections 5.2 and 5.3).

Meditation and Similar

I group a number of techniques together, because they are based on the meditation (mindfulness) principle. The Western world has now become thoroughly anamored of this approach to mental health. There is an embarrassment of choices in what type of meditation to adopt. You make your own choice, basically. I cannot honestly report that some are better than others. It's horses for courses. Being comfortable and enjoying what you do will prove far more beneficial than trying to practice a technique which does not sit well with you, just because it's supposed to be "better".

Buddhist Vipassana meditation is hugely popular in the West. It's all about 'being present', letting your mind run, and accepting whatever thoughts come up, while practicing detachment from each thought. Mindfulness is taught along with an awareness of the breath, though the breathing is often considered to be just one sensation among many others, not a particular focus.

Transcendental Meditation™ is more proprietary and you may have to swallow gobbets of Maharishi-worship to get accepted into its circle of followers. TM has been extensively studied, however; you can find details of its valued properties in *The Physiology Of Consciousness* by Robert Keith Wallace.[164] As neuroscientists have studied meditation, they've discovered some interesting ways in which it affects the physical structure of the brain. These include effects that can be seen in autonomic functions and neurotransmitters as well as changes in blood flow and brain wave activity.

But Herbert Benson's *Relaxation Response* does it just as well, with no cost to you (see next section).

Autogenic Training

Autogenic training is a mind control technique for autosuggestion and deep relaxation, developed by the German psychiatrist Johannes Heinrich Schultz (1884-1970) and first published in 1932. During each session, the practitioner will repeat a set of visualizations that induce a state of relaxation (see below).

Each session can be practiced in a position chosen amongst a set of recommended postures (for example, lying down, sitting meditation, slumped in a comfortable chair). The technique can be used to alleviate many stress-induced psychosomatic disorders and calm the response to pain.

Herbert Benson, MD, a Harvard professor also did significant research into this approach. He called it the Relaxation Response and wrote an influential book with that same title. Benson described the relaxation response as a physical state of deep rest that changes the physical and emotional responses to stress from the "fight or flight response" to a state of physiological calm (parasympathetic mode).

See section next section.

Autogenic training has been subject to clinical evaluation from its early days in Germany, and from the early 1980s worldwide. In 2002, a meta-analysis of 60 studies was published in *Applied Psychophysiology and Biofeedback*, finding significant positive effects of treatment when compared to controls over a number of diagnoses; finding these effects to be similar to best recommended rival therapies; and finding positive additional effects by patients, such as their perceived quality of life.[165]

Autogenic training was popularized in North America, particularly among practitioners, by Wolfgang Luthe, who co-authored, with Schultz, a multi-volume tome on autogenic training. Luthe was a firm believer that Autogenic training was a powerful approach that should only be offered to patients by qualified professionals.

However, I consider it perfectly safe for self-taught therapy.

Like many similar techniques (progressive relaxation, yoga, Chi'gong, varieties of meditation) autogenic training takes time to learn. But some biofeedback practitioners shortened the process by taking the most basic elements of autogenic imagery and developing "condensed" simplified versions that could be used in combination with biofeedback devices.[166] In 1963 Luthe discovered the significance of autogenic discharges, paroxysmal phenomena of motor, sensorial, visual and emotional nature, related to the traumatic history of the patient, and developed the method of "autogenic abreaction".

Luthe's disciple Luis de Rivera, a McGill University trained psychiatrist, introduced psychodynamic concepts into Luthe's approach, and developed "autogenic analysis" as a new method for uncovering the unconscious.[167] How It Works

It is not appropriate to try and give you a comprehensive guide to the training in a book of this nature but here is an outline guide.

Basically, autogenic training is a series of auto-suggestion commands (hence the name). The would-be participant lies down, on a sofa or bed, or sits comfortably in a slouching chair.

With eyes closed and feeling relaxed, he or she then recites along these lines, repeating each phrase several times, until it begins to take effect:

1. My left arm is heavy. My right arm is heavy. Both of my arms are heavy.

2. My right leg is heavy. My left leg is heavy. Both of my legs are heavy.

3. My body feels heavy. By body is sinking into the bed. My body feels like lead.

4. I feel warm. My arms are warm. My legs are warm. My arms and legs are warm.

5. My heartbeat is slow and regular.

6. My breathing is calm, relaxed and regular.

7. My forehead is cool.

From this point on, the instructions get more difficult. You should consult a text for further details.

I can report that I use this technique successfully myself, for deep relaxation, and you can soon train your body to respond to the instructions. I have even produced a "Mind Power CD" to help get you started: http://alternative-doctor.com/mindpowercd

I certainly think it's easier for us Westerners than trying to "wipe away thoughts" and "keep an empty mind", or other tricky conceptual auto-suggestions, as in meditation.

Relaxation Therapy

One of the best ways to calm and soothe troubled thoughts is by what I have introduced in this book as multi-media sensory stimulation (MMSS, section 3.10). It's a combination of binaural beats (different frequency in each ear), photic driving (flashing lights), slow stately music and ingenious "mind walks".

The great thing is the electronic device does all the work. You just have to follow the guided meditation imagery.

MMSS takes the participant down to low alpha and theta brainwave frequencies. These are unquestionably calming. Alpha is ultra-relaxation; theta is trance and dreaming. Once the experience is over, the calm and relation persists. As you grow accustomed to the modality, the effects last longer and longer, eventually many days.

I have also written up Herbert Benson's "relaxation response", a modernization (and free version), of what Transcendental Meditation purports to do.

Yoga, Tai Ch'i and Pilates are all, in their way, very relaxing therapies and will help quell anxiety attacks. Make them a part of your routine, if you are troubled by anxiety.

Finally, try flotation, if you've a mind to and can find a center near you.

Forest Bathing

Here's something that's new to Westerners, though not Japanese.

If you have not heard of it, or tried it, check out what is called *shinrin-yoku*.[168] It's Japanese for "forest bathing". No water, just soaking one's self in the calm tranquility of a woodland or forest, walking along slowly and drinking in the calm and beauty. Trees seem to have a specially soothing effect.

There's good science too: Numerous studies have found that spending time mindfully in nature not only soothes the body and mind, but also offers a substantial boost in natural killer (NK) cell activity. NK cells are responsible for keeping cancer cells in check and are a vital component of the immune system.

Qing Li Senior Assistant Professor at Nippon Medical School in Tokyo, has conducted a variety of experiments to examine the effect of forest bathing on mood, stress levels and immunity.

In two studies, small groups of men and women respectively were assessed before and after a two-night/three-day forest bathing trip. During the trips the subjects went on three forest walks and stayed in a hotel in the forest. Blood tests were taken before and after the trip, revealing a significant boost in NK activity in the subjects in both groups, which persisted as long as 30 days after the trip.

Dr. Li believes the increase in NK cell activity could be attributed to breathing air infused with the essential oils of trees called phytonicides. These compounds protect trees from disease, insects and fungus — while also helping to boost immunity in people.

Dr. Li also oversaw the second study, which compared the effects of forest bathing on various mental states. The Profile of Moods (POMS) questionnaire, which measures both varying moods and enduring mind states, was used test to gauge participants emotional states. The questionnaire was composed of various feeling words like sad, happy, considerate, friendly, etc. Each person indicated how mildly or strongly they experienced each feeling throughout the week. At the conclusion of the study, participants who engaged in forest bathing reported heightened vitality and lower levels of sadness, anxiety and hostility.

If you cannot break away for a full shinrin-yoku experience, don't underestimate the power of indoor plants and scenic views from windows. As *Mother Earth News* reports:

"Norwegian research shows that having a plant at or within view of an office workstation significantly decreases the risk of sick leave. A 2010 study from the University of Technology, Sydney, Australia, reported that levels of anger, anxiety, depressive thoughts, and fatigue all reduced over a three-month period, and not just by a little bit—these parameters were reduced by about 40 percent, while reported stress was down by 50 percent. On the other hand, those without the stress buffer of a visible plant indicated that stress levels rose over 20 percent during the study."[169]

Don't get me going on gardening; I love gardening! It's shinrin-yoku and more...

We Can Become Kinder and More Generous

Richard Ryan, a professor of psychology and psychiatry at the University of Rochester, believes communing with nature far exceeds the benefits of easing stress and improving health — it also greatly influences our values and overall behavior as we go about our daily lives.

"Stopping to experience our natural surroundings can have social as well as personal benefits," says Ryan. He adds that exposure to natural surroundings, compared to those of the man-made variety, helps to cultivate stronger ties of community and closer relationships, as well as increasing our generosity with money.[170]

Ryan should know. Along with a team of researchers, he conducted four experiments involving 370 participants who were either exposed to nature or man-made settings. They were instructed to notice colors and textures of the images on 19-inch computer screens, and to imagine the sounds and smells of the environments. For the first three experiments, half the group viewed images of buildings, roads and other cityscapes, while the other half observed natural landscapes like lakes and deserts. Both the urban and nature images were matched for color, layout, lighting and complexity. The fourth study involved participants that either worked in a lab with or without plants.

Once the experiments were completed, the participants answered a questionnaire which rated the importance of four life goals: wealth, fame, connectedness and community.

With all four studies, those exposed to the natural world consistently ranked close relationships and community higher than they had before the experiments. The questionnaire also assessed how deeply engaged the participants were in the images. The deeper the connection to nature, the more they appreciated community and closeness, whereas those who focused more on artificial environments rated wealth and fame higher in importance.

Levels of generosity were also put to the test. Two of the studies involved giving participants a $5 prize, which they could either keep or give to another anonymous participant, who would then be gifted an additional $5 bill. In turn, the anonymous participant could decide to return the prize money or keep it. In short, the first person had little reason to trust the second participant and also risked losing the money altogether.

Interestingly, those who were in contact with nature were more willing to share the money. And the more they were immersed in the natural environment, the better chance they would be generous with their winnings.

Why? Because nature helps us connect with our true, authentic selves, says study co-author Andrew Przybylski. An example is how the participants who focused on landscapes and plants said they felt a heightened sense of personal autonomy, such as "Right now, I feel like I can be myself."

Przybylski believes humans are essentially communal by nature, since we evolved in a hunter and gatherer social structure that depended on cooperation for survival. Natural surroundings also encourage introspection as we are removed from the distractions and pressures of man-made environments. "Nature in a way strips away the artifices of society that alienate us from one another," he says.[171]

2.5 Alzheimer's and Dementias

Once we used to talk about "senile dementia" as if going batty was a concomitant part of growing old. We no longer think that way. There are far too many active, alert and cognitively fully-functioning elders, who are clear in mind right through to the ninth decade, tenth and beyond and show no signs of dementia due to aging.

It's a vanished diagnosis; we no longer believe in such a phenomenon.

The one recognized surviving condition from this earlier era of age prejudice is Alzheimer's Disease (AD), an extensively studied brain function deterioration. While not fully understood, it is clear the AD is not aging, but is basically an inflammatory condition. As such, it is one of the many degenerative diseases that are based on inflammatory damage, others include arthritis, diabetes, arteriosclerotic (artery disease) and even cancer.

We don't have to age mentally. I'd love to think that my brain will be in good working order, right up to the day I die. I know I am my mind, the spirit within, and not my body or even my brain. Nevertheless, my communication point with the physical universe is my brain, so I know it is important to look after it.

No organ is more critical than our brain, which means that even subtle damage due to wear and tear will show up first in thought function; we begin to get slower in our movement and manners, easily muddled, more forgetful and eventually a little silly. Shakespeare summed up the final stage well in his Seven Ages of Man (*As You Like It*, Act II Scene VII): we go back to a kind of second childhood, where we are not fully capable mentally. This may be quite mild, where the patient is known to be a little "dotty" (short for dotage), or as severe as full-blown dementia. The "Seventh Age" applies to women also. In fact *women tend to suffer more from the dementias.*

You do not want to enter this final stage, for sure, and you do not need to. Many people dread losing their faculties as they get older and even, half-jokingly, ask someone to put a bullet to their head, rather than allow this to happen, so great is the abhorrence of becoming mentally inept. I urge you to follow the advice given in this section and with luck you never will.

Poor diet and lifestyle may not exactly *cause* AD but such folly will make any health condition worse. Conversely, eating well, taking sufficient exercize and supplementing needed nutrients will help your body fight any disease process more effectively.

The Picture Is Changing

The 1990s were labeled the "Decade of the Brain". Unfortunately, we learned little and solved nothing. The problem has grown till we have a new millennium of brain dysfunction, with Alzheimer's disease leading the field of causes.

Alzheimer's Disease (AD) is named after Aloysius Alzheimer (1864-1915).

In November 1901, Dr. Alzheimer, a German neurologist, made his first examination of a 51-year-old woman named Auguste Deter who was experiencing problems with memory and language as well as various psychological problems such as disorientation and hallucinations. These symptoms matched the definition of what was then called dementia, but she was very young to be displaying them.

The patient died on April 8, 1906. Since Dr. Alzheimer had never seen another case like hers, he obtained the family's permission to perform an autopsy on her brain. When he examined it, he observed extensive atrophy, especially in the cortex—the thin outer layer of grey matter that is involved in memory, language, judgment, and thought in general. He also noted what are now termed amyloid plaques and neurofibrillary tangles, which are characteristically associated with AD.

AD accounts for up to 80% of dementia cases. But there are other types, with other causations. For example loss of brain function may be due to extensive blood clots or brain hemorrhages, hydrocephalus (a drainage problem), Creutzfeldt-Jakob disease (a prion attack), Huntington's Disease (genetic), Wernicke-Korsakoff Syndrome (vitamin B deficiency) and end-stage Parkinsonism (partly pesticides and pollution).

I will not be addressing these rarer forms of dementia separately or individually. Suffice it to say it is worth processing any individual through a series of health improvements and benefits may be observed.

This comes down to the subject of inflammation: many diseases have an inflammatory component (including Alzheimer's) and if the fire of inflammation is quenched then brain cells, which had become dysfunctional, may be able to recover somewhat.

This is the chief explanation for a number of cases in which dementia has, for a time, been reversible.

Alzheimer's Statistics

It's a big problem! Worldwide, nearly 44 million people have Alzheimer's or a related dementia (Alzheimer's Disease International).

Two out of three people with Alzheimer's are women (Alzheimer's Association).

Only 1-in-4 people with Alzheimer's disease have been diagnosed (Alzheimer's Disease International). You have to be wary of claims like this. How do they know? If it hasn't been diagnosed, then how do they find it?

Alzheimer's and dementia is most common in Western Europe (North America is close behind).

1-in-9 Americans over 65 has Alzheimer's disease and one-third of Americans over age 85. (Alzheimer's Association)

Alzheimer's disease is the 6th leading cause of death in America (Centers for Disease Control). Yes, don't forget: people die of Alzheimer's, usually quite quickly (4 to 8 years)

So it's a pretty big deal for all of us.

The global cost of Alzheimer's and dementia is estimated to be $605 billion, which is equivalent to 1% of the entire world's gross domestic product.

There's a huge toll on the caregivers too, many of whom feel they have no choice but to give up their own life and become caregivers, till the Alzheimer's patient dies. Many become concerned for their own health, as a result of the strain of caregiving to a dementia patient, which can be very demanding.

Yet, despite the gloom, it is not widely known that Alzheimer's is a fairly preventable disease and can even be reversed to a degree, sometimes remarkably so. One has to approach it the right way.

Facts You May Not Know

The human brain has been described as the "3 pound universe", meaning that all our thoughts, actions, perceptions, emotions, desires and dreams are supposed to be contained in an organ weighing no more than 50 ounces, lodged inside the skull!

There are approximately 100 billion brain cells (neurones), each making between 5,000 and 50,000 hard-wired connections or "synapses". That means around 4 quadrillion connections! This awesome power needs a great deal of energy (a total of 25 watts, for those who are technically minded).

In fact our brain, which is only 2% of body weight, requires over 25% of our nutritional energy output. That makes the brain very vulnerable to damage and degeneration, from lack of oxygen, poor nutrition, toxic overload and chemical deposits, including drugs. It means we have to look after our brain with extra care.

At the age of 75 you still have 85% of the brain cells that you were born with, and the good news is that in 2002 scientists at the Salk Institute in La Jolla, California proved that brain cells can replace themselves. Previously it was always thought that loss of brain cells was permanent, but we can now potentially regenerate and revitalize our brains. This is great news.

Therefore, the more we can look after our diet, take the right nutrients and keep our minds active – the better our brains will work.

But here's the thing: our brains are 60% fat! After decades of the low-fat diet madness and folly, we have an epidemic of dementia. Do you think there might be a connection?

Pharmaceutical Drugs Don't Cut It

Drug treatment is controversial (which means basically useless).

Big Pharma has wet dreams about the huge market for any potential treatment for Alzheimer's. Accordingly, they lie. You will hear phrases like "scientifically proven" to prevent or slow Alzheimer's. It's all fudging.

Tacrine (Cognex), one of the most widely prescribed drugs was refused licensing in several countries, since there was no evidence it did any good, despite aggressive marketing persuading doctors to prescribe it. Aricept (donepezil) is just as useless. Tacrine was finally withdrawn in 2013 *because it is dangerous.*

Let me caution about any connection with the so-called Alzheimer's Association. It poses as a charitable foundation, helping spread knowledge and awareness of Alzheimer's. It is nothing of the sort. It's merely a pharmaceutical company front group. They are not there to spread truth but to promote Pfizer's drug aricept.

How do I know? When I was at the university in Colombo, Sri Lanka (2002) I was invited to speak to the newly-formed local Alzheimer's Association. I chose to speak about diet and lifestyle. There was a good buzz about this. But the International Alzheimer's Association got to hear about it and banned my talk. They didn't want people to learn you can get 10X the improvement from diet that you can with their lousy drug product.

Now we are hearing "it's important to screen and diagnose Alzheimer's early." Why? The industry's standard TV ad says "Alzheimer's can't be cured and can't be prevented." In fact without any effective treatment on the table, screening is worse than useless. It's potentially harmful to tell patients they are candidates for dementia. Prof. Jason Karlawish from the University of Pennsylvania feels it might motivate people to make healthy lifestyle changes. But it's unethical to do it just to drum up sales of medicines.

And that's all "screening" is really for... pump the patients full of drugs for more years, and make more money.

While we are considering medical drugs, let me deplore the stupid practice of giving powerful antidepressants to elderly patients (usually just to shut them up and make them more "manageable") Antidepressants, especially selective serotonin reuptake inhibitors (SSRIs), can significantly disrupt sleep architecture in elderly patients and may contribute to early signs of neurodegeneration that can progress to dementia, research shows.

SSRIs increase sleep latency in the elderly and decrease REM [rapid eye movement] sleep duration and are also associated with REM sleep behavioral disorders, including nightmares. See section 3.4 for more understanding of sleep architecture.[172]

Understanding Alzheimer's Better

The main reason there is no effective treatment is that we don't really know what causes Alzheimer's. No doubt you will have heard of tau protein, neurofibrillary tangles and the dreaded amyloid plaques. Amyloid beta does show up, true, but it's a wild assumption that this is therefore the "cause" of Alzheimer's.

One landmark study showed that up to 50% of people diagnosed with Alzheimer's do not have any of the supposed characteristic signs at autopsy—no amyloid plaques, no tangles, nada.

Lon White MD, a professor of geriatric medicine at the University of Hawaii in Honolulu, and his colleagues performed brain autopsies—the only surefire way of diagnosing Alzheimer's—on more than 400 elderly Japanese-American men. Only about half of those who had a diagnosis of Alzheimer's before death had the brain plaques that signal the disease.[173]

You need to be clear about this: the beta amyloid plaques are not proven to cause the damage. They are more likely markers for the damage. Amyloid plaque has been found in normal individuals, without any cognitive impairment. Yet so many articles have said, so often, beta amyloid causes Alzheimer's, that is seemed to have become "true".

In fact at least one line of enquiry postulates that amyloid plaques may be the body's defense reaction to inflammatory disease. In other words, the plaques protect us from further damage! This research group believes there is very strong evidence to suggest that certain viral infections could be at the root of the problem.

In January 2016, a team led by Shawn Gale, an associate professor in psychology at Brigham Young University, looked at the infection history of 5,662 young to middle-aged adults alongside the results of tests intended to measure cognition. The team tested for the burden of chronic infections, specifically immunoglobulin G antibodies for toxocariasis (cat or dog toxocara roundworm, sometimes known as visceral larva migrans (VLM)), toxoplasmosis, hepatitis A, hepatitis B, hepatitis C, cytomegalovirus, and Herpes simplex 1 and 2.

The team created a scoring index of infectious burdens and the higher that score, the worse the person performed on cognitive function testing (worse learning and memory skills, as well as slower information-processing speed than those with a lower score, even after controlling for other factors, like age, sex and financial status).

The important point about this study is that it was the first to quantify multiple infections and connect them to markers of early dementia. The result was not striking but it was definite.[174]

Other researchers, like Ruth Itzhaki, professor emeritus of molecular neurobiology at University of Manchester, UK, (where I qualified in medicine), believe microbes may play a much bigger role than suspected in Alzheimer's. In March 2015, Itzhaki and a world-wide group of researchers wrote an editorial in the *Journal of Alzheimer's Disease*, asking the scientific community to consider a proposed link between Alzheimer's and certain microbes, notably herpes simplex virus Type 1 (HSV-1), Chlamydia pneumoniae and spirochetes. The spirochetes are the spiraling ones that include those bacteria responsible for syphilis (Treponema pallidum) and Lyme disease (Borrelia bugdorferi).

Itzhaki and her lab published their first paper in 1991 finding a clear HSV-1 link to Alzheimer's. According to Itzhaki, over 100 published studies, from her lab and elsewhere, have since been supportive of the same link. Nevertheless, Itzhaki says, the work has received only a cursory nod from the greater research world and little funding. Out of the $589 million allocated to Alzheimer's research by the National Institutes of Health in 2015, exactly zero appeared to be spent on studying the proposed HSV-1 connection.

So they can go on saying "there's no scientific proof" because there isn't any; they are making sure of that.

Then, in June 2016, *New Scientist* reported a work by Rudolph Tanzi of Harvard Medical School.[175]

He reinforces the strong likelihood that Alzheimer's is, in fact, an infection caused by either Herpes Simplex or Chlamydia. The amyloid plaques that so mesmerize scientists might not be the cause of the disease at all but are the brain's response to the infection?

In other words amyloid plaques may be part of the immune response.

Wouldn't this typify the blundering stupidity of modern medicine: to try and get rid of the one good thing that's fighting the problem, on the crazy assumption it must be causing the problem? (without any evidence at all)

What You Can Do

The first point to grasp is that your brain thrives on activity! It's a use it or lose it thing. Science has shown that the number of connections in the brain can be increased, no matter the starting point, by simply making demands of the mind. More connections mean more brain power. Any kind of stimulus is valid, be it crosswords, conversation, creative hobbies, learning a language, sports or the arts, but doing what you love has the most benefits.

Daily exercise is important. It stimulates and tones up both body and mind. You know the old saying "healthy body equals healthy mind" (*Mens sana in corpore sano*). I couldn't agree more. Exercise releases endorphins, increases circulation and therefore oxygen supply to the brain. Endorphins are natural feel-good substances in our bodies. **Don't just think in terms of swimming, jogging or cycling. Walking is very good and non-stressful. Dancing is even better, since it has the added joy element, which reminds us we are young at heart and that life after all is great!**

A 2003 study from Stamford University showed that dancing especially was valuable for beating signs of dementia! Dancing can lower stress and increase serotonin levels, with an accompanying sense of well-being.[176]

Now it seems dancing can also make us smarter, or at least block the deteriorating brain function of aging, according to a study that was led by the Albert Einstein College of Medicine in New York City and published in the New England Journal of Medicine.

Here are the findings in a nutshell:

It followed senior citizens (75 and older) for a period of 21 years, looking at whether any physical or cognitive recreational activities influenced mind function. Researchers discovered that some activities had a significant beneficial effect on rates of dementia, including Alzheimer's disease. Other activities had none.

Activities studied were reading books, writing for pleasure, doing crossword puzzles, playing cards and playing musical instruments. And they studied physical activities like playing tennis or golf, swimming, bicycling, dancing, walking for exercise and doing housework.

One of the surprises of the study was that almost none of the physical activities appeared to offer any protection against dementia. There can be cardiovascular benefits of course, but the focus of this study was the mind.

However, there was one important exception: frequent dancing offered protection against dementia.

Here are the comparative results:

- Reading - 35% reduced risk of dementia
- Bicycling and swimming - 0%
- Doing crossword puzzles at least four days a week - 47%
- Playing golf - 0%
- Dancing frequently – risk reduction of 76%.

That's a huge lowering of risk!

Why Dancing?

Why is dancing better than other activities for improving mental capabilities? Because typical ballroom dancing, where steps and coordination count (sorry boppers!), means a lot of snap decisions, especially for the woman or "follower", who gets very little warning of what's coming next.

But men, you can also match her degree of decision-making if you choose to do so.

Here's how:

1. Really pay attention to your partner and what works best for her. Notice what is comfortable for her, where she is already going, which signals are successful with her and which aren't, and constantly adapt your dancing to these observations. That's rapid-fire split-second decision making.

2. Don't lead the same old patterns the same way each time. Challenge yourself to try new things each time you dance. Make more decisions more often. Intelligence: use it or lose it.

Those who fully utilize their intelligence in dancing, at all levels, love the way it feels. Spontaneous leading and following both involve entering a flow state. Both leading and following benefit from a highly active attention to possibilities.

The essence of intelligence is making decisions. The best advice, when it comes to improving your mental acuity, is to involve yourself in activities which require split-second rapid-fire decision making, as opposed to rote memory (retracing the same well-worn paths), or just working on your physical style.

One way to do that is to learn something new. Not just dancing, but anything new. Take a class to challenge your mind. It will stimulate the connectivity of your brain by generating the need for new pathways. Difficult classes are better for you, as they will create a greater need for new neural pathways.

Quick Thinking Is Crucial

Healthy, well-functioning seniors who undertake a type of computerized cognitive training that targets processing speed have a 29% reduced risk for dementia after 10 years, with those completing the most training sessions having the greatest benefit, new results suggest.

Cognitive training that focused on memory or reasoning alone did not significantly reduce the risk for dementia; only speed of reaction (note again what I said above about quick decision making in dancing).

Participants were randomly assigned to one of three types of cognitive training — memory, reasoning, or speed of processing — or to a control group that received no cognitive training.

This was a long study: 10 years, and followed 2785 original participants. Testing and re-testing was carried out at 1,2,3,5 and 10-year intervals. During the decade-long follow-up, 260 participants developed dementia.

Compared with the control group, the risk for dementia was 29% lower in the speed training group. But memory training made no difference to whether an individual developed dementia or not.

The authors noted that the attrition rate in the study, at 5.5% per year over the 10 years, falls within the typical range for studies of older adults with a long-term follow-up.[177]

What's the take home? Fast gaming is probably the way to go. Online computer games will probably come on stream during the life of this book, some specifically targeting seniors and getting them to interact, according to the dictates of this study.

Lifestyle Changes

A 2015 randomized controlled trial, published in *The Lancet,* demonstrated how a comprehensive prevention program can reduce the risk of dementia in those who are at high risk. In Finland 1,260 adults, aged 60 to 77 years old, participated in the Finnish Geriatric Intervention Study to Prevent Cognitive Impairment and Disability. Half were randomly assigned to the intervention group while the other half served as controls. All were at high risk of dementia.

The intervention consisted of regular meetings over the two-year trial period with various health professionals to address diet, exercise, brain training exercises and metabolic risk factors. At the end of two years, the intervention group scored 25 percent higher overall on the Neuropsychological Test Battery (NTB) — a standard test to evaluate mental functioning — than the control group. They scored even higher on certain parts of the test.

Executive functioning scores (the brain's ability to organize and regulate thought processes) "were 83 percent higher in the intervention group, and processing speed was 150 percent higher." That's impressive.

According to professor [Miia] Kivipelto, 'Much previous research has shown that there are links between cognitive decline in older people and factors such as diet, heart health, and fitness. However, our study is the first large randomized controlled trial to show that an intensive program aimed at addressing these risk factors might be able to prevent cognitive decline in elderly people who are at risk of dementia.'[178]

Nutrition

I have mentioned the very strong possibility that low-fat eating may be driving the Alzheimer's "epidemic". Step one then is put back fats into your diet right now. Saturated animal fats are totally fine. You can't live without them. We need fats.

Fresh whale or seal blubber would be ideal! Since you can't buy that at the local supermarket, a good substitute is coconut oil. Decades of relentless phoney propaganda by the food industry and Big Ag (trying to push corn oil and peanut oil, etc. for their own profit) have made people scared of products like coconut oil and butter.

You'll find the ignorant hysterics online, of course. Long-chain saturated fatty acids, like the ones that make up most of the fat in coconut, palm kernel, and palm oils, do in fact raise LDL cholesterol. These saturated fats are called palmitic, myristic, and lauric acids. They also make up most of the saturated fatty acids in meat, poultry, and dairy fats like milk, butter, and cheese.

But these days we know better than to worry about LDL. It's *what sort of LDL?* The small particulate size is the dangerous fraction. Coconut oil and butter do not raise that.

But the old prejudices die hard and, despite the fact that the saturated fat story was a complete criminal fabrication by a science crook called Ancel Keys, old fools that were suckered by the false science are not going to admit they were wrong.

Studies purportedly telling us that saturated fat is bad NEVER distinguish the fat sources. But there is the world of difference between fresh coconut oil and the rancid week-old fat used for cooking burgers and French fries!

Moreover, today's saturated animal fats, from miserably unhealthy and half-starved cattle, loaded with pesticides, hormones and other pollutants means that "fat" is not really being measured at all.

So the die-young message "avoid fats" will continue, till the old guard dies off or retires.

Meantime, your brain is made up of 60% fat remember! Unsaturated fat, that is. Take plenty of EFAs (EPA and DHA, avoiding omega-6s as much as possible). Your Mom was right, all those decades ago: fish is good for the brain. Only Big Ag and Big Food have perverted everything, till you can't trust food any more.

Enjoy your butter.

Mushrooms (Fungi)

This group of foodstuffs may have special relevance for Alzheimer's and other dementias.

First, the "lion's Mane" mushroom (*Hericium erinaceus*). It is a powerful stimulant of nerve growth factor, with lots of good science showing it can generate more brain cells.[179]

My good friend Eric Cerecedes told me a fascinating story about this, one of many:

You know about 10 years ago I had a close family friend that was stricken with Alzheimer's. His name is Dick, and Dick degenerated very quickly. Within a couple of years of his diagnosis he was not able to carry on a conversation or form memories. He could not dress himself or take himself to the bathroom anymore. He was depending on his wife to meet most of his basic needs.

My brother who is a tissue culture specialist and fungal researcher had done some research on *Hericium erinaceus*. He found some studies in Japan that demonstrated that this mushroom was very effective against Alzheimer's, and helped to even reverse some of the symptoms. So we got Dick on an Alzheimer's regime, making sure that he was on a healthy diet, as well as taking the extract of the Lion's Mane mushroom daily. Somewhere between month four and five, Dick got up, he got himself dressed, and he took himself to the bathroom for the first time in over a year, and day by day, Dick's slowly but surely, had a full recovery from Alzheimer's.

He was forming memories again, having coherent conversations, driving a car, and by the end of his life he was taking care of his wife instead of her taking care of him. Dick did die a couple of years ago, but the beautiful ending in that story is that he died with all of his senses and that's more than any of us could have hoped for him.

In seeing that, Eric quit his job in business in Los Angeles and moved to Southern Oregon to start a medicinal mushroom educational outreach program. His company is called Mycoformulas (you can find the link in the Valuable Resources section in the back of the book). Other mushrooms with a strong traditional reputation for healing of all kinds include *Ganoderma lucidum* (Reishi), *Grifola frondosa* (Maitake), *Trametes versicolor* (Turkey Tail) and Cordyceps sinensis

Chaga (*Inonotus obliquus*) is particularly valuable in this context. Known as "The King Of Medicinal Fungus", it is purported to reduce inflammation, boost the immune system and fight viruses. It's also one of the most powerful antioxidants known, second only to raw chocolate. In other words, it's a brilliant anti-inflammatory.

But the star remains *Hericum erinaceus*. It is the Alzheimer's fungus!

If you prefer, you can take tablets or capsules (make sure you get the mycelial form of the mushroom extract). Dose: about 250 – 500 mg daily.

Or you can use it as a tea infusion.

Beta Glucans

While on the subject, consider beta glucans. These polysaccharides are unusual heavy-weight sugars (named from glucose) are powerful extracts of mushrooms or yeasts that stimulate the immune system. If there should be an infective element to Alzheimer's, such as a Herpes virus or Chlamydia bacterium, then helping the immune system suppress that infection should logically be beneficial.

These versatile compounds are also used for high cholesterol, diabetes, cancer, and HIV/AIDS. Beta glucans are also used for colds (common cold), flu (influenza), H1N1 (swine) flu, allergies, hepatitis, Lyme disease, asthma, ear infections, aging, ulcerative colitis and Crohn's disease, fibromyalgia, rheumatoid arthritis, and multiple sclerosis.

In fact, they are among the most powerful curative medicines known, with over 158,000 PubMed studies verifying it.

Healthcare providers sometimes give beta glucans by IV (intravenously) or by injection into the muscle (IM) to boost the immune system in people with cancer, HIV/AIDS and post-operatively, to prevent infections.

It has been reported, however, that when administered intravenously, beta-glucans may cause dizziness, headaches, nausea, vomiting, diarrhea, constipation, hives, flushing, rash, high or low blood pressure, or excessive urination; even lung inflammation.

You see, many formulas being sold rely on generic science. A lot of competitors market very impure products containing under-performing and shabby ingredients.

My colleague AJ Lanigan has developed what has to be the best oral beta-glucan formula in the world: Beta-1, 3D Glucan:

A large 2008 JANA study carried out by Dr. Vaclav Vetvicka at Louisville University showed that Better Way Health's Beta-glucan (Beta 1,3D) has the highest proven immunological benefits: Eight (8) times more effective than any mushroom based beta-glucan and 160x more effective than many of the popular Internet products being sold.[180]

Another 2010 study published in *Open Glycoscience* was the most comprehensive study ever done on immune system supplements. It compared the world's top 16 immune supplements: Immutol, Maitake Gold, PSK Krestin, Wellmune, etc. - Compared to all these, Better Way Health's Glucan #300 was found to have the highest biological activity and it was not even a close call! Glucan #300 had 8x more immune response than the 2nd place immune supplement. That makes it hands down the best immune system supplement in the world.

Check the **Valuable Resources** section for more information (and a free download)!

Foods To Feed Your Brain.

Oily fish, flax seeds (linseeds) are rich in omega-3 fats which nourish nerve fibers. Eat oily fish at least twice weekly (do your best to get uncontaminated sources). Linseeds after being crushed can be sprinkled over cereals, into desserts or blended with fresh juices.

Eat plenty of fresh fruits and vegetables, which are high in anti-oxidants that protect the brain from degeneration.

Dark blue foods, such as blackberries, blueberries and bilberries, are rich in particularly powerful antioxidants called *anthocyanins*. Scientists at Tufts University in Boston recently found that eating a half a cup of fresh blueberries daily helps to reverse brain aging, thanks to their high anti-oxidant activity.

[Dr. Keith's champagne note: this divine drink contains an antioxidant called tyrosol, which is even richer in antioxidant activity than blueberries!]

Green tea is high in antioxidants but black tea also has plenty of catechins, which work as antioxidants.

Foods to eat less of…

Sugar over excites brain cells until they become exhausted, at which point sweet foods no longer give you an energy boost but make you feel tired. This includes all sugars: maltose, dextrose, white and brown sugar, corn sugar (really just HFCS) and honey.

Eliminate all refined white flour cakes, waffles, pancakes, breads, and junk take away meals, most of which are high in sugar, fat and salt (and sugar turns to a hard fat if not burned up during exercise).

At all costs eliminate artificial sweeteners such as Aspartame and Splenda, which are found in many manufactured foods and drinks. These excitotoxins over-stimulate the brain, which can trigger insomnia, anxiety and feelings of tension.

Reduce alcohol intake. In small quantities, it is a boon, increasing social contact and bonhomie, which is good for the brain and our emotions. But we must remind you, as always, excess alcohol can be very damaging.

Any foods which are bad for your arteries are bad for your brain, which depends on an efficient blood supply for essential nutrients. In essence that means avoid manufactured foods; eat only whole foods, organic if you can get it.

More Stuff You May Not Know

Certain studies have shown that exposure to electromagnetic radiation significantly increases the risk of Alzheimer's, or makes it rapidly worse. This means working with or near computers, VDUs and similar equipment. But also, of course, it means that mobile phones are adding to the risk.

Good scientific studies have tied Alzheimer's disease to plasma homocysteine levels. Increased amounts of this important bio-marker in the blood spells trouble for the heart and for the brain. However homocysteine levels can be readily brought to normal, using vitamin B6, B12 and folic acid supplements. I usually add TMG (trimethyl glycine) 1,000 mg daily.

An important study at Heidelberg University, Germany, showed that in a large proportion of Alzheimer's cases, the mechanism is that of failure of small blood vessels in the brain (this would lead to brain starvation and degeneration). Chelation, is known to be very good at restoring the function of older blood vessels. For this reason it is an important treatment for heart disease, strokes and anti-aging. But the great benefit to Alzheimer's can be understood.

Another part of the puzzle is exposure to toxic metal poisoning. Aluminium was once thought to be a main offender for Alzheimer's. Actually, fewer people think that today, but the aluminium hypothesis is making a comeback. Prof. Christopher Exley at Keele University UK has been able to test several autistic brains and several "dementia brains" (yes, I know, it's a silly expression) and found some of the highest aluminium levels ever found in human tissue.[181]

Mercury poisoning is also a likely culprit. But whichever is correct, the good news is that chelation can remove these toxic metals from the tissues. This has been done effectively for over fifty years. Modern switched-on doctors have recognized the value of chelation for Alzheimer's and other degenerative disorders caused by metal poisoning, however standard chelation (with EDTA) is little use for removing aluminium and mercury.

Get Infected With Friendly Bacteria

Now researchers have come up with a whole new direction for dementia. Throughout this book, you'll read repeatedly about the health benefits of good intestinal bacteria and the damaging effect of disruption of the microbiome in our gut (dysbiosis).

In fact disorder of our intestinal flora is the most potent cause of general inflammation known (see my book *Fire In The Belly*). Not surprisingly then, healthy bowel flora can have a powerful impact on Alzheimer's, primarily an inflammatory disorder.

There's one microbe in particular, known as *Mycobacterium vaccae* (or *M. vaccae*), that could be very helpful in settling down this unwanted brain inflammation. This bacterium abundant in soil. When we're outdoors we breathe it in the open air... So that could be one good reason to spend time in Nature (see also Forest Bathing section in 2.4).

We'll see later that science is homing in on the connection between our gut and brain function. Some researchers even go so far as to call the gut the second brain. Since over 90% of the body's serotonin comes from there, you'll see they have a point.

A 2013 study published in the journal *Behavioral Processes* provided more evidence for this theory when researchers Dorothy Matthews and Susan Jenks fed a group of mice live M. vaccae bacteria and then had them run a maze. A control group ran the maze without the benefit of the microbe.

The results were stunning. Mice that ate the bacteria before and during the trials "completed the maze twice as fast as controls and with reduced anxiety-related behaviors."[182]

You'll start hearing of the "old friends" or the "hygiene" hypothesis of stress-related diseases. This theory states that, because we spend less time in nature and overuse antibacterial soaps and other germ-killing aids, our bodies no longer reap the benefits of friendly microbes, like M. vaccae.

The hypothesis gets its name from the "strategy of 'reintroducing' humans to their old [intestinal] friends to promote optimal health and wellness. Without them our bodies fall prey to the negative effects of stress and chronic inflammation, and this adversely affects our bodies' own ability to prevent diseases.

In a 2016 study published in the journal *Trends in Immunology*, researchers "immunized" mice with M. vaccae and found that their exposure to the microbe (or infection, if you will) prevented stress-induced colitis and reduced fear, anxiety, symptoms of inflammation and poor stress management in the test animals.[183]

You will immediately see why WHAT WE EAT is of such crucial health importance, even though mainstream doctors completely ignore it, or even dismiss it as unimportant.

The Serotonin Factor

The reason for the animals' decreased anxiety in the above studies is that ingestion of M. vaccae stimulates the release of serotonin in the brain. Higher levels of this neurotransmitter is said to elevate mood and decrease anxiety.

But serotonin is not just the "feel good" neurotransmitter; it's also essential to synaptic functioning (gaps between brain cells). Your neurons need serotonin to communicate with each other. This molecule also plays a crucial role in memory and learning.

Serotonin production naturally slows as we age. Research suggests that this decrease could be linked to depression, decreased cognition, memory problems and Alzheimer's disease later in life.[184]

Autopsy study of brains of people with Alzheimer's disease have shown serious serotonin deficiencies. Low serotonin is not so much a specific risk factor for cognitive impairment and Alzheimer's as it is a sign that overall brain health and function are compromised. Likewise, boosting serotonin production may not necessarily prevent mild cognitive impairment or Alzheimer's. Instead, low serotonin and the symptoms it causes should be seen as red flags that brain health is suffering, which increases the risk for Alzheimer's.

Of course this does not mean the SSRIs actually work as supposed. Trying to block its re-uptake is a desperate measure, from a corps of scientists who basically don't know what they are doing! (or why!) But Big Pharma will continue to try and hoodwink the community with "solutions" that are worthless.[185]

Dig Deep

Spending time in green places, city parks and uninhabited woods alike, increases your exposure to M. vaccae. Get outside and breathe the fresh air as often as you can (see Forest Bathing in the previous section).

Stop washing your hands and sterilizing the kitchen counter obsessively.

Eating fruits and vegetables directly from the tree, shrub or vine also helps you to ingest beneficial quantities of this microbe. As long as they're grown without pesticides and herbicides, you'll be pretty safe to eat them without washing. (I'd be wary of vegetables grown in or near the ground, especially in manure-rich soil. Those I'd wash.)

Dig a little deeper and you'll discover that gardening or otherwise closely interacting with the earth gives you even more M. vaccae.

There has been a growing understanding in the healthcare sector about the importance of the healing environment, ever since US experimental psychologist Roger Ulrich's groundbreaking 1984 study proved that surgery patients with a view of nature suffered fewer complications, used less pain medication and were discharged sooner than those with a view of a brick wall.

Since then, research has been building, suggesting that gardens can specifically improve the health of people with dementia in a number of ways, from encouraging cardiovascular exercise, stimulating the appetite and increasing vitamin D levels, to improving mood, relieving stress, and providing an activity to share with family and carers.[186]

Photobiomodulation

What if there was a way to really stimulate the brain to re-grow the missing and dysfunctional cells it needs for good performance? Is it even possible? What if it had already been shown to greatly benefit Alzheimer's cases, allowing certain individuals to regain their contact with loved ones and the outside world? Would that be exciting?

Well, it's here.

Instead of attacking—yes, attacking—biomarkers and treating the symptoms, we want to work on the biological healing process.

The body's healing ability is almost miraculous. We can help it along in a most unusual way. It has been shown that light at 810 nm (that's near infra-red) is especially helpful in restoring brain function in dementia and stroke patients. It also helps veterans (PTSD) with traumatic brain damage.

This new specialty is called *photobiomodulation* (altering metabolism with the use of light forms).

All living things require light just as they need food, air and water. In the 6th century BCE Herodotus observed this, noting that exposure to sunlight was required for normal bone growth. Heliotherapy or treatment with sunlight, was used by the ancient Egyptian, Greek and Roman physicians to address many conditions and has been practiced since the dawn of time.

The discovery of the powerful healing properties of red laser light was discovered by Endre Mester (1903–1984) He was actually trying to cause skin cancer; he took rats and shone red laser light on shaved patches of skin. To his astonishment, the hair grew back twice as fast on the backs of the rats which had been "dosed" with the red laser light than it did with the controls.

Near-infrared light has gained increased attention for its ability to activate anti-inflammatory processes and is now widely used in veterinary medicine to treat sprains, bone fractures, and to speed the healing of wounds. Over the last ten years, there has been an assemblage of animal studies focusing on the use of transcranial near-infrared light therapy (NILT) to treat brain injury from stroke or trauma.[187]

So what about human patients? Dr Margaret Naeser, research professor at Boston University School of Medicine, has worked with this and found improvements in movement and function in about 66% of stroke patients. She went on then to show this can also improve cognitive function. Dementia cases were making marvelous reversals.

Initially, as described, the work was done with low-level lasers ("cold" lasers). It has since been understood that the light need not have the penetration or coherence of lasers. Light is just light, after all! The crucial factor is the wavelength: 810 nm. This in turn defines frequency of vibration.

As Prof. Naeser points out, light therapy has been around for a while "but it's always been used on the body, for wound healing and to treat muscle aches and pains, and joint problems. We're starting to use it on the brain."

As it happens, Professor Naeser is also a licensed acupuncturist and has conducted past research on laser acupuncture to treat paralysis in stroke, and pain in carpal tunnel syndrome.[188]

How exactly is the brain-repair effect happening?

Work from the University of California, San Francisco, shows that brain stem cells can divide and multiply, under the influence of near infra-red light. The cells seem to replicate themselves. What is even more amazing is that the new brain cells start to move around, find each other. They start to link up and form new neural networks just like brain tissue.

It's even been filmed, cells caught in the act!

Check out the link for an incredible video in the **Valuable Resources** section!

I find it endlessly fascinating. Remember, it's less than 20 years ago doctors and scientists were teaching—making a big thing out of it being a "scientific fact"—that you can't grow new brain tissue. That's disgusting and shows how little understanding of nature they had. Nature can fix almost anything! I've built a career on that.

Practical Details

Dr. Anita Saltmarche, in Toronto, Canada and Dr. Michael Hamblin at Harvard Medical School have shown definitively that 810 nm LED lights, applied directly to the head, at the right frequency, have a powerful biological restorative effect. This works directly through the skull. So you will hear it called *Transcranial Light Therapy*.

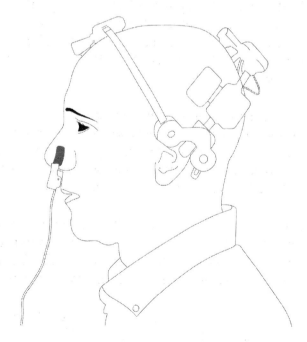

What's great is that brain scans show that the brain responds immediately, after just one treatment. And from then on, it goes on improving.

The cost of devices that can do this in the home, for example the VieLight Neuro headgear (see illustration), is ridiculously small ($2,000 or less) when you compare this sort of technology with the $10,000s and $100,000s of standard medical gear. Most households can afford something like this and if it can repair brain tissue—of course it can—then everyone in the household should be using it, not just patients with Parkinson's, Alzheimer's or PTSD!

No doctor visits are required. There are no additional costs, having your own unit. It's battery powered so no suppressive FDA regulations and licensing issues apply.

The Neuro is pre-programmed and runs for about 25 minutes, before switching itself off. Recommended use is not more often than every second day.

Now, before I finish, let me give you another dose of super-science, without trying to overwhelm you.

You may not have heard of the Default Mode network in our brains. This is what kicks in when we are not actively using our brains.

The concept of a default mode network was developed after researchers inadvertently noticed surprising levels of brain activity in experimental participants who were supposed to be "at rest"—in other words they were not engaged in a specific mental task, but just resting quietly (often with their eyes closed). Although the idea that the brain is constantly active was clearly expressed by Hans Berger in the 1930s, it wasn't until the 1970s that brain researcher David Ingvar began to accumulate data showing that cerebral blood flow (a general measurement of brain activity) remains high even during resting states.[189]

In the early 2000s, Raichle, Gusnard, and colleagues published a series of articles that attempted to more specifically define the areas of the brain that were most active during these rest states. It was in one of these publications that they used the term *default mode* to refer to this resting activity.[190]

A number of diseases, like Parkinson's and Alzheimer's, autism, MS, schizophrenia and depression, are associated with a dysfunctional default mode. It's absolutely fascinating to report that the characteristic amyloid plaque lesions of Alzheimer's are found at the same locations as the hubs or nodes of the default mode network. That must be telling us something important but nobody, as yet, knows what it is!

What we are finding is that it is possible to dramatically reverse some of these conditions. Brain tissue can recover a lot. Brain cells are just cells, like any other in the body. They know what to do; they know how to heal. We just have to help them!

I'm very excited about this new technology. It has enormous potential for us all to increase our mental performance, not just for patients to recover from dysfunctionality. I have my own device and use it often.

Let's wrap this up with an awesome recovery story, using the VieLight Neuro. Here is an email I got from one of my subscribers (lightly edited for compactness):

Dear Prof. Keith,

Our daughter Diana had a catastrophic brain stem stroke at age 28 and was one of the lucky survivors, albeit with a high degree of disability but fully cognitively functional.

She also continuously battled brain imbalances causing her to have overstated emotional outbursts, i.e., laughing and crying. Frequent crying sessions are of course very hard to handle, both for her and for us.

It usually took 5 – 6 weeks of concentrated effort and exercises to get better brain balance and to get her emotionally stable.

Then we bought Vielight Neuro Alpha, after watching your video on its capabilities, because she was again slipping into overemotional outbursts. After just the second session with Vielight Neuro the change and improvement was remarkable. She stabilized almost instantly and has remained that way. It was so fast!

Now we use Vielight Neuro Alpha for her about three times per week and she continues to be stable, though interestingly, over the Christmas break, being busy in other directions, we missed a few sessions, and she reminded us of it as she was getting teary again.

I thought to give you this feedback for your records and that you would like to know.

Best regards
Michael

This tale highlights a very important point I seek to make over and over, which is that *Nature heals*. Nobody is truly busted or broke, as doctors like to think. We have awesome powers of re-growth and recovery! (see section 4).

Brain-Wise Supplements

The star brain nutrient is the antioxidant glutathione, a naturally occurring amino acid within the body. It is a powerful brain and liver food, which helps those organs detoxify and take care of themselves. But as we age glutathione levels fall, and toxins such as heavy metals and pesticides reduce levels even further. Glutathione is manufactured in our cells from a number of precursors such as Alpha Lipoic Acid (ALA); Acetyl-L–Carnitine and N Acetyl Cysteine (NAC).

In a 2002 published study, rats fed on extra ALA and Acetyl-L-Carnitine lived 50% longer than normal rats and enjoyed greatly improved overall health. The animals were so vigorous that media headlines referred to them as the "dancing rats".

Bruce Ames, a cell biologist at the University of California, Berkeley, reported in the Proceedings of the National Academy of Sciences that he fed elderly rats two chemicals, acetyl-L-carnitine and the anti-oxidant alpha-lipoic acid. Both are normally found in mammal cells, and both are sold in health shops. Then he tested the animals for memory and stamina.

"With these two supplements together, these old rats got up and did the macarena," he said. "The brain looks better, they are full of energy: everything we looked at looks more like a young animal."[191]

After the age of 50 I suggest you take 200mg of ALA, and 500mg of either NAC or Acetyl L Carnitine on a daily basis.

N-acetyl-cysteine (NAC) has surprisingly robust science in connection with brain function.

Researchers from The University of Melbourne examined the effect of NAC as a maintenance therapy for bipolar depression. Individuals with moderate depression were asked to take 1gram (1,000 mg) of NAC twice a day for 2months.

An 8 point reduction in depressive score was observed at the end of 8 weeks with improvement in functioning and quality of life.

A 2014 study evaluated NAC's effect in major depressive disorder. This study was published in *The Journal of Clinical Psychiatry*, 2014. Patients were given NAC or placebo in addition to conventional treatment for 12 weeks. The follow up lasted till 16 weeks.

Till 12 weeks, no significant differences were observed between NAC and placebo. In patients with high depressive scores, treatment differences were observed from week 6. At week 12, improvement in 'impaired functioning' scores was observed with NAC treatment.[192]

So professional lairs, such as Paul Offit MD, are seriously misleading when they claim "supplements don't work", "no scientific proof", or similar. These critics obviously never read the literature; they just make up opinions, which favor their products, and ignore useful natural remedies, which they see as a threat to their greed.

Phosphatidyl serine and phosphatidyl choline help to protect nerve fibers and keep the brain fit and sleek. Take a minimum of 50mg daily of either, or both. Once we would prescribe lecithin—usually derived from soya beans—because it is rich in phosphatidyl serine and choline. We know lecithin increases levels of choline acetyltransferase [ChAT], which is interesting, because ChAT is responsible for the synthesis of the neurotransmitter acetylcholine, which is essential for memory and brain function and, when elevated, helps work against a number of neurological disorders like Alzheimer's disease.

But these days we worry about soya products. These can act as anti-nutrients, goitrogens, xenoestrogens and enzyme disruptors.

Even more alarmingly, test animals subjected to long-term consumption of lecithin were found to be "hypoactive, had poor postural reflexes, and showed attenuated morphine analgesia;" meaning that it lessened the pain-killing effects of morphine.[193]

This tells me there are things unknown about soya lecithin and it is recommended that you ignore vigorous marketing ploys and if you take it at all, dose only once a week.

A better idea would be to get your lecithin from other sources, such as liver, red meat, whole grains, legumes, and egg yolks (in fact, the term "lecithin" is derived from the Greek word for egg yolk, *lekithos*). So yet another way that the low-fat frenzy has hurt people—avoiding egg yolks is not, and never was, healthy. You need lutein and zeaxanthine for healthy eyes and the lecithin for your brain.

Also helpful are glutathione, N-acetyl cysteine and alpha lipoic acid. These are powerful brain anti-oxidants and have remarkable effects on mental performance and cognition. So much so that otherwise healthy individuals notice considerable improvement too!

Ginkgo Biloba – a herb proven to improve memory, increase circulation and acts as a brain stimulant. 500mg of standardized extract daily. Remember that herbs are potent medicines and not always without side effects - take for 6 weeks, then stop for a month and then begin again. In a very important study published in 1997 by the Journal of the American Medical Association, *Gingko biloba* was shown not only to prevent Alzheimer's degeneration but actually improved many of the cases, compared to the placebo (all the more remarkable, in that the AMA has always been opposed to natural and nutritional therapies!)

Vinpocetine - This to me is the *herb extraordinaire* for memory issues. It is an extract of the wonder plant *Vinca minor* (periwinkle); from the same source we also get two anti-cancer chemo-therapeutic agents (vinblastine and vincristine). In humans vinpocetine has been shown to:

- dilate brain arteries (more nutrients)

- reduce the tendency of blood to clot (thus protecting against heart disease and stroke)

- speed up brain metabolism

- act as an antioxidant

- aid recovery after stroke

A 1987 study in the *Journal of the American Geriatric Society* showed unequivocally that vinpocetine protects against dementia and improves those who already have it. Good enough reasons for vinpocetine to be classed as a major anti-aging substance.[194]

A study published in the Lancet Jan 20th 2007, has shown daily folic acid (800 mcg daily) significantly improves cognitive performance in older adults — specifically as it relates to memory and information processing.[195]

More general advice on whole-body healthy supplements is covered later in the book.

Parkinson's Disease Footnote

It can't be said that Parkinson's disease (PD) is the same, or even similar to, Alzheimer's. There is no association with amyloid or neurofibrillary tangles. But both are neurodegenerative diseases and a great deal of what is written in this chapter would apply to PD as well as AD. For example, transcranial light stimulation can help.

Parkinson's disease is characterized by tremors, loss of balance and decreased mobility. It affects roughly one million people in the United States. It's not a fatal condition, but as it progresses it usually leaves its victims completely disabled.

Much-loved comedian Billy Connolly is now struggling with this disease. Film actor Michael J Fox has had it for years now, not to mention the late Mohammed Ali.

Statistically, Parkinson's disease affects more people than Lou Gehrig's disease (ALS), muscular dystrophy and multiple sclerosis combined. Men are at greater risk. It strikes three men for every two women.

There is a large body of evidence linking PD and pesticides.[196]

Now there is a new risk factor that has emerged: my old enemy... Milk!

I can't say anything good about milk. I was recorded once by the BBC saying if I were to ban one food on Earth it would be milk and that—at a stroke—I would cure over 100 million sick people! There's a link to a site in the **Valuable Resources** section in the back of the book. Thing is, what is it about milk that damages the brain? The culprit identified by a study published this year (2017) thinks low-fat dairy is the problem (including reduced fat yogurt, frozen yogurt, and skim and low-fat milk). Maybe this is yet another unhealthy aspect of the low-fat craze; not just Alzheimer's?

But could it be pesticides as well? I found a 2015 study that linked milk consumption to PD in a male Hawaiian population. It is speculated that it could most likely be through dairy contamination with pesticides.

Researchers found that loss of neurons in the substantia nigra (part of the brain associated with Parkinson's) was highest in people who did not smoke BUT who consumed greater amounts of milk. They also correlated milk intake to brain levels of a pesticide called heptachlor epoxide, which was found in the milk supply in Hawaii in the early 1980s.

The latest study, published in the June 2017 issue of the journal *Neurology*, studied 129,346 people for 25 years. Their principal finding is: "Of the total participants, people who consumed more than one serving a day of low-fat dairy, particularly low-fat and skim milk, had a greater risk of PD compared to those who consumed one to three servings per month. Though low-fat and skim milk were the biggest culprits, sherbet and frozen yogurt were also associated with an increased risk."[197]

One of the theories is that the link may be because milk proteins can decrease the amount of uric acid in the body. Uric acid is produced from the natural breakdown of protein foods and is usually filtered out through the kidneys. Low levels of uric acid have been associated with an increased risk of Parkinson's disease, especially in men.[198]

However, my wife Vivien points out that people in Starbuck's these days all want "low fat" and skimmed milk, in the belief these are healthy choices. But then they swallow Starbucks' sticky syrups and GMO-rich cakes, with corn syrup. Is it really the milk that's doing it or just cumulative ignorance and bad habits ?

Statins Too

Statins are the biggest earners for the pharmaceutical industry. The science is riddled with contradictions and hidden (concealed) data, attempting to prop up the myth that we should all take these deadly junk pills.

The drugs companies pushed for the American Heart Association to expand guidelines for statin use, and recently they obliged.

Unfortunately, the AHA, the drug companies and doctors won't tell you that taking these drugs every day can increase your risk of developing Parkinson's disease.

In a study published in the journal *Movement Disorders*, researchers used MarketScan, a large U.S. insurance claims database, to see if there was a connection between statins and Parkinson's disease.

They discovered "statin usage was significantly associated with PD risk." This applies particularly to lipophilic statins, which go by the generic names atorvastatin, lovastatin and simvastatin. Drugs in this category cross the blood-brain barrier more easily than other kinds of statins, which may account for their devastating effect on the brain.[199]

It's a well-established medical fact that statins do not decrease the risk of heart attack in people who have never had one, and also that they don't decrease the risk in women. They do decrease the risk of a second heart attack in men who have already had one (very slightly; but not nearly as much of a decrease as brushing your teeth three times a day. I'm not kidding!).

Yet the medical profession continues to push these drugs with religious zeal. Actually, as Lee Euler jokes (Awakening from Alzheimer's), that's a slander on religion, as the resurrection of Jesus Christ is backed by quite a bit more evidence than are the benefits of statin drugs. Chances are pretty good your doctor will get angry with you if you refuse to take them. That's one good reason to seek out an alternative or integrative doctor. There are plenty of other reasons.

2.6 Hyperactivity, Autism And Minimal Brain Dysfunction

Right! Adults do not have a monopoly on biological or functional brain disorder. Let's look at a group of problems which are of great concern in respect of youngsters.

Let me start by saying that I deplore the ignorant postures of certain members of the online marketing profession—people who call themselves "health researchers"—meaning they have no medical qualifications whatever. They just get their information by Googling and sell "eBooks", which are often filled with misleading nonsense.

A cadre of these individuals has started to put it about that hyperactivity disorder, attention deficit disorder and other examples of brain dysfunction in children do not exist; that they are simply an invention of the pharmaceutical industry, designed to sell drugs like Ritalin and Adderall.

This is where their boundless clinical ignorance brings down the truth. They have never worked in an office or facility where buzzed children are patients. I have. I have seen children absolutely "wired", running around in an exhausting state of overstimulation, the poor parents at their wits end, not knowing what to do.

I remember looking out of my study window one day to see one of my nurses chasing a child around the lawn, trying to catch him for his next shot (part of a series of food allergy testing). He had been triggered by a minute dose of the food and now needed the "neutralizing dose". It took her several minutes to catch him. This was a case where I could diagnose hyperkinetic syndrome at 600 paces!

I am proud to have been among the pioneer doctors who fought to get this condition recognized and so be effectively studied and solved. I particularly resent fools trying to walk backwards, because of their agenda, and plunge parents back into the nightmare of a hyperkinetic child, with no sympathy and no solution.

When I say studied and "solved" of course, I mean properly solved, not doped up with drugs. The causes of ADD and ADHD are few and can be listed as follows: food allergy and intolerance, chemical sensitivity, heavy metal toxins, vaccinations, stealth pathogens, parasites and certain metabolic difficulties.

There is no abnormal brain chemistry and there is no "Ritalin deficiency".

Casebook

Timmy was a young Irish boy, brought to me in 1986 as a result of my appearance on Gay Byrne's radio show in Dublin, Ireland. To describe him as hyperactive I think would be to understate the case. For the entire one hour interview with his parents, he leapt up on my desk and ran across it between the parents and me; jumped down and climbed on the examination couch along the next wall; ran along that and then jumped down and went across the top of the sideboard near the door; leapt off that and ran along the row of chairs opposite the examination couch; finally, back onto my desk and across it....

And when I say climbed up or on, I'm talking about furniture that was almost head-height to him. He was like a miniature hurdler!

This went on for the entire sixty minutes, occasionally interrupted by the anxious parents, who would grab Timmy and hold him down; but then he would wriggle free while they answered some difficult question for me.

I estimate this lad carried out some fifty circuits of my office during that time. It was distracting and exhausting to watch. The furniture was significantly damaged by footmarks and scuffs. I felt for the misery of his parents, having to put up with this, hour after hour, day after day.

The solution, fortunately, was very simple. I could see the diet Timmy was being fed contained plenty of likely trigger foods. I explained how an exclusion diet worked, double-checked the parents could cope with it, and sent them home with a follow-up appointment one week later.

When he came back, Timmy was an utterly transformed child. He sat quietly through the entire consultation, reading a book, and didn't move, except occasionally to adjust his posture to something more comfortable. The parents of course were overjoyed and nobody but the warm Irish know how to thoroughly express their gratitude for help received.

We booked Timmy into the testing room, to find out what the exact triggers were and the rest, as they say, was history...

Another autistic child was equally memorable. If I say the furniture had to be nailed down, that would usually be a jokey expression. In this case, the parents assured me it was true. This four year-old had managed to tear a door off its hinges, he was so strong when in one of his rages.

So don't tell me that ADHD is an invented condition, created by Big Pharma, merely to sell drugs. Humbug!

The Clinical Basis

ADD and ADHD not only occur—they can be predicted to occur!

If you refer to the list of the stages of excitation and depression during allergic and hyper-sensitivity reactions drawn up by Dr. Theron Randolph (see Ups and Downs 2.3) you will probably see that we can predict that some individuals will be markedly 'accelerated' and made restless, irritable and badly behaved because of marked stimulatory effects from food.[200]

Others would be suppressed and slowed down. Where there are learning and co-ordination difficulties but no real brain damage, the term minimal brain dysfunction suggests itself.

ADHD is said to affect predominantly boys, with a ratio to girls of about 5:1. However, I always believed that girls are affected just as often but that their response tends to be different: they are more moody, withdrawn and unhappy. A certain amount of reserve is conditioned into females, whereas boys are encouraged to be more boisterous and extro-vert.[201]

There has since been research to prove that I am right. The symptoms of ADHD present-ed in female children and adolescents are different from male, which may explain the supposed lower prevalence rates of ADHD in females; some studies have indicated that girls with ADHD may be up to twice as likely as boys to have the inattentive type of ADHD and may suffer more from internalizing symptoms and inattention, in contrast with the hyperactive and aggressive symptoms shown by boys.[202]There has been much controver-sy about the connection between diet and hyperactivity and many doctors, particularly those with a psychiatric leaning, often refuse to accept the existence of this link. Instead they prefer to blame mother as 'neurotic', insisting that the child's difficulties are imagi-nary or, if not, that they are being caused by maternal concern.

Two follow-up studies (one in males, one in females), which examined the persistence of ADHD in patients who had received an initial diagnosis when aged 6–17 years, reported that 11 years after the initial diagnosis, 35% of males and 33% of females continued to meet the criteria of the Diagnostic and Statistical Manual of Mental Disorders 4th edition (DSM-IV) for ADHD. In other words, persistence is almost identical between genders.[203] [204]Minimal brain dysfunction in children is probably one of the commonest early-life allergic effects. It may lead to antisocial acts, temper tantrums, poor concentration, learn-ing difficulties and emotional unhappiness. Dyslexia is an interesting and unusual con-dition which may respond dramatically to the clinical ecology approach. Some young-sters afflicted with these problems have a very hard time in life; everyone thinks they are naughty, stupid or lazy and they get no help and may even be scolded or punished for things they have no control over.

Naturally, if undetected these difficulties may roll on into adult life. There the condition shifts emphasis often, causing more inner neurosis and unhappiness. Patients may brood and feel melancholy; life doesn't seem worth living and many patients have said they have on occasion contemplated suicide.

This subject of "brain allergies" dominated my allergy practice for over two decades; until I retired in fact.

Background

While the medical profession, psychiatrists in particular, are obsessed with labeling a collection of symptoms with some fancy title, my preferred idea is to approach mental disorders in terms of functional causes. That way, the path to recovery becomes obvious.

For example, according to my great mentor, the late Dr. Theron G. Randolph, more than half of the so-called psychosomatic reactions are in reality undiagnosed allergic reactions. Even Charles Dickens, the Victorian novelist, knew about this effect; in his book *A Christmas Carol* he had Ebenezer Scrooge address an apparition (dead spirit) as follows: "You may be an undigested bit of beef, a blot of mustard, a crumb of cheese, a fragment of an underdone potato. There's more of gravy than of grave about you, whatever you are!"

This association between foods and strange mental disturbances is not surprising, given that the brain is the central location for the management and interpretation of perceptions. If something affects neurological function, it could result in almost any symptoms you could name, from fatigue, mood swings, anxiety, feeling unreal, spacey, confused, unable to concentrate, poor memory, inability to handle stress, and bad dreams, to (so-called) depression, psychosis, uncontrollable violence, schizophrenia, mania and hallucinations, with many intermediate types and mixtures of symptoms. Throw in attention deficit disorder, hyperkinetic syndrome, autism spectrum disorder (ASD) and learning difficulties and we cover a lot of kid's psychopathology too![205]

But instead of worrying about fancy names, like paranoia, say, or bipolar, we should be diagnosing wheat allergy; instead of mood swings or dissociation, let's address the egg allergy; catatonia or panic attacks could be a manifestation of mold or hydrocarbon allergy. There are many such examples from my case files (see for example, the Irish Potato Boy, section 2.8).

By far the most interesting discovery in psychiatric medicine, though most psychiatrists are unaware of its existence, is in this realm of 'brain allergy', whether due to real allergy, intolerance, low–grade poisoning, etc. The effects can be subtle, amusing, bizarre, dangerous or disastrous, in varying combinations.

Proof of the connection between diet and brain dysfunction has been very slow in coming. Most so-called "research" is actually geared towards opening up a vast new market in dosing children with advanced and powerful medications.

One of the early pioneers was Dr. Ben Feingold, very much a 'conventional' allergist. He tried the effect of excluding aspirin-related foods (salicylates) from the diets of hyperactive children. He claimed that the results were very good. Others tried to reproduce what he did and said it made no difference. However, Feingold went on to improve his results by also banning food additives, such as colorings, many of which are chemically related to aspirin (salicylates). You may have heard of this 'Feingold diet'. Its place is limited; a full exclusion diet is far more effective, followed by challenge testing to identify culprit foods.

Then, in 1983, a trial on migraine in children at the Great Ormond Street Hospital was conducted by a team under Professor John Soothill. It showed that 93 percent of migraines were caused by food allergy. Even more interestingly, *the children on low-allergy diets showed a dramatic decline in their behavioral disorders* – 100 percent, in fact. This never gets talked about but is probably more significant than the discovery about migraines. The important point about this trial is that it was conducted with vigorous scientific protocol and is impossible to dismiss, though some doctors still try.[206]

One of Professor Soothill's team, Dr Joseph Egger of Munich, later went on to study hyperactivity as a separate issue. In a subsequent study published by Egger and Soothill again *all hyperactive cases responded to a low-allergy diet* (part of a double-blind challenge study on low-dose desensitization vaccines), fully confirming this approach to treatment. There can now be no argument as to the connection between diet and hyperactivity.[207]

Yet doctors, pediatricians and psychiatrists continue to regard drug dosing as the first line of treatment, not the last desperate solution. According to *ADDitude*; ADHD News, July 2010, 15% of children were not even screened before starting medication.

That's disgusting and a measure of today's psychiatry. There are no real qualifying tests... so we'll just drug the kids anyway.

Testing

One of the complaints in this day and age is that ADD and ADHD are being "over-diagnosed". How this claim can be argued, without having figures for the "real" incidence is difficult to fathom.

One can say that it's being over-treated but that's another line of enquiry altogether.

Also, it must not be forgotten that today's world-at-large is becoming ever more frenetic, with everyone's attention distracted by advertizing "noise", intrusive electronic gadgets, relentless TV and movie over-stimulation. I read only this morning that in children's films versus those aimed toward adults, deaths amongst major characters were 2.5 times more common, and 2.8 times more likely to be murders. Movie parental characters fared particularly badly—they were five times more likely to die in children's films.[208]In a sense, everyone in this celebrity-oriented, consumer-driven, gadget-crazy, frenzied 21st century society is hyperactive! It could be said that the whole population is shifting in a direction which, 20 years ago, would have been considered ADD. Children are just more sensitive to disturbance; that's all.

According to WebMD, there's no single test to diagnose ADHD. Instead, doctors rely on several things, including:

- Interviews with the parents, relatives, teachers, or other adults
- Personally watching the child or adult
- Questionnaires or rating scales that measure symptoms of ADHD
- Psychological tests

With children, the doctor will talk with the parents about ADHD symptoms they have seen. The doctor will want to know what age the behaviors began and where and when the child shows symptoms. The doctor may ask for a behavior report from the child's teacher, report cards, and samples of schoolwork. If he/she is smart, the doctor will also conduct a detailed diet inventory, on the look out for processed foods, sugar (itself an extreme brain excitant), colorants and additives and antinutrients.

With adults, the doctor may want to talk with a spouse or other family members. He'll want to find out if they had symptoms in childhood. Knowing if an adult had ADHD behavior as a child is important for making a diagnosis.

To rule out other conditions, a doctor may ask for tests, including:

- Hearing and eyesight
- A blood test for lead levels
- A blood test for diseases such as thyroid disease
- A test to measure electrical activity in the brain
- A CT scan or MRI to check for brain abnormalities

What Doctors Look For

To diagnose ADHD, doctors most often use guidelines established by the American Psychiatric Association. The group has identified 3 types of the disorder:

1. Inattentive Type: A person must have at least 6 out of these 9 symptoms, and few symptoms of hyperactive-impulsive type:

1. Doesn't pay attention to detail or makes careless mistakes
2. Doesn't stay on task
3. Doesn't listen
4. Doesn't follow instructions or finish schoolwork or chores

5. Trouble organizing tasks or activities

6. Avoids or dislikes doing things that take effort or concentration

7. Loses things

8. Easily distracted

9. Forgetful

2. Hyperactive-Impulsive Type: A person must have at least 6 out these 9 symptoms, and few symptoms of inattentive type:

- Fidgets or squirms a lot

- Gets up from his seat a lot

- Runs or climbs at inappropriate times

- Has trouble playing quietly

- Always "on the go" as if "driven by a motor"

- Talks excessively

- Blurts an answer before the question has been completed

- Trouble waiting his turn

- Interrupts others

Whereas these sorts of ratings do have a place, I would always listen very carefully to what the mother has to say. She is probably more attuned to anything slightly off-center with her child than any "objective" test.

Valid Tests

To assess your child, professionals may use the Conners' rating scale. It was big in my day (1980s–1990s) but is not totally exclusive. Actually, it is a set of three questionnaires; one for the parents, one for teachers and one for self-assessment (where the child is old enough to report).[209]

Alternatively try this test yourself, from the ADD/ADHD Support Site:

1. Gives up easily on tasks, assignments and self-interests.

2. Poor reality testing skills, and avoids reason or logic.

3. Poorly developed skills of integration, interpolation (bringing things into the current concept) and extrapolation (expanding the idea outwards, to include other relevant concepts).

4. Poor skills of attention and concentration, unable to sustain focus of interest.

5. Difficulties in short term and long term memory acquisition and management.

6. Difficulty in making up their mind, or making choices without undue anxiety.

7. Poor planning abilities, unable to follow through consistently or complete tasks.

8. Difficulty in differentiating between competing, extraneous stimulati.

9. Easily distracted from tasks, conversations or social interactions.

10. Often over-stimulated and over-sensitized to their surroundings.

11. Poor listening skills, often interrupts others, abruptly changes topic.

12. Overly excitable, reactive and easily muddling up topics from one situation to another.

13. Inability to manage emotional responses, temper tantrums.

14. Easily frustrated, emotional labile/unstable leading to immediate changeable moods, behavioral inconsistencies.

15. Often hyperactive, fidgety, overwhelmed with feelings of restlessness.

16. Inability to maintain appropriate social conduct, often disruptive in school.

17. Experiences difficulty in following instructions and guidance.

18. Impatient, difficulty in delaying gratification.

19. Overly demanding may become self-destructive and aggressive.

20. Poor sleep patterns, often not rested, angry or despondent upon rising.

Cited with permission

Autism

Autism is a very big topic and, of course, very current right now. The big question being asked is whether there is any connection between childhood vaccinations, especially measles and pertussis, and the subsequent development of autism spectrum disorder (ASD).

I have a particular niche in this field, being the first (1983) or almost the first, to report the development of severe ASD (it was then called disintegrative psychosis) immediately after the measles vaccine. It should be emphasized that these children were entirely normal in development until vaccination. Then suddenly, inexplicably and sadly, the child began to go backwards in development, lose mental and motor skills and turn into a socially isolated individual.

However, the debate is still wide open. For years many people have considered mercury in vaccines to be the cause of the skyrocketing incidence, but that doesn't hold up: since mercury has been removed from vaccines in some territories (California, for example) the incidence of autism has continued to rise.

Dr. Andrew Wakefield carried out studies that showed convincingly that live attenuated measles virus inhabits the tissue and intestines of autistic children. Orthodoxy now claim that Wakefield was guilty of fraud; to prove their case, they brought in fraudulent evidence! Go figure. Just be aware that Wakefield's evidence holds up to scrutiny amongst honest doctors.

But vaccinations may not be the cause at all! Some kids have autistic symptoms before their first vaccine. Kids get autism who have never even had a vaccination. What other explanations could there be?

Acetominophen (Tylenol/Paracetamol)

Another theory I brought to public attention in 2015 is that acetominophen (Paracetamol/Tylenol) may be destroying childrens' detox pathways.

In 2013 a landmark paper was published in *The Journal Of Restorative Medicine* by William Shaw, PhD, director of the Great Plains Laboratory, gathering evidence of a definitive link between acetominophen/paracetomol and autism. I should remark I was shocked mainly because this drug (as Panadol) was in the UK 20 years ahead of the widespread use of Tylenol in the USA.[210]

The abstract almost speaks for itself. Let me walk you through the key findings:

It appears that the marked increase in the rates of autism, asthma, and attention deficit with hyperactivity throughout much of the world may be largely caused by the marked increase in the use of acetaminophen in genetically and/or metabolically susceptible children, and the use of acetaminophen by pregnant women.

Toxicity of acetaminophen may cause autism by overloading the defective sulfation pathway catalyzed by phenolsulfotransferase, which is deficient in autism, leading to overproduction of the toxic metabolite N-acetyl-p-benzoquinone imine (NAPQI). Increased levels of NAPQI reduce the ability to detoxify a host of toxic chemicals in the environment, increasing oxidative stress, which leads to protein, lipid, and nucleic acid damage from free radicals.

We know for certain that autism kids (which I was treating successfully as early as 1982 with a holistic dietary and detox approach) are susceptible to toxic overload. So anything which clobbers the ability to detox will result in a rapid and nasty toxic accumulation in these kids (including mercury, where present, but only secondary to the loss of elimination).

Epidemiological evidence also supports the association of increased acetaminophen usage with autism, asthma, and attention deficit with hyperactivity. These marked increases in the United States coincide with the replacement of aspirin by acetaminophen in the 1980s.

Do bear in mind that association does not mean causation. But if you have a model which would explain the findings, then it becomes the current number one hypothesis, as in this case.

The anomalous hair mercury concentrations of children with autism are consistent with exposure of growing hair proteins to NAPQI derived from acetaminophen, which competitively inhibits the reaction of mercury with hair sulfhydryl groups.

This is why people think that mercury is involved. But as I said, kids without any mercury have autism. It's not mercury, it's the build up of any toxins. Heavy metals (don't forget lead causes severe brain damage) are just part of the picture. That's why no statistical correlation is found. It's not the problem, whatever the out-of-date, fact-shy conspiracy theorists want to believe.

Finally, large-scale faulty production of acetaminophen products, such that the labeled values were exceeded by the true concentrations, in addition to contamination with bacteria and unwanted chemicals, may have greatly increased the chances of children receiving overdosages of acetaminophen and potential toxins for perhaps as long as a decade.

High Vaccination Rate Low Incidence Of Autism? Go Figure

One of the puzzling aspects of autism is the marked increase in the incidence of autism that began in the United States in the early 1980s and has appeared to increase continuously since then. The current estimate (November 13, 2015) according to a National Health Interview Survey (NHIS) is 1 in 45. The highest incidence of autism has been reported to be South Korea, where the rate is now reported to be 1 in 38 among boys. It has been definitively proven not to be due to more aggressive diagnosis; it's a real increase.

Yet, the incidence of autism in Cuba is 0.00168% of the population compared with an estimate of as high as 0.50% of the US population. That's over 400 times higher! Yet vaccines are compulsory in Cuba, which has one of the most highly vaccinated populations in the world (99.7%).

So once again, that's the death-knell to the vaccination and mercury theory of autism. It is simply not supportable by any intelligent thinker.

What is highly significant is that, here in the USA doctors routinely advise acetominophen/paracetomol as a prophylactic for the fever that commonly accompanies vaccination, even up to five days beforehand. In fact some kids get their first autistic symptoms before vaccination.

If high fever continues after vaccination in Cuba for more than 2 days, the parents are advised to visit the physician's office where the drug metamizole is most commonly prescribed and NOT acetominophen/paracetomol.

Here's the bottom line from the published article: there is clear evidence that increased acetaminophen use in genetically vulnerable children appears to be a major cause of the epidemics of autism, attention deficit with hyperactivity, and asthma.Mercury does not show up and there is no correlation with mercury levels in children, because it's just one of thousands of toxins which can accumulate. Blood levels don't count: it's how fast the child can remove toxins and with a detox system poisoned by acetominophen/paracetomol, the child is in big trouble.

You can read the full *Journal Of Restorative Medicine* article (which has 83 relevant citations) for more facts. But I'd like to add this. Even after the paper was submitted for publication, yet another study came out, supporting Shaw's research and also making the connection between acetominophen/paracetomol and autism:

Bauer and Kriebel, working at University of Massachusetts- Lowell, reported that prenatal use of acetaminophen was strongly correlated with autism/Autism Spectrum Disorder prevalence, using all available data for the period 1984 to 2005. In addition, the authors found that after acetaminophen became commonly used to treat circumcision pain after 1995, there was a strong correlation between country-level autism/ASD prevalence in males and a country's circumcision rate. A very similar pattern was seen among US states and when comparing the three main racial/ethnic groups in the US.[211]They keep saying the jury is out. Well, it's time the mercury dodos were ousted and replaced by intelligent dispassionate citizens. We need real answers, not pet theories.

We still don't know and whatever our pet theories, nothing conclusive has been settled. I will not pursue the debate further here.

What we do know is that children with autism spectrum disorder (ASD) respond generally very well to the food allergy approach, chemical clean up, heavy metal detox and targeted nutritional supplements. It's not a lost cause; far from it. In fact some children recover so well as to return to normal schooling.

Orthodox Treatment

Not surprisingly, doctors who don't understand the diet and nutrition connection in childhood hyperactivity and disturbed behavior often resort to treating with drugs. It's the last thing these kids need. These are very heavy medications that greatly over-burden the body's systems, especially in a child: amphetamines (Adderall, Vyvanse) or methylphenidates (Concerta, Daytrana, Ritalin). Both classes of drugs are highly addictive stimulants.

Moreover, they don't work as supposed.

The 1994 *Textbook of Psychiatry*, published by the American Psychiatric Press, contains this review (Popper and Steingard): "Stimulants [such as Ritalin] do not produce lasting improvements in aggressivity, conduct disorder, criminality, education achievement, job functioning, marital relationships, or long-term adjustment."

A 1998 review conference convened by the National Institute of Mental Health entitled "NIH Consensus Development Conference on Diagnosis and Treatment of Attention Deficit Hyperactivity Disorder [ADHD]", found that Ritalin has not been shown to have long-term benefits. In fact, the panel stated that Ritalin has resulted in "little improvement on academic achievement or social skills."[212] Yet there is a thirst to prescribe Ritalin and Adderall and the like, as if this were THE definitive treatment and its effectiveness was well-proven in science.

More than a decade after a national US scandal regarding the over-prescription of Ritalin and similar drugs to millions of children diagnosed with attention deficit hyperactivity disorder, or ADHD, the Federal Centers for Disease Control and Prevention now reports a *far higher rate of diagnosis* than a decade ago.

An astounding 19 percent of high school-age boys – ages 14 to 17 – in the U.S. have been diagnosed with ADHD and about 10 percent are taking medication for it. Ten percent of high school-age girls have likewise been diagnosed.[213] There is no valid rationale for these medications, except they are powerful stimulants. You may think it strange that a child who is hyperactive and mentally agitated should benefit even slightly from a strong stimulant. Surely a sedative would be better?

In fact you need to understand this: most hyperactivity/hyperkinetic disorders are because the brain is under-functioning. Once again, let me refer you to the table of Ups and Downs scale of excitement, suppression and addiction (page2.3).[214]

The most extreme outer-end of this range of complaints is a dopy, dysfunctional state which can include narcolepsy (dropping asleep). Knowing this tendency the brain, if you like, shakes and agitates the person back to wakefulness. The movement is to fight falling asleep or narcolepsy state. As one wit of my acquaintance put it, "Nobody can fall asleep while jogging."

Note the side effects of Ritalin and similar drugs, which are:

- Paranoid delusions

- Paranoid psychosis

- Hypomanic and manic symptoms, amphetamine-like psychosis

- Activation of psychotic symptoms

- Toxic psychosis

- Visual hallucinations

- Auditory hallucinations

- Can surpass LSD in producing bizarre experiences

- Effects pathological thought processes

- Extreme withdrawal

- Terrified affect

- Started screaming

- Aggressiveness

- Insomnia

- Since Ritalin is considered an amphetamine-type drug, expect amphetamine-like effects

- Psychic dependence

- High-abuse potential DEA Schedule II Drug

- Decreased REM sleep

- When used with antidepressants one may see dangerous reactions including hypertension, seizures and hypothermia

- Convulsions

- Brain damage may be seen with amphetamine abuse

As I reported in section 1.3, for every symptom on this list there is at least one published scientific paper confirming it.Given that the 1998 NIH conference mentioned above found no real benefit from Ritalin and the like, would you want your child to risk these horrific symptoms?

A Better Idea...

There is simply a better way to turn off this massive brain disorder: to stop the excitation/ depression curve by completely stopping whatever it is that over-stimulates brain tissue, be that foods, chemicals, allergies, stealth pathogens or heavy metal toxicity.

Start with a diet intervention. You can find out more about how to do this in section 5.2, my own book **Diet Wise**, the associated video educational series **Diet Wise Academy**, or if you are still hungry for more: Richard Mackarness *Not All In The Mind* is recommended, Jonathan Brostoff's *The Complete Guide To Food Allergy and Intolerance* , and

Doris Rapp's *Is This Your Child? Discovering and Treating Unrecognized Allergies In Children and Adults.*

You can find these recommendations in the Valuable Resources section at the back of the book.

In my experience, fully 90% or more of children respond extremely well to a proper exclusion diet. The "recovery rate" (no further trouble) can be as high as 100%, as noted by the Great Ormond Street Hospital migraine study of 1983. Subsequent challenge testing, if done conscientiously, will identify the culprit foods. *Note that it is not necessary keep a child on a full exclusion diet indefinitely.* This is only a diagnostic step. The actual trouble will turn out to be a few trigger foods and only those need to be avoided, or substituted, long-term.

If the results are not fully what you hoped, then go on to the second and subsequent stages of my protocols.

Chemical Sensitivity

Food is not the only inflammatory excitant. Chemicals of all kinds can do it too. I have had my child patients made sick by father's after-shave, felt tip pens and perfumes used by the teacher, paints and cleaning fluid used on the school premises. It's very sad when the child is diagnosed as naughty, inattentive or in some way intellectually handicapped, when all that is wrong is that the youngster's brain has been knocked out by chemical inflammation.

See section 5.3 for advice on identifying and treating chemical sensitivities.

Heavy Metal Overload

Our environment is overloaded with poisonous metal substances (mercury, aluminium, arsenic, beryillium, lead, etc.) which, but for our mining and industrial ingenuity, would not naturally be there. We may be clever at the industrial extraction of these substances but little attention is being paid to the toxic potential of the metals we have brought into our world.

The problem is these metallic substances are extremely toxic *and irritant*. Even well below levels which would be considered poisonous, such substances are capable of causing a *highly detrimental inflammatory process* in the human body.

See section 5.11 concerning heavy metal detox.

Neurofeedback

This is very much a frontier program. It is getting great results for children in the ADD/ADHD category.

Basically it's a system for measuring tired or underperforming parts of the brain and then waking them up! The initial testing, using what is known as the 10/20 system, identifies parts of the brain that could be performing better. The child is then asked to play a computer interactive game in which he or she is made to move objects, float them, set fire to them or in other ways interact with the software simulation.

The wiring up is arranged in such a way that the parts of the brain which needed activating are the ones which produce the positive result in the computer sim. Without knowing or worrying about what part, the child has only to follow instructions and make the right changes and, by arrangement, that part of the brain which needs activating has come to life.

After a few weeks of training, the picture has considerably changed. Remember, I said that amphetamine and methylphenidates work by stimulation of quiescent parts of the brain. Neurofeedback does the same thing—but without any of the worrying side-effects.

The child no longer has to jiggle, twitch, fidget and move around, just to stay awake!

Other Nutrient Factors

Vitamins and minerals can also play their parts. Children deficient in zinc, for example, tend to experience more behavioral disorders and these can extend into their adult lives.

According to nutritionist Melvyn R. Werbach, M.D, writing for Orthomolecular News, "aggressive behavioral syndrome" is marked by restlessness, irritability, impulsivity and a proneness to violence. Diagnostically, it overlaps the DSM III-R diagnoses of Attention-deficit Hyperactivity Disorder, Conduct Disorder, Oppositional Defiant Disorder and Antisocial Personality Disorder.

The importance of psychological factors (upbringing, life experiences, etc.) is well known. By contrast, the contribution of nutritional factors to such behaviors is often unrecognized, and therefore not properly addressed.

Nutritional factors are neglected for a number of reasons:

1. It's a new specialty and much of the literature on nutritional treatments has yet to evolve beyond the early stages of scientific investigation

2. Physicians learn so little about nutritional medicine during their training that they feel too uninformed to include it in their practices

3. Sub-optimal nutrition is generally believed to be rare in industrialized societies - even though up to 50% of the population may fail to ingest the Recommended Dietary Allowance for one or more vitamins or minerals.

4. Nutritional factors are neglected, in part, because marginal nutritional deficiencies are not believed to affect behavior despite growing evidence to suggest that that belief may be false.

Deficiencies of several vitamins are known to be associated with irritability and aggression. These include niacin (B3), pantothenic acid (B5), thiamine (B1), vitamin B6 and vitamin C.

The scale of the problem is not really known. Moreover, as Werbach says, under laboratory conditions, adverse behavioral changes precede any measurable vitamin deficiencies, which will make the process of recognizing and establishing a link between the two very difficult.

While few clinical studies have been published to prove a relationship between the aggressive behavioral syndrome in humans and nutritional inadequacy, Lonsdale and Shamberger, writing in *The American Journal of Clinical Nutrition*, reported on twenty people eating "junk food" diets who were found to have biochemical evidence of marginal thiamine deficiency. Their subjects, and particularly the adolescents, were impulsive, highly irritable, aggressive and sensitive to criticism.[215]

Following thiamine supplementation, their behavior improved concurrent with laboratory evidence of improved thiamine status, suggesting that marginal thiamine deficiency may have contributed to their aggressive behavioral syndrome. You can find a helpful link to the rest of this article in the Valuable Resources section at the back!

Genetic Testing

Finally, one cannot leave the subject of childhood brain dysfunction without some discussion of genetic testing and what it has to offer.

As I hinted above, there a many instances of brain dysfunction which are caused by subtle (or complex) disorders of normal cell metabolism, such as phenylketonuria. But there are many less obvious examples of metabolic dysfunction, which will only come to light with careful and extensive genetic testing for unfavorable variants.

In a 2013 paper (published January 2014), genetics researchers identified 25 missing or duplicated stretches of DNA that are found occur in some patients with autism. These variants, say the researchers, are "high impact"; although individually rare, each has a strong effect in raising an individual's risk for autism.[216]

These may emerge as predictive markers, meaning they can be tested for and may become part of a clinical test that will help evaluate whether a child has an autism spectrum disorder.Surprisingly (or perhaps not) research is beginning to uncover evidence for clinical and biological links between autism/Pervasive Developmental Disorder (PDD) and schizophrenia, with particular attention to childhood onset schizophrenia.

You might consider getting a limited genome test (laboratories do not try to cover ALL possible alternatives). After all, our gene structure does not change throughout life, though we are certainly able to alter the *expression* of those genes.

2.7 Alcoholism and Addictions

Alcohol and drug addictions probably kill more people than any other psychiatric disorder. It takes an enormous toll.

In the USA alone, alcoholism related deaths accounted for approximately 88,000 deaths per year from 2006–2010, and accounted for 1 in 10 deaths among working-age adults aged 20–64 years. This figure usually includes motor accidents due to drivers being intoxicated.

More than 64,000 died from drug overdoses in 2016, including illicit drugs and prescription opioids—nearly doubled in a decade. Source: CDC.

Just in ballpark figures, that's 150,000 deaths per year. Compare that to suicides: In all, 42,773 people died from suicide in 2014, compared with 29,199 in 1999.

Since the 1970s, neuroscientists have been asserting that dopamine plays an essential role in the brain's processing of rewarding experiences. Dopamine was, as the thinking went, the "pleasure neurotransmitter"—the substance responsible for producing sensations of pleasure in the brain, regardless of whether that pleasure comes from enjoying a good meal, having sex, or snorting cocaine. This understanding, according to a 1997 article in *Time* magazine, made the answers to questions about what causes addiction, "simpler than anyone has dared imagine." The article goes on to claim that dopamine "is not just a chemical that transmits pleasure signals but may, in fact, be the master molecule of addiction."[217]

This simplistic view is nonsense, in fact. Although it should be said that there is a great deal of evidence that indicates dopamine release is correlated with pleasure, there is also substantial evidence that suggests dopamine isn't responsible for *creating* the feeling of pleasure.

Important note: Let me clear up an important point. People think that drugs "do" things to your brain and that feels nice. Some even argue the fact that, because drugs mess with the brain and that changes how you feel, then it PROVES that the brain is where our thoughts lie.

These positions are not correct. Let me set you straight: Drugs, including "safe" recreational drugs like marijuana and alcohol, are actually poisons. They knock out brain cells, by disturbing their smooth metabolic functioning. The nice feeling (or thrilling experience) you get is just BEING YOU. With the motorized, electronic brain humming away, you get stuck with the physical paradigm. But when the brain is rendered less capable, then the real YOU emerges and it feels wonderful, to be a creative free spirit.

I liken it to living in a cupboard or closet, dark and closed in. Then one day someone leads you out into the fresh air. It feels light, wide open and free. That's the feeling of unfettered spirit. You "unhook from the brain" and become, for a short time, exterior to the physical universe.

So the artificial situation is without drugs. You take hash, coke, LSD or whatever and escape into the wild psychic yonder!

NOT RECOMMENDED, by the way. There are better ways to do this. I am simply countering the oft-heard argument that, since drugs alter brain function, that proves we are just a brain.

This section covers the last of my "Suffering Seven". Let's start with alcoholism and I'll kick you off with something startling, fascinating and almost totally unknown anywhere else in the world…

Most alcoholics are not addicted to alcohol, they are actually addicted to a foodstuff. The alcohol is just a jet-propelled "fix". Take whisky: it's made of grains, typically barley or wheat. A whisky addict is probably hooked on the wheat. How do I know?

Administer a shot of pure alcohol (ethanol) to an alcoholic with severe withdrawal symptoms (*delerium tremens* or the DTs) and nothing happens! The cravings continue unabated. But administer a subcutaneous shot of wheat extract and the patient calms down, the symptoms lessen or vanish, the desire for a tipple vanishes!

I tested and proved this for myself so often in my facility that I am in no doubt about this hidden truth. It makes all the difference to beating alcohol addiction. If you don't simultaneously ban wheat from the diet, the patient is most unlikely to ever break his or her dependence on whisky.

If you have a problem with drink therefore, I recommend you embark on a full exclusion diet, as part of going on the wagon (see section 5.2). You'll find more success if you do—fewer cravings and an easier withdrawal phase.

Let's dive into the whole subject of addiction. We'll look at alcohol first but a whole host of lessons can be learned which apply to other addictions too…

Sunshine In A Bottle

That's what the Italians call it. Ethyl alcohol (ethanol) is consumed in vast quantities all over the world, indicating just how pleasurable most people find mild degrees of intoxication. There is little doubt that a meal without wine or beer doesn't have the same warm glow that is so important to easing social tensions. The problem comes when this goes too far; excessive intake impairs your health.

Short-term side effects of drinking, such as hangover, are said to depend on 'impurities', particularly the presence of other alcohols such as butyl and isoamyl alcohol, which are known as congeners. Brandy contains the highest percentage of congeners and this gives it its rich aromatic smell – enhanced by gently warming, which increases vaporization of these secondary alcohols.

Doctors like me gradually uncovered the fact that allergic reactions to foodstuffs contained in intoxicating drinks such as yeast, wheat, corn, sugar and other ingredients are also a major cause of the negative after-effects of drinking.

The great doyen of clinical ecology, Theron Randolph, likened alcoholic beverages to 'jet propelled food allergy' and it's valuable to remember that phrase. Food allergics seem to suffer far worse reactions to drink than the rest of the population; indeed, for years I have regarded this as a fast rule-of-thumb criterion for food allergy. Wheat, for example, may be tolerated in some forms by a wheat-allergic, but when a small tot of whisky is drunk, it can put the patient in bed!

All alcoholic beverages contain yeast by definition. Also, there are many potential 'additives' you'd rather not hear about, including sulphites and other antiseptics, "letting down" agents in wine such as ethylene glycol (anti-freeze), asbestos, clay, seaweed, polyvinylpyrrolidine, citric acid, tannic acid, fumaric acid, sorbates, arsenic and monosodium glutamate. This doesn't mean all drinks include these substances, of course; simply that they may.

The real trouble seems to come from the foodstuffs themselves. For that reason I have reproduced Theron Randolph's important table of ingredients for most of the common alcoholic beverages. Remember, this is only a guide; individual products vary greatly. This is meant to help you to know what to look for.

The foodstuff is the key to making alcoholic drinks. Brewer's yeast (*Saccharomyces cerevisiae* or *S. uvarum*), needs sugars or starch to ferment. Thus high sugar-content foods, such as grapes, other fruits, honey and sugars are chosen for fermentation; or very starchy foods, which will easily turn to sugars that can be fermented (wheat, corn, barley, rice, potato, etc.)

Distilled spirits contain far higher levels of alcohol but still retain sufficient of the characteristic food to impart flavor and, of course, will also transfer any food allergy reaction.

● Always present
○ Sometimes present

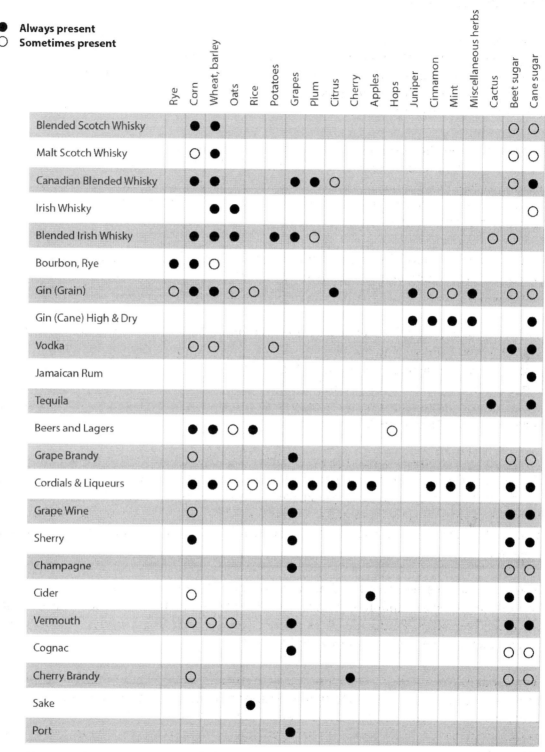

	Rye	Corn	Wheat, barley	Oats	Rice	Potatoes	Grapes	Plum	Citrus	Cherry	Apples	Hops	Juniper	Cinnamon	Mint	Miscellaneous herbs	Cactus	Beet sugar	Cane sugar
Blended Scotch Whisky		●	●															○	○
Malt Scotch Whisky		○	●															○	○
Canadian Blended Whisky		●	●				●	●	○									○	●
Irish Whisky			●	●															○
Blended Irish Whisky		●	●	●			●	●	○								○	○	
Bourbon, Rye	●	●	○																
Gin (Grain)	○	●	●	○	○						●		●	○	○	●		○	○
Gin (Cane) High & Dry													●	●	●	●			●
Vodka		○	○			○												●	●
Jamaican Rum																			●
Tequila																	●		●
Beers and Lagers		●	●	○	●							○							
Grape Brandy		○					●											○	○
Cordials & Liqueurs		●	●	○	○	○	●	●	●	●	●			●	●	●		●	●
Grape Wine		○					●											●	●
Sherry		●					●											●	●
Champagne							●											○	○
Cider		○									●							●	●
Vermouth		○	○	○			●											●	●
Cognac							●											○	○
Cherry Brandy		○								●								○	○
Sake					●														
Port							●												

Please note that yeast occurs in all alcoholic beverages

Certain general observations will also help you make the right choice. Beers and stouts are the worst tolerated of all. Dry cider and dry white wine (including champagne), without contaminants, are the best tolerated. Red wine is usually disastrous since it may contain large amounts of histamine. Spirits are surprisingly well taken, considering their strength, but people vary.

The virtual "definition" of an alcoholic is someone drinking half to a full bottle of spirits, per day. That's a very heavy addiction.

Alcohol and Sexual Misbehavior

Over the years I had a number of interesting cases where a food allergy reaction provoked unseemly behavior in a patient; women in particular. One woman behaved very inappropriately in a coffee challenge test; for another it was ice cream.

These were older ladies and could look after themselves in the main. But I am concerned for teenage girls and younger women: this effect needs to be more widely known. One lass clearly reacted badly to vodka and orange. She got drunk quickly, got up on the table and started taking her clothes off, on more than one occasion. Surprisingly, it wasn't the vodka that made her tipsy; it was an allergy to the orange! See, food allergy has the same excitatory then suppressor effect on the brain as alcohol does—both are poisons. At first it shuts down the inhibitory center, which is why people get frisky and misbehave. Then as the poisoning gets worse the whole brain shuts down and lying under the table fast asleep is a common ending!

In another case it was definitely the vodka. The young patient was smart and suspected as much; vodka tended to make her lewd and suggestive. So in 1987 I carried out a double-blind experiment and filmed the results. Sadly I have lost the recording of that day or, more exactly, my first wife wiped the tape, but the shoot was certainly memorable.

I gave the patient 10 microshots: 6 were saline blanks and four were as follows: whisky (barley malt), gin (wheat and juniper), vodka (corn) and brandy (grape), all randomly mixed and without visual clues (blind). With camera running, we recorded her reactions. On the fourth injection, she became very giggly and claimed she was going to whip the trousers off the cameraman. Another of the shots made her very depressed. And one made her talkative and cheerful, but without being suggestive or aroused.

When we broke the code, sure enough: the fourth shot was the vodka. She was right. I warned her off it, of course. The one that made her depressed was gin and I warned her off that too. Whisky was the best drink for her (if she wanted spirits).

Looking back there was an ethical issue here, which I overlooked in my enthusiastic research. Moreover there was a negative outcome. With her permission we released the findings to the press, as a dire warning to other young women, to figure out the foodstuffs in their alcoholic drinks. But for years afterwards fools and miscreants would try spiking her drinks with vodka. The man she eventually married was very angry with me and I don't blame him.

Now—to understand the link between food allergy and addiction, we need to bring in another fascinating and little-known piece of science theory...

Hans Selye's General Adaptation Syndrome

Hans Selye's hypothesis of stress adaptation is one of the most important learnings in all of health. It's on a par with the need for exercize, hygiene, whole foods and vitamins. Here is the *whole secret of addictions and withdrawal symptoms*. The fact that so much experience matches the theory suggests that it is 'true'. It's just that very few people know about it and even fewer have figured out the important applications. So listen up now...

Briefly, stage one is the first encounter with the "insult" (challenge), when the body reacts and alarm signals herald the onset of some adversity (a stressor). These signals we know as symptoms; some unpleasant response that entails a desire to limit the exposure by escaping from whatever is causing the symptoms.

Avoidance brings the reaction to an end and the symptoms go away. But if the individual does not desist and instead keeps on, eventually he or she might learn to tolerate the stressor and find it doesn't worry him or her too much. For example, someone moving to a much hotter climate might feel very unwell at first, but with persistence learns to tolerate heat at a level that would have been dangerous to him or her on first arrival. We call this adaptation process stage two.

It might be possible to go on coping with a stressor to which we are adapted for a long time, perhaps indefinitely. But usually the adaptation eventually runs out and the stressor begins to produce symptoms once again. This is stage three.

But this time, the consequences are more serious. The individual concerned no longer has any powers of resistance. His or her body has run out of fight and the stress can become overwhelming. This is the stuff of coronary heart disease, perforated ulcers, cancer and strokes. When the effect is less threatening to life, increased allergies can certainly be a possible outcome. If stage two is 'adaptation', this stage could be termed maladaptation.

A good example, illustrating the theme of addiction, would be tobacco. Those who smoke will doubtless remember that their first attempt was accompanied by unpleasant consequences: headache, dizziness and nausea are not uncommon (stage one). But by persisting, the would-be smoker gets used to tobacco and the symptoms are no longer experienced; he or she is adapted (stage two). Finally, as the addiction takes hold, the individual will find that unpleasant symptoms come on with a vengeance when going too long without a 'fix' for the nicotine craving. This is stage three and one of the hardest of all addictions to break.

Alcohol Addiction

Now you understand more of the underlying mechanisms of alcohol dependence, you may be ready to answer the big question: are you an alcoholic?

It is generally agreed that at least one of the following symptoms are necessary for such a diagnosis:

- Drink alcohol four or more times a week
- Have five or more drinks containing alcohol in one day
- Not be able to stop drinking once you've started
- Need a drink early in the morning to get yourself going
- Feel guilty or remorseful after drinking
- You are secretive and hide your drinking levels from others
- Heard a relative, friend, co-worker, or doctor express concern about your drinking or suggest you cut down

Excessive drinking can lead to addiction and delay the desire to seek treatment and interfere with the effectiveness of therapy or medication once on a treatment plan.

Other Addictions

There is little to add to the science of addictions; Hans Selye has covered all the bases. Be it tobacco, heroin, crack, alcohol, spray cans, uppers, downers, or medicinal drugs, the same essential phase three mechanism is at work. Going too long without the next dose will set up unpleasant withdrawal symptoms which depending on severity may be very difficult to endure.

Here are some tips to help you break the addiction:

Avoiding "innocent" addictions, while battling bad ones, will often help. Give up tea, coffee and sugar at the same time as avoidance of your addictive substance. Caffeine dependence might seem a very small problem but it does seem to "prime the system", so to speak and makes other withdrawal symptoms appear worse.

You might like to go on a strict exclusion diet, as I suggested above, as part of a generalized avoidance regimen. The extra discipline can help. In any case, choose only organic wholefoods, uncontaminated with pesticides, drink unchlorinated, unfluoridated water; preferably filtered by reverse osmosis, followed by an activated carbon filter.

You would also do well to avoid any kind of chemical stimulant. Be on the alert for perfumes, paints, cleaners, solvents, sprays (including dreaded "air fresheners"), deodorants and other cosmetic scents. The Scott-Mumby general rule is: if there is sufficient to cause a scent or odor, there is enough to trigger symptoms.

You need a good nutritional program. My advice is to get started days ahead of the beginning of abstinence. Addictions are extremely stressful.

Addressing The Past

When in med school, I remember the senior lecturer in pharmacology stepping onto the rostrum and saying, no hesitation, no ifs and buts: "In all cases of alcoholism there is an underlying psychosis." It was a bit of a whack on the jawbone.

I've never forgotten that moment, though it was over 50 years ago and even though I don't entirely agree with what he said. But I hold it to be true that in every case of alcoholism or addiction, there is some underlying emotional pain which, if addressed and eliminated, would make the addiction substance unnecessary.

To that end I would call your attention to the brief description of Punk Psychology® which appears in section 3.12. It's the simplest, fastest, easiest to understand and most effective way of cleaning up pain and emotional charges from the past.

To ignore this major element in the onset of addiction is to set yourself up for a fail.

Dosing on drugs or alcohol soon ceases to be a pleasure and remains only as a means of shutting out the unwanted misery. If there is no buried misery, or it has been defused and scrubbed, you'll find getting rid of the addictive substance much easier. It's only logical, as you can see.

2.8 Crime, Violence and Delinquency

The Appleton School Experiment

Appleton Central High School in Wisconsin, was once a dangerous place to learn. A police officer was on permanent duty, to try to forestall violence and even gun crimes. Then a remarkable dietary experiment took place, which should be known and copied by schools worldwide (but isn't).

The soda-filled vending machines at the school were replaced with new ones offering only juice, water and energy drinks. Natural Ovens and Bakery, a local company, took over the cafeteria and offered fresh fruit and vegetables, whole grain breads and entrees free of additives and chemicals, instead of pizza and fries.

As a result, the poor discipline statistics plummeted. The principal LuAnn Coenen reported that, since the new regimen was implemented, there were zero weapons on campus, zero expulsions from the school, zero premature deaths or suicides and zero drugs or alcohol on campus.

With the departure of junk food, she also saw the departure of vandalism, litter and the need for police patrolling her hallways.

In classrooms, teachers suddenly felt like they were getting through. Students were on task, they were attentive, they began to concentrate for longer periods of time.

Not surprisingly, grades went up too. Appleton Central High School was no longer "bottom of the class"!

It had transformed from a dangerously violent, frenetic and essentially dysfunctional institution into a calm, emotionally positive and productive learning environment.

This is a very stern lesson. Bad diet has a high mortality rate: *junk food can send people crazy, turn them violent and people get killed*. Fact.

Food Allergy Can Also Lead To Violence

For many years, around Thanksgiving and Christmas time, I would remind (warn) my readers that there is a huge spike in murders at these festival times. Cynics could argue it goes back to the first ever Thanksgiving, which was to celebrate the safe return of the Massachusetts militia from slaughtering 700 innocent Pequot Indians.

While certainly, as one wit put it, there is too much DNA in the room at such family gatherings, it is also a time when we all classically over-eat and over-drink. You will find abundant evidence throughout this section, and the rest of the book, that excess of poorly tolerated or inflammatory foods can cause severe psychological disturbance, including rage, violence and murder.

I Make Medico-Legal World History

In 1986 I became the center of world media attention for a series of patients who had made their way through my practice facility. There was May (not her real name), who repeatedly attacked her husband with knives. Fortunately no murder or mutilation was committed. We traced that to a brain allergy (section 4.7).

Then came a teenage lad Jason, who would attack his teachers and was strong enough to really hurt them or possibly do lasting harm. There was concern and he came to me. I found he had a wheat allergy (not gluten, wheat allergy) and that made him violent. He was in the habit of eating half a loaf per day (6 – 8 slices). When made to desist, he calmed down and became a sociable, likeable lad.

As a result of that story in the press, I was asked to evaluate another youth. He had attempted to strangle his step-father and had been charged with attempted murder (afterwards commuted to a lesser charge). Judge Peter Gibson, from the Ballymena Crown Court in Northern Ireland referred the case to me, to see whether food allergy might be making Tony violent.

Indeed, that was the case. Beef, strawberries and onion played their part. But his outstanding reaction was to potato. It made him extremely unstable and aggressive. His threatening manner when given a tiny shot of potato allergen really frightened my nurses, who were pretty hardened, I have to say.

As a result of the emerging fascination, Channel 4 News came to my clinic and spent a half day shooting footage, including a re-staging of Tony's potato test. The program was duly televized. Yet again Tony became wildly aggressive, sweating, shaking, clenching his fists and making violent threats—this time seen by the whole nation (with permission, of course).

The story had a happy ending. Tony pleaded guilty to the lesser charge; Judge Gibson gave him a conditional discharge; and the condition was that he stick to the Scott-Mumby diet! A kindly and intelligent judge saved the lad from jail time, by asking the right questions of the right person.

So I made medico-legal history. For the first time, anywhere in the world, a court accepted evidence that food allergy could drive a person to uncontrolled violence and even attempted murder.

As a result of the Irish "Potato Boy" story in 1986, I was quoted (Channel 4 News) as saying I could empty out half the prisons of the world, if I could only control the diets fed to inmates. It received a lot of comment.

Later a (Yorkshire cop) got on the bandwagon, with the same message, but has never seen fit to mention me, as the chief early pioneer in this field.

The Science Of Criminality

Centuries of research, aimed at reducing the incidence of criminal violence has largely failed. Literally hundreds of psychoanalytic techniques, behavior modification systems, and experimental drug therapies have been attempted, and none has proven to be effective. The sad truth is that most violent criminals become recidivists, whether they participate in rehabilitation programs or not.

The lack of progress in combating crime and violence has resulted from several factors. First and foremost, there is no clear understanding of the basic causes of violence and antisocial behavior. Criminologists still debate whether the predominant cause is psychological, sociological, biological, or something else. Another barrier to progress is the fact that criminal violence is not a single condition, but rather a diverse set of afflictions. The inadequacy of classification methods for separating criminals into appropriate groups has hindered progress for over a century.

A Scandinavian study utilizing adoption records focusing on cases in which a biological parent or adoptive parent evidenced criminality. Their evaluation showed a strong relationship between criminality of biological parents and their sons.[218]

Another adoption study found that sons whose biological parents had a criminal record were four times as likely to have a serious criminal record, compared with those without familial criminality. This effect far exceeded the effects of environmental factors studied including adoptive parent criminality, child abuse, and poverty.[219]

Now the Health Research Institute has observed distinctive chemical imbalances in violent subjects and has developed the classification system, based on hair chemistry as shown in the accompanying table.[220]

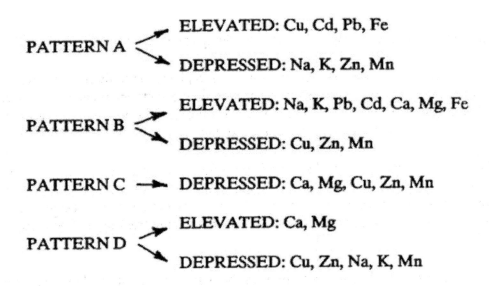

Patterns Of Chemical Imbalances Observed in Criminals

The Type A and B patterns were discovered in a sibling experiment involving 24 pairs of brothers, ranging in age from 8 to 18 years. Each of the sibling pairs included an extremely delinquent, violent brother and a brother who was well-behaved, with no history of behavioral or academic problems. The violent siblings were found to possess the Type A or Type B imbalances whereas the sociable controls did not.

Subsequent testing of general delinquent populations revealed that C and D type hair-chemistry patterns are common to persons exhibiting low-to-intermediate aggressiveness.

Two recent double-blind experiments in California (with 90 and 198 subjects, respectively) have confirmed the high incidence of the A/B/C/D patterns in criminal populations and their low incidence in the general population. These distinctive patterns have been found in violent subjects of all races, age groups, and socioeconomic levels. Studies of mass murderers and serial killers (including Charles Manson, Henry Lee Lucas, James Huberty, and Patrick Sherrill) have revealed intense A or B patterns to be present in most cases.

Clinical studies of violent persons exhibiting the A/B/C/D hair-chemistry patterns have been performed by Carl C. Pfeiffer, MD, PhD, and others at the Brain Bio Center in Princeton, New Jersey and elsewhere.[221]

You can read more about Pfeiffer's work in section 5.7.

Treatments

The important question in this respect is: did nutritional corrections show any benefit?

Approximately 200 Type A, B, C, or D subjects have been placed on individualized treatment programs designed by Carl Pfeiffer, to correct the specific chemical imbalances observed. This needed care: the optimum treatment for a Type A person, for example, would probably worsen the condition of a Type B person.

Confidential surveys of parents, teachers, and counselors show that more than 75 percent of the treated subjects report a "significant improvement," with best results obtained with children. Since this information is anecdotal, these treatments must be regarded as unproven until double-blind, controlled experiments measuring treatment effectiveness is done.

The "nature vs. nurture" debate still continues in the field of criminology. However, the evidence is mounting that both factors are important ingredients in forming criminal personality. The principal cause of violent crime appears to be a biochemical predisposition triggered by environmental stress. The eventual solution to this critical societal problem may lie in the fields of biochemistry and nutrition.

Omega-3s and Jail Time

It's not just about vitamins and minerals. Defective levels of essential fatty acids also show up often as a factor in relation to crime. A 2014 study, for example, showed marked benefits from supplementing omega-3 fatty acids, something we know protects the brain for neurological damage due to free radicals and excitotoxins.

The results showed a generalized reduced anxiety, improved mood and better emotional stability in criminal inpatients after a long-term intervention with Atlantic salmon oil, providing vitamin D, eicosapentaenoic acid (EPA) and docosahexaenoic acid (DHA)

In the usual manner, 95 male forensic inpatients were randomly assigned into a winter fish group (Atlantic salmon three times per week from September to February) or to a control group (no fish, just chicken, pork, or beef three times per week during the same period).

Heart rate variability (a measure of calm or stress) and self-reported improvements were assessed before the trial and at the end of the 23 weeks dietary intervention period. The Fish group showed significant improvements, including a decrease in anxiety-state.[222]

Diet And Prison

If hospital diets are an unhealthy joke, prison diets are a dangerous departure from common sense.

Thing is, you only have to turn on the nightly news to see that serious crime is on the upswing. It's tempting to suppose it's mostly drug-related violence and rival gang shootouts. But is it?

According to Orthomolecular News (April 30, 2016), we are witnessing an increasing number of random murders. What motive could there be for a young adult, with or without a police record, to suddenly go berserk and commit multiple murders? Many perpetrators are found to have psychiatric problems, sometimes, ironically, fueled by treatment with psychotropic drugs coupled with alcohol. Certainly, it's not as simple as easy access to guns and lack of economic opportunity.

There is always a search for motive in a murder case. In urban areas like Chicago, the popular thinking is that the motive is either derived from gang warfare, a sense of hopelessness, or partially generated by bad cops. In earlier Chicago days, mobsters' clear-cut motivation was money acquisition and the power it generated. That's why Willie Sutton robbed banks.

But is that the real story?

"I am absolutely convinced that there is a direct link between diet and antisocial behaviour, both that bad diet causes bad behaviour and that good diet prevents it." - Lord Ramsbotham, Her Majesty's Chief Inspector of Prisons.[223]

Knowing what we know about certain vitamin deficiencies and their relationship to mental disease, while considering how substandard the typical American diet is, one can't help considering this association. B12 deficiency, as a cause of dementia, has been accepted in the medical literature for many decades.[224] [225]

Dr. Abram Hoffer, the psychiatrist who also had a degree in biochemistry, made the brilliant connection of niacin and schizophrenia. Niacin treatment not only worked, but he provided a plausible explanation of how it worked.

[see section5.7]

"The UK prison trial at Aylesbury jail showed that when young men there were fed multivitamins, minerals and essential fatty acids, the number of violent offences they committed in the prison fell by 35%."[226]

Attempts to explain mental problems by levels of serotonin, dopamine or norepinephrine, individually, is no explanation at all, since neurotransmitters work in balance with each other. None are metabolized properly if their B-vitamin cofactors are deficient. Corrective measures may ensue from larger doses of these B-vitamins. By co-factors I mean zinc, magnesium and other minerals which make vitamins work.[227]

Pyridoxine has the widest range of individual variation—certainly much more of it is required than the pitifully low RDA, a minimal standard even of which many Americans don't achieve. Wheat germ and wheat bran are food sources rich in pyridoxine. A donut just doesn't cut it.

Speaking of donuts, how many of us have witnessed a sudden outburst of anger, and even violent behavior, in an individual under the influence of low blood sugar? Hypoglycemia results from a previous huge load of high fructose corn syrup or other sugars, and/or in conjunction with too much alcohol. (see section 5.8)

"Those who received the extra nutrients committed significantly fewer offences compared with placebo... the Dutch Ministry of Justice (in) their double-blind study reported a 48% difference."[228]

We need to measure the blood levels of vitamins in criminal perpetrators. We also need to provide nutrition supplements with customized recommended treatment doses. Every prison should have an orthomolecular physician. Studies have already been conducted on violent crime perpetrators. We already know enough to bring great improvements.

A straight lift from Orthomolecular Medicine News Service, by Ralph Campbell, MD, April 30th, 2016.

For more information on this fascinating topic, see the **Valuable Resources** section.

PART 3
EVERYMAN PSYCHOLOGY

Ok, we've had an emotional introduction to the problems we have with incompetent and criminal psychiatrists. Hopefully enough to prevent you ever consulting with one, or taking any member of your family to be drugged to oblivion!

But let's not commit the absurd folly of saying the person could not possibly be suffering from genuine psychological distress factors. That too needs to be excluded or corrected if necessary, even while searching for probable physical causes.

Stress is universal in human life and a poor response to it is not always optimum.

We are all, to a degree, living stressful lives. Some of us are more easily able to cope than others. Each and every individual has a different ability to handle excess stress but if you can sidestep it or artificially reduce it then you will be a much happier person. Also you will gain massive confidence in your ability to handle problems.

This part contains some exceptional understandings of the functioning human mind and powerful methods to get it under control, instead of letting it run wild.

3.1 Is Grieving An Illness?

Psychiatrists and family doctors jump to say yes, to offer "anti-depressants" which will close down your feelings but will not solve the grieving.

In 2012, for the first time, the American Psychiatric Association reference guide to mental disease, the DSM (Diagnostic and Statistical Manual of Mental Disorders) included the concept of "bereavement". What does this mean? That feelings or outbursts accompanying the passing of a family member or close friend—such as crying, insomnia, fatigue, confusion and profound sadness—may now be viewed as a treatable illness rather than as a normal reaction to life's most shattering moments?

Big Pharma, via their cronies in the APA, is hoping to make this one stick, so they can sell more drugs.

Needless to say, not everyone agrees with this shift in thinking. Some say the grieving process should not be interrupted; it's natural and healthy.

"To me, grief is a normal condition, not to be tagged with a diagnostic code and to be treated," stressed Dr. T. Byram Karasu, chairman of psychiatry and behavioral sciences at Albert Einstein College of Medicine and psychiatrist-in-chief at Montefiore Medical Center in New York City. "Everyone loses someone in their lives at some point. So, this would be classifying everyone at some point. No one would be immune to this."

"And that does not make sense, because grief is a normal and very healthy behavior," said Karasu, who also chairs the APA's National Task Force on the treatment of depression. "One has to feel joy as well as pain and depression, otherwise life is not worth living. And one should not interrupt the grieving by medication or psychotherapy. You have to feel the loss, and only by feeling the loss and recovering from it will the person become a better person. Interrupted grief will remain unfinished business."[229]

Karasu's stance is in line with those expressed by the editorial board of the British medical journal *The Lancet*, which lays out its opposition to the new clinical approach in its Feb. 18, 2012, issue.

"Grief is not an illness," the journal's editors argue, noting that a diagnostic change in the APA's forthcoming manual would empower clinicians to interpret any post-loss despair that endures beyond a two-week window as a troubling sign of sickness rather than a standard sign of coping.

The Lancet team suggests that, instead, an intense but normal bout of grief can last six months to a year, depending on the very individualized nature of the particular relationship that has been severed by death.

"Medicalizing grief, so that treatment is legitimized routinely with antidepressants, for example, is not only dangerously simplistic, but also flawed," the authors noted.

Let's look further at stress, not as a disease process but as something we are all subject to from time to time.

Here I would like to share my own rather clever definition of stress, it's enormously useful: *stress is the difference between what you've got and what you wanted!*

Thank about that for a moment. If you wanted riches and you are broke, that's a life of misery. But if you never cared for money and would rather work in the service of others, then you will not find your circumstances stressful due to shortage of money.

Stressors vary enormously, of course. Over the years I have regarded relationships, difficulties at work, financial crashes, viral illnesses, exams, lack of sleep, bullying and peer pressure all as possible sources of stress and strife.

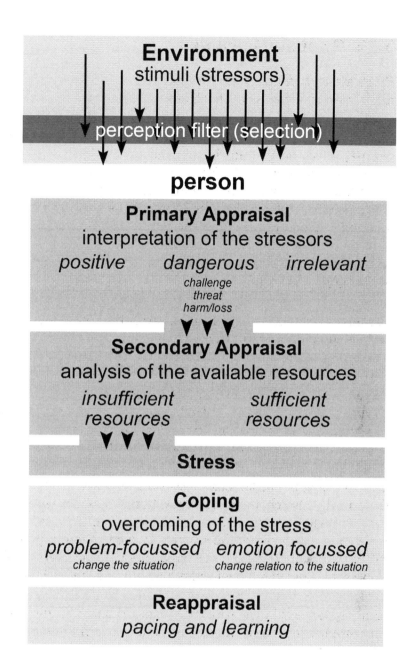

In theory, once the stressor is removed, our bodies return to a neutral state. This perfect biological system is interrupted when we experience stressful life events that then become chronic stress. A state of heightened, chronic stress can lead to an increased risk of illness, many of which can be very serious. This correlation has been verified time and again in the research.

3.2 Objective Measure

Unfortunately, there is no real objective test for stress. Stress means different things to different people and what may be stressful one person can seem like excitement and adventure to another. But that is not to say some estimation cannot be made. For example, Holmes and Rahe's "Social Readjustment Rating Scale (SRRS)" is a workable attempt to quantify stress objectively.

In 1967 Thomas Holmes and Richard Rahe combed through the medical records of over 5,000 patients to see if there was a connection between illness and the most stressful life events. They found a remarkably strong correlation and were able to rank stressful situations in the form of a "life events scale", predicting how likely is was that a person would fall ill subsequently.

Rahe tested the reliability of the stress scale again in 1970. He assessed 2,500 U.S. military members (sailors) and asked them to rank their most stressful life events. He then followed these sailors for six months, tracking their visits to the dispensary, to see if there was a correlation between their reported "life stress" and their visits to the doctor. The study once again proved the reliability of the scale. There was the exact same positive correlation between reported stress and illness as found in the original examination of medical records: the more stressful the event, the higher likelihood of illness.

Moreover, this result held true cross-culturally (looking at Japan and Malaysia in addition to the United States). It's also true among different groups within the United States (African, Hispanic, and White Americans).

The results were tested again in 1997.

So one of the first things we can do in fixing mental health problems without toxic drugs is to estimate just how much stress the individual has been subjected to. You can plot this scale on yourself, if you wish to.

The actual hit list has changed only slightly over the years. Here are the top forty social stressors, with the scores assigned to them.

Each event is assigned a "Life Change Unit" score. These are then added together over a year and used to predict illness. For adults, the most stressful life events and their "Life Change Unit" scores are as follows:

Life event	Life change units
Death of a spouse	100
Divorce	73
Marital separation	65
Imprisonment	63
Death of a close family member	63
Personal injury or illness	53
Marriage	50
Dismissal from work	47
Marital reconciliation	45
Retirement	45
Change in health of family member	44
Pregnancy	40
Sexual difficulties	39
Gain a new family member	39
Business readjustment	39
Change in financial state	38
Death of a close friend	37
Change to different line of work	36
Change in frequency of arguments	35
Major mortgage	32
Foreclosure of mortgage or loan	30
Change in responsibilities at work	29
Child leaving home	29
Trouble with in-laws	29
Outstanding personal achievement	28
Spouse starts or stops work	26
Beginning or end school	26
Change in living conditions	25
Revision of personal habits	24
Trouble with boss	23
Change in working hours or conditions	20
Change in residence	20
Change in schools	20
Change in recreation	19
Change in church activities	19
Change in social activities	18
Minor mortgage or loan	17
Change in sleeping habits	16
Change in number of family reunions	15
Change in eating habits	15

A score of 300 or higher puts a person at risk of illness. 150-299 shows a moderate risk of illness and a score of less than 150 predicts only a slight risk of illness.

CzernySmith Assessments also do a good online assessment service. For a modest fee you have a detailed report, or for slightly more ($200) you can have a report and some professional coaching on dealing with stress.

3.3 Other Ways To Deal With Stress

"Pull yourself together; you'll get over this," is not a successful strategy for dealing with stress, although it has its adherents, particularly among family doctors.

A better approach is to do something to diminish the stress levels, or combat them meaningfully in a biological sense. By the latter, I mean change our physiological response to stress, so that its effects are less damaging.

A simple example of this would be Herbert Benson's "Relaxation Response". It's a sort of meditative physiology, without the oriental mystery and pseudo-religious beliefs that seem to get attached to meditation.

The Relaxation response is actually the direct opposite of the familiar "fight or flight" of urgent physiological changes that leap into action when a creature senses danger. First described by Walter Bradford Cannon over 80 years ago, this model states that animals react to threats with a general discharge of the sympathetic nervous system, preparing the animal for fighting or running away. More specifically, the adrenal glands produce a cascade of hormones, notably adrenalin and noradrenalin (US: norepinephrine and epinephrine). Later cortisol, which is very damaging, enters the picture when stress becomes chronic.

The Relaxation Response, on the other hand, is characterized by eat, sleep and chill out. It's a mental, physical and emotional response leading to a place of deep rest.

Herbert Benson, a Harvard University cardiologist, distinguished himself by demonstrating, scientifically (with instruments and recordings), that there is no magic or transcendental mystery to the Maharishi's Transcendental Meditation™

That in fact there is no need for a mantra or chanting "Om". Just repeating a simple word, or even just the number "One", over and over, has identical effects... and it's free! Catholics might want to try the "Hail Mary" prayer. Just keep it simple.

Here are the steps, following instructions in *The Relaxation Response*, pages 162-163:

1. Sit quietly in a comfortable position (don't lie down, this is not sleep).

2. Close your eyes.

3. Deeply relax all your muscles, beginning at your feet and progressing up to your face. Keep everything relaxed.

4. Breathe gently through your nose. Become aware of your breathing. As you breathe out, say your chosen word or just "one", silently to yourself. For example, breathe in ... out, "one",- in ... out, "one", etc. Breathe easily and naturally.

5. Do this for 10 to 20 minutes, once or twice a day but at least once. You may open your eyes to check the time, but do not use an alarm. When you finish, sit quietly for several minutes, at first with your eyes closed and then with your eyes opened.

6. If you can't sit still that long, do it while you are exercizing. Say your word on each foot fall if you're running, or with each stroke if you are swimming.

Don't even worry about whether you are successful in achieving a deep level of relaxation. Maintain a passive attitude and just let relaxation come at its own pace. When distracting thoughts occur, that's not a failure either. Just try to ignore them by not dwelling upon them and return to repeating your word, phrase or "one."

Don't try this within two hours of a meal, since the digestive processes seem to interfere with the elicitation of the Relaxation Response.

With practice, the response should come with little effort.

There is no reason to get involved with mantras. It could be counter-productive and lead to inner disturbances. Far better to use a soothing, gentle sound, preferably with no meaning, or association, to avoid stimulation of unnecessary thoughts. The word "one" is as good as any. Or just a "Hmmmm" humming sound.

As Benson says, it's hard for people to accept this simple technique: "It's so easy. The main problem we're having now in this context is its simplicity. Our culture feels that unless something is expensive, mechanical, complicated, it must not work. But if you make it more complicated you destroy its essence, which is passivity and simplicity."[230] There are scores of other ways to summon the relaxation response, as well, said Benson at the American Psychological Association's 2008 address. "Anything that breaks the train of everyday thought will evoke this physiological state."

That includes participating in repetitive sports such as running, letting go of tension through progressive muscular relaxation, practicing yoga, knitting, crocheting, even playing musical instruments.

"You know how when you play an instrument and you become 'one' with that instrument and the time flits away? That is the relaxation response," he said. "You know the high you get from running? That is the relaxation response coming about by the repetitive motion of your footfall."

Low-Dose Exercize

Interestingly, low-intensity running and other simple but enjoyable exercizes have been shown to benefit depression sufferers greatly. "After adjustment for a range of confounders, those who reported undertaking no exercise at baseline had a 44% increased odds of developing case-level depression compared with those who were exercising 1-2 hours a week," the investigators reported.

They also determined that had everyone exercised at least 1 hour a week, 12% of the cases of depression that were identified at follow-up could have been prevented.

Yet, interestingly, exercize had no beneficial effects on anxiety states and other disorders. Moreover, "Most of the protective effect of exercise is realized with relatively low levels of exercise, with no indication of any additional benefit beyond 1 hour of exercise each week," the investigators note.[231]

Here's another study, with much the same conclusion:

Mats Hallgren, PhD, and colleagues at the Karolinska Institute in Stockholm, Sweden, investigated the effects of exercize, such as yoga or aerobics, on mild to moderate depression.

At the end of 12 weeks, they found that the severity of depression was significantly lower among patients who participated in any one of the exercise interventions compared to those who received usual care, and that the benefits of exercise were seen regardless of how intensely the patients exercised.

Furthermore, the benefits of exercise on depression were maintained up to twelve months, even when not continued at the optimal rate.

"Exercise is medicine for depression, even when the 'pill' is small," Dr Hallgren affirmed.[232]

The low levels of exercize needed to have this effect means more is not necessarily better. So Dr. Benson's suggestion that low-level repetitive exercize has powerful meditative qualities might be correct.

3.4 Rest and Sleep

And while we are now on the subject of simplicity and relaxation, let's look at sleep.

Without question, proper sleep is one of the most healing and restorative physiological tools we have to overcome stress. Sleep deprivation does the opposite. Stress causes hyperarousal, which can upset the balance between sleep and wakefulness. Stress causes insomnia by making it difficult to fall asleep and to stay asleep, and by affecting the quality of your sleep.

Sleep, on the other hand, can calm down stress. It's one of the most relaxing and restorative things we can do to combat our modern over-active world.

Most of us have had the experience of lying in bed late at night, unable to sleep as stress loops invade our thoughts. A growing body of scientific research indicates that stress can have profound effects on sleep. Compared to those not experiencing insomnia, insomniacs have a greater number of stressful life events in the previous year. More recent research indicates that, in particular, it is the person's *perception of stress* that influences insomnia.

But is also cuts the other way: lack of sleep can raise your stress levels significantly.

A recent study built from this reasoning and examined the effect of sleep on stress. Participants took an exam that was mildly stressful. Compared to those experiencing a typical night of sleep, those in the sleep deprived condition experienced higher levels of stress.

Outside of the laboratory context, other researchers have similarly shown that a lack of sleep leads to stress and psychological strain.[233]

Understanding Your Sleep Cycles

Sleep is traditionally divided into "sleep cycles" of about 90 minutes each. There are four stages of sleep and we cycle through each. Stages 1 and 2 are REM sleep, so-called (from rapid eye movements, which characterize that level of sleep).

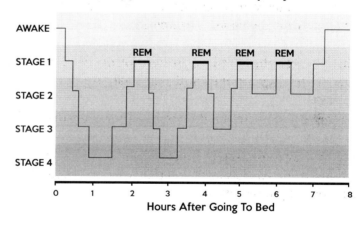

In the US, stages 3 and 4 are combined to form what is lumped together as "deep sleep". In the rest of the world, the stage 3 and 4 terminology is used. It takes a full cycle to go down from stages 1 and 2, to deep sleep, and back up. There are five sleep cycles per night (making a total of 7 ½ hours, rather than 8 hours).

What we do know is that the first part of a sleep cycle is about restoration and repair. There are no rapid eye movements in this phase (non-REM sleep). The brain waves at this time are slow and rhythmical, like breathing. These cycles have to do with processing short-term memory and converting it to long-term.

Conclusion? You need to be in bed well before midnight and fast asleep for maximum brain health (see next section). 10.30 is a good bedtime!

Study the chart: you'll see that the first two sleep cycles are quite deep. After that they become shallower.

Non-REM Sleep vs. Alzheimer's

Matthew Walker PhD, director of the Center for Human Sleep Science at the University of California, Berkeley, has done signal research and found that disruption of the non-REM sleep cycle is associated with a build-up of amyloid protein, the toxic substance that forms plaques and damages brain tissue.[234]

No-one can yet say that these plaques cause Alzheimer's disease—in fact they probably don't—but they only show up in cases of dementia and that must be significant.

Other key research, by Maiken Nedergaard at the University of Rochester, New York, revealed the importance of what is called the *glymphatic system* in the brain. It's like the lymphatic system in the rest of the body but unique to the glial cells of the brain—hence the strange name.

Turns out that the glymphatic system is a waste disposal network that flushes our brains of nasty toxins built up through the day, including amyloid protein. But it only works effectively in the stage of deep non-REM sleep; 10 or 20 times more efficiently, in fact.

What I am trying to tell you is there is now a well-established link between poor sleep cycles, especially missing out on non-REM sleep, and the later development of Alzheimer's disease.

We need our deep sleep. It's both a preventative for dementia and, once established, it can slow down the progress of the disease. Getting too little sleep across your lifespan will markedly increase the risk of developing dementia.

Unfortunately, sleeping pills are ineffective here. They do not and cannot create the right kind of deep sleep I am talking about. To cure insomnia you need the restful induction of theta brainwaves that can be achieved by MMSS devices (see section 3.10). If your sleep has been poor for many years, start catching up NOW!

3.5 Flower Remedies To Adjust Psychology

Here's a strange thing, if you haven't already met it: the idea that flower "essences" can adjust your thinking and help you through tough times.

It goes back to an English physician (OK, with a Welsh name) who developed a new discipline. Dr. Edward Bach (pronounced like batch) was a homeopath and is rightly famous for the development of a number of bowel "nosodes" (a nosode is a homeopathic preparation made from obnoxious or toxic materials, such as bacteria, designed to dislodge a condition within the body).

But he was perhaps not so comfortable using remedies derived from hostile sources. He wanted something purer, gentler and simpler. He eventually hit on the idea of flower essences.

Like any good physician, Dr. Bach knew that attitude of mind plays a vital role in maintaining health and recovering from illness. After identifying 38 basic negative states of mind and spending several years exploring the countryside, he managed to create a plant or flower based remedy for each one.

Bach was what we would call a "sensitive", he touched flowers and he got vibrations or "messages", as to what the plant would heal. It all sounds a bit woo-woo but there is no question: Bach's flower remedies work and work well.

Wanting to make his flower essences more available to the general public, Bach enlisted the help of Nelsons Homeopathic Pharmacy in London back in the 1930s. Under his instruction, they began to make and sell stock remedies from the mother tinctures he supplied. In 1990, this relationship was formalized, and since then Nelsons (the Pharmacy's parent company) has been responsible for all the bottling and distribution of the Bach remedies.

Today, Nelsons produces millions of stock bottles each year from its warehouse facility in Wimbledon, London, and the Bach® Original Flower Remedies are sold in over 70 countries around the world.

His premier formulation, called "Rescue remedy" (made from Cherry Plum, Clematis, Impatiens, Rock Rose and Star of Bethlehem) should be in every medicine cupboard. It can be obtained from virtually any pharmacy and whole food store. It's good for shock, trauma, fear, panic, tension and mood changes.

The original Bach natural remedies have been used confidently in Europe for over 100 years. If you like celebrity endorsements, Jennifer Aniston says it keeps her cool under pressure; Cate Blanchett and Salma Hayek have been fans for years; Roberta Flack uses the soothing effect of "Rescue Remedy®" for menopausal hot flashes.

There's also a sleep formulation, with added white chestnut, which could be particularly valuable to those under stressful circumstances.

- **White Chestnut:** To help ease restless mind.
- **Star of Bethlehem:** For trauma and shock.
- **Clematis**: For the tendency to "pass out", and unconsciousness, being 'far away' and not present mentally.

- **Cherry Plum:** Fear of mind giving way, verge of breakdown, anger.
- **Impatiens**: For irritability, tension and fidgetiness.
- **Rock Rose:** For frozen terror and panic.

Flower essences have proved to be of great help in restoring "the will to live", overcoming the shadow of this extreme diagnosis, giving strength to the organism and helping the patient to respond positively towards any chosen treatment regimen, by altering the mental landscape. Flower essences can bring optimism, courage, determination and strength.

As Dr. Marina Angeli, a psychiatrist in Athens, Greece, put it: "Flower essences have proven to be very important in cleansing and rebalancing mental-emotional states, giving space to the person's soul to bring him/her back to life again, by unblocking the energy system to a point where it is able to nourish and cure the body."

Please note: this is not the same as saying flower essences themselves may in any way effect a cure. Only nature and the mental determination of the patient can do that.

There are books on flower remedies, which give far more detail on the actions of each of Bach's remedies than I can incorporate here. Suffice it to mention:

Olive

Bach described Olive as the remedy for "those who have suffered much mentally or physically and are so exhausted and weary that they feel they have no more strength to make any effort." The remedy helps to restore enthusiasm for life. It helps you tap into a higher source and thereby find new energy and restoration at all levels.

Elm

Elm is for those who "suddenly feel overwhelmed by their responsibilities and feel inadequate to deal with them or keep up with events; this is often brought about by taking on too much work without taking care of oneself. As a result they feel depressed and exhausted, with a temporary loss of self-esteem." The remedy helps you find balance in your life, setting realistic expectations and goals. It also helps you to be open to receiving assistance from others and from the Higher Self.

Walnut

Walnut is a remedy specifically to help in dealing with change of any sort: divorce, marriage, change in career, menopause, or any revolution in circumstances. Some workers use Walnut for dealing with jet lag and what I call "travel shock" (the general effects of moving from country to country). Walnut can help you navigate through change in a positive way, following your inner direction, while at the same time protecting you from negative external influences.

Mimulus

Mimulus brings courage in the face of known and understandable fears, such as flying, a hospital visit, a confrontation over some unpleasantness in the family, or an illness, such as cancer. Those with marked Mimulus traits tend to be physically delicate and wilting, with a tendency to blush easily, stammer, or suddenly become speechless. Others talk too much from sheer nervousness.

Other Flower Remedy Ranges

It only remains to mention there are other flower essence ranges. But I have no experience of these and so am unable to make comparison or recommendations.

Ones that you may come across include The Ranger Of Light essences, the Findhorn range, Himalayan Flower Enhancers and Australian Bush Flower Essences.

If you want to learn more about flower essences, I suggest you start with Edward Bach, "The Twelve Healers," in *The Bach Flower Remedies*.

3.6 Talking

In this day and age of sound bites, quick fixes, hearty slogans and media mottoes there seems less and less time for the one truly powerful mode of communication: talking!

Yet there is no question that being able to share our burdens will lighten the load. We have sayings like "A problem shared is a problem halved."

But this misses the really important point by a mile, which is that talking about a problem changes our own perception of it, the structure of the difficulty alters, we gain new insights and new ways of coping. It is our own view of what we are experiencing that begins to dance and transform, as we spread it out in front of us to view, prior to sharing it with others.

So, yes, we need someone to talk to. But the idea that the someone needs to be a wiser person is a big misunderstanding. He or she just needs to be a good listener; to keep us talking!

Researchers from California have proved that sharing your feelings helps to beat stress but also that *sharing with someone in the same situation as yourself yields the best results.*

This could be because sharing a threatening situation with a person in a similar emotional state 'buffers individuals from experiencing the heightened levels of stress that typically accompany threat'.

Lead researcher Professor Sarah Townsend, believes sharing experiences could help people deal with stress in the workplace.

'For instance, when you're putting together an important presentation or working on a high-stakes project, these are situations that can be threatening and you may experience heightened stress.

'But talking with a colleague who shares your emotional state can help decrease this stress.'

'Imagine you are one of two people working on an important project: if you have a lot riding on this project, it is a potentially stressful situation,' added Professor Townsend.

'But having a coworker with a similar emotional profile can help reduce your experience of stress.'

The findings were published in the journal *Social Psychological and Personality Science.*[235]

3.7 Meditation

Not everything about meditation is as fuzzy, soft and holistic as teachers and practitioners want you to believe. There have been severe negative outcomes, which get swept under the carpet. For example, in a new study published in PLOS One, "The Varieties of Contemplative Experience," researchers found that meditation didn't only deliver positive reactions — it could also produce negative or "challenging" ones, such as fear, involuntary body movements and panic.[236]

These negative types of results are often under-reported in literature. The 2017 study authors interviewed almost 100 people who practiced meditation, as well as teachers from three main traditions (Theravāda, Zen and Tibetan). They discovered that meditation affects seven main aspects: cognitive, perceptual, affective (i.e. emotions and moods), somatic (relating to the body), conative (i.e. motivation or will), sense of self and social.

The subjects reported a variety of reactions, both positive and negative, and they lasted anywhere from as soon as the person started practicing to 25 years into their practice.

While the introspective nature of meditation is meant to bring up difficult thoughts (as with people who re-experienced traumatic memories) and is certainly meant to be a challenge, many believe they'll automatically reap the benefits right away. But the practice isn't as simple as sitting down, closing your eyes and letting the good vibes flow — your mental state, your teacher and even your physical location can make a difference.

"This is a good example of how a contextual factor can affect associated distress and functioning," Jared Lindahl, one of the study's co-authors, said in a press release. "An experience that is positive and desirable in one situation may become a burden in another."

Similarly, people have been questioning the use of apps and other technology, which impose meditation imagery that has the potential to be disturbing. Moreover, these apps often coerce the listener to meditate for a certain amount of time or at a specific point in the day, which might also ironically create stress with regards to a habit that's meant to be calming.

All that said, meditation and particularly mindfulness do have a place in staying healthy in mind. The difference: meditation generally means slowing down and trying to still the mind, by the use of breathing exercizes and calming but deliberate thoughts. Mindfulness, on the other hand, simply means to pay attention to what you are doing in the NOW; to remain self-aware and alert and break out of automatic thinking patterns that trouble our thoughts.

In my own Supernoetics® writings I use the expression "see yourself being yourself." Georges Gurdjieff called it "self-remembering". Its origins can be found in the sutras of Patanjali and others.

Important note: this is not the same as feeling unreal or de-personalized or, as patients sometimes phrase it, "seeing myself down a long tunnel." That's something called dissociation and it concerns psychiatrists and psychologists. I'm talking about stepping out of the stream of reality but seeing yourself still as part of that stream. It's not scary: just the difference between feeling bored (say) and *seeing yourself being bored*! (that's me, being bored, rather than "I am bored").

If you plump for meditation, or mindfulness exercizes, make sure you and the teacher know the difference in what you are doing. However, here is an approach to relaxing and de-stressing that has been proved to have the same physiological benefits as many years of meditation, yet it can be achieved in just a few minutes.

Here's a useful and simple trick that is a kind of meditation exercize that can help you conquer moments of intense and unwanted emotions...

3.8 An Unusual Technique For Raw Emotional Pain

I've told this story before... often. But it is instructive!

Many years ago I discovered—after my first wife left suddenly and unannounced—a way to handle unpleasant emotions. I was pretty wrecked by the experience (divorce is one of the heaviest stresses of all, as the Holmes-Rahe Life Events Scale tells us). But I found that if I lifted up on high and looked down on myself, weeping, that I didn't feel the same emotions that were tormenting the "Keith down there." I was amazed!

I was like an outsider, watching "him" and seeing what he would do. In fact I felt sorry for him but realized that "he" was learning things that he had never faced before. It would make him a better doctor, I knew, because he/we would understand the suffering of others far better.

It was the first really shattering experience of my life. Up until then, I had just been having a ball, changing the world with my medical breakthroughs and riding over problems and upsets like a person charmed (though others might say I was arrogant, shallow and insensitive).

Now I was forced to confront raw pain and, like all pain, it hurt and changed my mentality. My whole attitude to life changed for the better (I have actually been able to *thank* my first wife for the formative experience).

I could see all this from above and thought it was a good thing. You know, I do believe the "me up here" was looking forward to the learning sessions, when "him down there" would start with a sigh and quickly find himself in tears. It was a cleansing and I could see it doing him good.

He loved his wife, or thought he did, and believed that, at the age of 50, he would never find another woman. I could see the folly of this installed belief, that was making the loneliness particularly poignant, but I had no way to tell "him" to not be foolish.

If I descended to his platform, then I felt the full force of all the negative emotions that were natural in this situation (though disempowering and pointless). So this executive self chose to remain aloof and largely uninfluenced by the unpleasantness going in "downstairs".

Higher Wisdom

Slowly it dawned on me that being free of emotional turmoil would allow me to make far better executive decisions... and that's what happened. After a period of several years living in Spain and licking my wounds, I started back on the road to a new medical career. From that point on I achieved more, faster, with more reward, than at any other point in my life.

By the age of 60 I was born again with more mental powers and physical energy than I had had when I was younger. At the age of 70, I launched my real life mission (Supernoetics®). Most folks are getting ready for the grave at age 70; I was just getting started!

Everything now seems to go my way. It can be slow, sometimes. But I get what I want with the force of an unstoppable tsunami. Everything bows before me.

If ever I run into a problem situation or can't think what to do, I take a ride "upstairs" on the glass elevator and look for the solution from a place of calm and freedom and mental power: theta being!

I'm going to teach you how to use this technique to transform your life and start getting the things you want, when you want them.

Not only that but your emotions will improve, you'll feel healthier, fitter and younger than ever in your life. You will experience a clarity of mind and vision that you never thought possible.

How It Works

Life isn't easy. We were not born with an instruction manual (I'm trying to write a Supernoetics® one now!)

Generally, when things are going well, they continue and feel good. But sooner or later, you will encounter a difficulty; it's inevitable. Thing is, because of our emotions, we blunder around destructively and make everything far worse than it needs to be.

First of all, you make your own emotions—deliberately—did you know that? The idea that "someone upset you" is corny and simply not true. In any given situation, you upset yourself, in response to something you didn't like. So the first big step is to stop creating negative emotions; life will be a lot more pleasant!

But at the same time, when we are upset in some way, we lose our standards of clarity and wisdom. When emotions run rampant, we act, feel and think in stupid ways. You know that's true. If you can't admit it for yourself, then you know from watching others that it's what happens. Angry, fearful or miserable people are irrational. They do silly things that only seem to contribute to their pain!

In this unfortunate state, you may not handle a distressing set of circumstances in the correct manner and later seriously regret the way you processed it. Your emotions take over and you find yourself unable to think through the situation with a clear head.

Sound familiar? Well, the trick is to separate your emotions from the actual problem state, so you can process things in a clear-headed manner.

Sound impossible? Well, it's not really... we just take a ride in the Glass Elevator! (section 3.15)

You'll not only separate yourself from the confusion and dismay, you'll be able to come up with decent solutions, instead of messy ones that don't work.

In a deeper sense it shows that you are YOU; you are not the problem, the emotions, the turmoil. Life has trained you to think you are. But it's very important to grasp as soon as possible that you are none of these things. You are a serene being, with lots of hostile experiences to content with, but separate from them. You must not identify with those hostile or negative experiences. That's the first rule of mental health. YOU ARE NOT YOUR EMOTIONS, even though we say we are: "I am angry", "I am sad," etc.

Learning To Look Down

If you've ever climbed a mountain, you'll know the world looks very different from on high. Somehow, problems seem more remote, the everyday world far away. It's inspiring! You are out of things. But this is a very unnatural state of affairs. Just think what would happen to the whole world, if everyone took to being hermits and just meditating on mountain tops.

One of the difficulties with the mindful and meditative approaches to life is that it can get unreal. You leave your troubles behind and try to convince yourself you have no worries. It's detachment and that's a word you hear a lot in esoteric scriptures.

I say it's artificial and much of the appeal is this idea of leaving things behind, rather than deeper spiritual insights. Life is a mechanism. You have to operate the mechanisms skillfully, not just be a spectator. That takes knowledge. In Supernoetics® we live our knowledge, we do not just accumulate it!

We are intensely practical in Supernoetics®. We have solutions. And this simple "glass elevator" hack is one of them. It won't take you long to learn to do it and gets phenomenal results.

It's easy to do. Ideally you would need to sit quietly. But you can do it standing and on the go, if needs must. The more authentic the experience, the more peaceful and empowered you'll feel.

If you can sit down and relax, so much the better. You can assists the process by listening to music. Adding binaural beats, flickering theta lights and creative mind images helps even more, but I don't recommend the uncontrolled flight of drugs. You don't need anything so heavy. If you can't easily find your viewpoint looking down on self, then pretend! Remarkably, it works just as well. The answers come just as easily. In fact I'll let you into a little secret: pretending to have another viewpoint is the same are the real experience. You only think you are inventing it. You'll do it anyway.

Like towards the ceiling or imagine floating towards the ceiling. "See" yourself hanging up there looking downwards and say to yourself ....

"There's (your name) down there. I wonder how he/she is going to handle this? I wonder what he-she will do?"

Look downwards at yourself objectively, as if you were a totally different person and merely an observer. Because you are looking at a "different person"; you are looking at the creature self, which is not the spirit of YOU. The first thing you will notice, that tells you this is working, is that you feel little if any emotion for that person down there.

This elevation will emotionally divorce yourself from the problem. Persevere with this for several minutes then let it go. Try it again later if a solution doesn't immediately pop into your mind.

Basically, the Higher You can see aspects of the situation that the struggling creature self probably cannot. As you watch the drama unfold, ideas and solutions will pop into your mind. The down-there you may get its own ideas. You can help by prompting and guiding. But don't try to take over.

Somewhere along the line, the right path will open before you, as if revealed by a dream, or maybe even by another self. Don't forget the model of the Complex of Self—the fact that we are really an aggregate of many spiritual entities and viewpoints.

There is always one enterprising being in there, that's trying its best to help. You need to be alert and listen to this possibility (see Spiritual Rescue Technology 3.16).

The Lag

The answer may not come at once, or not as quickly as you hoped. No worries: just get on with your routine.

Often, at some point later during the day, the answer will suddenly pop into your head. It may be something totally unexpected... right out of left field. The solution you are looking for of course is one of those "lateral thinking" insights that we call a *cognosis* in Supernoetics®.

You can also do this via sleep. As you settle down last thing at night, say firmly, *"During sleep tonight my Higher Self will come up with the answer I am looking for."* Say it and believe it.

I've had dozens of people learn this simple hack and make it work. It can take several days to develop as a new skill or habit. But it is worth it. Generally, anything which reduced emotional excesses and raises objectivity will help in the journey through life.

Excess emotion can be a soul destroyer and can totally disrupt our lives if not controlled. Our jails are filled with individuals who have let their emotions take control.

At the very least you could end up diagnosed as a borderline psychotic case. Best not to go there!

Under Pressure?

You can try a shortcut, if you have to think or act quickly. Challenge yourself with this question: *If I were all-wise and watching myself have this experience, what would I tell myself to do?*

It's not a delusion. It comes from a very deep philosophical wisdom, that we know everything; we are ultimately wise; we just have to believe in ourselves.

You'll come up with brilliant ideas, as soon as you learn to let go and float along with these insights! It's as much about rising above turbulent emotions as deep insight. With negative emotions out of the way, you can see more clearly and rapidly get to the answers or solutions you need.

That's where Supernoetics® piloting comes in (section 3.12).

3.9 Gestureism (Not to be confused with gesturalism in art)

This is a word I made up today! Just an idea. But hey, consider this:

Almost everyone knows, or hears sooner or later, that it's impossible to feel depressed if you look up. If you have never verified this for yourself, get up, go outdoors and try it!

You can follow up with looking down and you will see at once why we call depression being "down". Hang your head, slump your shoulders, and it starts to feel depressing in just moments! (finish up by going back to looking up and feeling more cheerful, then you can resume reading this text).

I noticed many years ago, for myself, that if I simply add a dance gesture to what I am doing, that I immediately feel happy and cheerful. It works whether I am chopping vegetables, cooking, shopping or if I do it in the middle of my exercize walk.

I'm not really interested in how it looks. This is just for me. This is about my own kinesthetic response, not voyeurism. I enjoy myself in these moments.

The word Gestureism came to me one moment when I put my hands up high (like a prophet) and made my shoulders work a little harder. I felt good and just after a long morning of writing for this book, I was a little stiff. It was, if you like, a moment of self-nurture. It was—in a word—delicious!

So now I am reminded of a quirky piece I wrote back in the 1990s: "Dancing For Joy While Driving a Car". I have decided to reproduce it here.

I suppose this piece ought to come with a severe health warning! Nevertheless, I share it with you from a position of love and exhilaration.

There have been (many) times in my life when my joy simply bubbled over; it effervesced, like sparkling wine overflowing the bottle when shaken.

Sometimes the thrill has overtaken me while driving the car.

I danced. Carefully, of course, with sufficient attention on the road and other traffic—but I danced at the wheel. Peripheral vision comes to the rescue; peripheral vision is how you drive home safely, without even noticing the stop lights or other vehicles. How you can't even remember the turns you made because they are on automatic.

It can be enhanced by good "caffeine music".

I rarely do it with a passenger but one Swedish girlfriend went home with a tale and, apparently, told all her friends. She wasn't scared she told me, but everything about common sense and social training cried out for her against what should be a crazy thing to do.

Yet she saw the delight! She felt it too!

Never do it on busy roads, especially in the city. I am talking about lonely roads in the backwoods or mountains. Scotland was always great for inspiring scenery and wild, empty places.

And, of course, it's modified dancing; it's what you can do while driving a car at 70 mph. Flexing your legs, wriggling your butt and twisting the body from side to side. If you don't believe me, try it in your car next time, before you start the engine, of course!

The music is part of this. I'm thinking of tunes like Din Din Wo (little child), by Senegalese singer Habib Koite; it's a default track that comes with Windows Media Player...

Yeah! Or the greatest dance rocker of all time, The Jean Genie by David Bowie, and my personal dance favorite: Land Down Under by Ozzie group Men At Work.

By the way, you just can't do this to Mozart or Bach. I've tried!

I tell you what: it sure beats boredom and travel fatigue. Trouble is, I don't think you can do it to order: you have to want to do it, the rhythm and desire has to well up from inside in a totally irresistible way. I think that high level of spirit energy protects you. Otherwise you are just a crazy hothead in charge of a dangerous vehicle.

Don't forget sensible dancing either. That works!

Some day I'll write the book "Gestureism". Meanwhile, have fun with the concept. Use it as a tool to lift your spirits.

3.10 Multi-Media Sensory Stimulation MMSS

Now we come to one of the most important techniques in the book, a marvelous technological way to relax, chill out, de-stress and get to a place joy and delight. I call it "multi-media sensory stimulation" or MMSS for short.

Basically it is a mixture of four sensory modalities that are, each one separately, capable of producing beneficial psychological change:

1. binaural beats

2. light entrainment (called flicker following)

3. soothing slow music

4. gratifying mind imagery

These can be mixed in various ways in various electronic devices. The one I favor most is called the Kasina, from MindPlace.com. Several of my own audio-visual tracks are provided on that particular device. One other worth mentioning is the Brain Tap, developed by Patrick Porter at Brain Tap Technologies.

To understand how this works, let's start with brainwave frequencies. This is not hard to understand in principle.

Brain Wave Frequencies

When we are awake and busy in mind with our everyday activities, our brains "vibrate" at between about 14 and 25 Hertz. Because these vibrations can be picked up on a brain scan monitor as wavy lines on a chart, we use the term brain waves, instead of vibrations. These are true frequencies, measured as Hertz (cycles per second).

Frequencies of 14 – 25 Hertz we call beta activity or beta state. It means arousal. Alertness.

If the frequency lies between 8 and 13 Hertz, we call that an alpha state. It is characterized by a relaxed, semi inward-looking calm. Daydreaming if you like. Very relaxed but aware.

Frequencies between 4 and 7 Hertz we call a theta state (alpha, beta, delta and theta are letters of the Greek alphabet). Theta means a trance-like state, dreaming, deeply introverted—but not unconscious. The person would still come to and answer a spoken question. Like in meditation.

Delta, on the other hand denotes a state of sleep or unconsciousness. Delta waves are from around 1 Hertz to 3 Hertz. A person in delta would not respond, unless woken.

It should be noted that every time we all go to sleep, we descend from beta, through alpha and theta, to a delta state. On waking we reverse this and gradually stir as we are aroused, up through theta, then alpha and into beta, alert and ready for the day (well, most of us!)

From this simple explanation, you would guess that alpha states are very desirable; relaxing, good thinking time! Theta is deeper and profoundly relaxing. That can be even better to calm the mind and limit the effects of stress.

So how do we get to alpha or theta?

A good question. In olden times the answer would have been just to meditate. Practice mind control, till you could get there at will. It was difficult but trained meditators learned to do in in a few years. Today we use electronic technology, as with the Kasina and other devices, to rapidly plunge the individual into a slower, more relaxed brain state. We do this by...

Brain Entrainment

Since the late 20th century, thanks to stereo technology from Sony, Panasonic and other developers, we have had the capability of playing separate frequencies into each ear. Without making this too technical, it has been found that the brain will detect *the difference* between these frequencies and tune to it. So if the right ear gets 450 Hertz and the left ear gets 440 Hertz, the brain will *detect* the 10 beats difference and tune to that: alpha frequency.

This tuning into a set frequency we call brain *entrainment* and it happens automatically and quite quickly—within minutes.

But it's even more interesting. What has been found is that all parts of the brain start vibrating at the entrained frequency. We called this state *integration* or *synchrony*. This is a state of true coherence (all resonating together) and does not happen in nature. It is very powerful.

Because it is generated by sounds differing in each ear, this technology is described as binaural beats (*binaural*: in two ears).

But wait! Sound isn't the only way to generate brain entrainment. There is a far older method, using flickering lights. We call this photic driving. Lights flickering at 10 beats per second, or 5 beats per second, will entrain the brain to alpha or theta, respectively. What's more, it's very powerful.

You may even have experienced its effect, without recognizing what was happening. If you have ever had the experience of feeling sleepy, or even nodding off, in front of a fire with flickering flames, you were probably sent into a theta relaxed state. Typical wood or coal fire flames dance at around 3- 5 times a second. You only have to look into the heart of the fire for a few minutes and it will start working. This is well-known magic.

Ptolemy (90–168 AD), a mathematician, and astronomer living in Alexandria, was the first to document the use of light to change mind patterns, while looking through a spinning, spoked wheel toward the sun.

French psychiatric Pierre Janet (1859 – 1947) noticed the calming effect of flickering lights. He treated agitated patients at the hospital of Pitié-Salpêtrière in Paris using a device with a rotating disc in front of a kerosene lamp. Holes in the disc caused the light to flicker and he could set the rate to a calming effect by altering the speed of rotation of the wheel. By all accounts, it was highly successful at reducing anxiety and hysteria in patients.

In modern times, William Grey Walter (1910-1977) also caught on to the effect of flickering lights and he gave us the term photic driving.

During the psychedelic 1960s, Brion Gysin (1916-1986), a painter and a poet, became interested in the hallucinations that could be caused deliberately by photic driving and designed his own stroboscope or "dream machine", as a means for spiritual enlightenment.[237]

Putting It All Together

OK, what happens if we put binaural beats and flickering lights together; does it work better?

The answer seems to be yes.

But I go two steps further than that. We can use calm, soothing music in addition to binaural beats and flicker following. So-called slow Baroque works best but any soothing gentle music, such as New Age harmonies and sounds, will work just as well.

We can arrange that the music is plainly audible, while the binaurals are tuned down to subliminal, meaning not heard consciously but still effective at the subconscious level.

Add to that some reassuring, even inspiring, creative imagery and we have an effect which is truly mind altering. I have recorded a number of awesome tracks which I call mind walks. With me to gently guide you, you can imagine a visit to Atlantis or old Avalon (King Arthur's isle), flying above the earth, travelling in deep space among the stars or doing love and gratitude!

The summation effect of music, voice, sounds and flickering lights I call multi-media sensory stimulation. It's the most powerful way I know of relaxing, healing, soothing and taking attention off the bitterness and worries of life. Half an hour in an induced theta state is truly restorative.

But there are even more benefits, would you believe...

All The Science

The first big step in science came with a ground-breaking paper entitled "Auditory Beats in the Brain" by Dr. Gerald Oster of Mt. Sinai Medical Center, published in the October 1973 issue of *Scientific American*. Oster introduced the first use of the term binaural beats in this article.

Robert Monroe (of the Monroe Institute of Applied Sciences) was also investigating binaural beats, which he used to induce "out of body" experiences.

In thousands of experiments, using an EEG machine to monitor subject's electrical brain wave patterns, Monroe verified that he could indeed entrain brain wave patterns using binaural beats.

There is now so much exciting science to show the manifold benefits of induced-alpha and theta states. Consider the following *proven* benefits:
- Weight loss
- Stress busting
- Giving up addictions
- Improved sexual prowess
- More creativity

- Kids enjoying this technology can shed ADD and ADHD.
- Improved moods
- Lowering blood pressure
- Learning a language
- Breaking dysfunctional patterns
- Improved memory/study scores
- Pain relief without drugs
- Coping with cancer and other diseases

Cranial Pharmacy Model

We can alter real-time brain chemistry, using brain entrainment.

Dr. Margaret Patterson and biochemist Dr. Ifor Capel at the Marie Curie Cancer Memorial Foundation Research Department in Surrey, UK, showed that certain frequencies in the brain dramatically speed up production of a variety of neurotransmitters: different frequencies triggered different healing brain chemicals.

I call it "cranial pharmacy".

A 10 Hz (alpha) signal boosts the production and turnover rate of serotonin, the well-known chemical messenger that increases relaxation and eases pain.

Catecholamines (like epinephrine), vital for memory and learning, respond at around 4 Hz (theta).

Acetylcholine is an important neuropeptide for higher mental processes as learning and memory.

Recent studies show that insufficient acetylcholine causes memory loss and reduces learning and intelligence, and confusion and memory loss in Alzheimer's disease have been linked, at least in part, to a lack of acetylcholine.

In fact, Acetylcholine has also been associated not only with a greater number of neurons in the cortex but also with greater brain size, with humans having the highest density of acetylcholine in the brain. So any means of inducing more of it is vital in a text such as this, dealing with holistic methods of restoring mind function.

Moreover, UC Berkeley researcher Mark Rosenzweig has shown a direct connection between acetylcholine and intelligence.

Hormonal Responses

Dr. Vincent Giampapa, MD, of Longevity Institute International, revealed that alpha, theta, and delta brain wave patterns dramatically affects production of three important hormones related to both increased longevity and well-being: cortisol (tuning it down), DHEA (Dehydroepiandrosterone Sulfate), and melatonin.

Informal studies, reported by Bill Harris of the Centerpointe Institute, claim that in 3 days, over 68% of participants using brain entrainment had an average increase of DHEA levels of 43.77%!

Several people had increases of up to 90%!

I notice with amusement that several meditation sites are claiming these figures were achieved by meditation only, which is fairly typical of the false claims that abound on the Internet. And of course, once one starts it, everyone copies the unfounded claims to support their own story.

DHEA levels are a key determinant of physiological age and resistance to disease. When DHEA levels are high, the body is at its peak—vibrant, healthy, and able to combat disease effectively. A 1986 study published in the *New England Journal of Medicine* found that a 100 mcg/deciliter increase in DHEA blood levels corresponded with a 48% reduction in mortality due to cardiovascular disease—and a 36% reduction in mortality from all causes![238]

Moreover, DHEA acts as a buffer against stress-related hormones (such as cortisol).

Cortisol we want LESS of, and it went down an average of 46.47%, with positive changes in 68% of the people, and with several people having decreases of 70 or 80%!

Melatonin levels increased an average of 97.77%, with positive changes happening in over 73% of the people!

Take these figures with a pinch of salt but you get the idea: brain entrainment, with or without meditation practices, is highly beneficial for general health and enhanced states of mind.

Cortisol is a hormone naturally produced by the adrenal glands and is perhaps the #1 aging "stress" hormone. It also interferes with learning and memory and is, in general, bad news for your health and your wellbeing.

Alpha and theta states are known to reduce cortisol levels, so it is only logical that brain entrainment would help.

Melatonin is the hormone that helps to create restful sleep. During sleep many important rejuvenating substances are created in the brain. Lack of quality sleep can dramatically decrease the quality of your life and greatly accelerate the ageing process.

So there is something going on here in the physiological connection between brain activity and hormone secretions. See section 5.9 for more on the critical HPA axis.

OK, enough technology. Go find out more about MMSS here: section 3.10.

3.11 The Science Of Loneliness

Before we go any further, let's examine the problem of loneliness. It's not usually diagnosed as a psychiatric disorder. But it is certainly a mental health issue.

Thing is, loneliness is very common; shockingly so.

Those who read my intimate and philosophical writings (Supernoetics) will know that I give special emphasis to LOVE (vitamin L). Love is not just something to give and get but love is who or what we are.

The sense of togetherness and belonging, being valued and appreciated, is crucial to our wellbeing.

Put another way, *loneliness is pathological.* And that's exactly what science shows. I'm not talking about elderly and isolated people, or those who society finds ugly or repellant. I mean anyone can be lonely, even in the middle of crowds, and it's really sickening. Loneliness is a public health disaster, linked to a slew of chronic illnesses.

Humans were not designed to be solitary creatures. We evolved to survive in tribes; the need to interact is deeply ingrained in our genetic code. So much so, says John Cacioppo, the director of the University of Chicago's Center for Cognitive and Social Neuroscience and author of *Loneliness: Human Nature and the Need for Social Connection,* that the absence of social connection triggers the same, primal alarm bells as hunger, thirst and physical pain.

Cacioppo has conducted dozens of studies and meta-analyses on how loneliness affects the mind and body. It's a bigger problem than you might think.

In the UK, for example, the Co-op and the British Red Cross found that more than 9 million adults are always or often lonely. The percentage of Americans who responded that they regularly or frequently felt lonely was between 11% and 20% in the 1970s and 1980s [the percentage varied depending on the study].

In 2010, the American Association of Retired Persons (AARP) did a nationally representative study in 2010 and found it was closer to 40% to 45%. And a recent study done on older adults out of University of California, San Francisco put it as high as 43%.

And yet we barely talk about it.

Why?

It is not hard to find plausible reasons. More people live alone, and the number of single-parent households is rising. Education and work mean that many of us live far away from our families. Marriages and relationships break down and it seems many hopefuls just give up. At the same time, technology has changed the way we work, shop, socialize and entertain ourselves, largely serving to reduce the amount of face-to-face contact we get. People seem to spend more time interacting with their electronic "toys" than with fellow humans!

This adds up to an epidemic of loneliness. Yes, epidemic, since chronic loneliness is very damaging to people's mental and physical well-being. As a public health problem it is up there with smoking and obesity, yet it hardly registers in the public mind. Doctors too are mostly ignorant of the weight of this phenomenon.

I introduced it in my compendium book *"Get Healthy For Your Next 100 Years"* (happily now re-issued under the title *"How To Live Beyond 100 Years"*), as one of the major causes of early death.

The sense of belonging is so precious to us that if we do feel alone, we tend to die early. Companionship keeps you alive! In a 19-year study, women who reported feeling lonely most of the time had a 76 percent increased risk of heart disease. Chronic loneliness, like stress, may trigger inflammatory and hormonal changes that promote cardiovascular disease.

It could also be, of course, that people living alone don't look after themselves properly, eating poorly and not taking enough care of personal health issues.

Either way, there is a new term, "emotional longevity," coined by Norman B. Anderson, Ph.D., the CEO of the American Psychological Association, and the author of the book titled, *Emotional Longevity: What Really Determines How Long You Live.*

Emotional longevity, says Anderson, is about connections—connections between biology and social relationships; among biology, beliefs, and behavior; and between biology and emotions. We have long believed some of these connections are important, and science has now confirmed them as such, but other connections are much more surprising.

One of the strongest contexts for getting and receiving warmth and support is marriage. More than 100 years of research finds that a sound marriage is good for your health. Married people live longer and have fewer chronic diseases than do single, widowed, or divorced people.

Divorced people live somewhat longer than unmarried people but less than those who remain firmly married. So, one may jokingly quote the poet Tennyson: "Tis better to have loved and lost than never to have loved at all"!

Something Has To Be Done

If anything, the trends driving increased loneliness have become even more apparent, and our scientific understanding of its impact has become much clearer. We also know how to intervene, quite easily and cheaply. Curing loneliness might just be the most cost effective public health intervention available.

There are answers. They just need implementing.

There may not be much we can do about social trends driving the epidemic, but our collective denial of it definitely needs to change. There are welcome signs that this is happening. Before she was murdered in 2016, British MP Jo Cox was working to create a national commission on loneliness. That has now been realized posthumously, bringing together MPs and various campaigns to raise awareness.

In her maiden speech to the UK House of Commons in 2015, Cox famously said "we have far more in common with each other than things that divide us".

Yet the archetype persists of old, odd and infirm people being the "lonely ones" and that it is something that does not affect the rest of us.

Prepare for a shock then:

More young people (18 – 34 years) feel cut off and lonely than old people. Here's the simplified demographic...

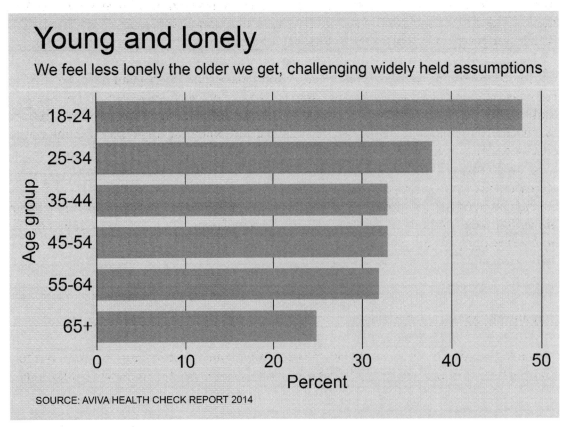

SOURCE: AVIVA HEALTH CHECK REPORT 2014

Why does it affect young people more? According to John Cacioppo, we all need different amounts of social contact. It is this, rather than the objective amount of social contact we have, that determines how prone we are to emotional isolation.

The environment plays a large role too. Some people, such as teenagers and those with certain mental health problems, may be especially prone to loneliness because they can tend to misread social cues.

You would think that trawling FaceBook, as youngsters do, might make them feel connected. But actually the opposite effect is likely: a young surfer rambling through FB pages might feel left out from all those exciting "other lives" they are seeing. It's unlikely that someone of average IQ is going to realize that what they are seeing on social media is highly curated (an internet term, meaning cherry-picked or edited for content).

Loneliness Is Bad For Our Health

A meta-analysis of nearly 150 studies found that a poor quality of social relationships had the same negative effect on risk of death as smoking, alcohol and other well-known factors such as inactivity and obesity. Correcting for demographic factors, loneliness increases the odds of early mortality by 26 percent. That's about the same as living with chronic obesity.

One apparent reason is that loneliness lowers willpower, so we are more likely to indulge in self-defeating behavior. We may take risks and make bad decisions – from choosing unhealthy food, to avoiding exercise. Feeling socially isolated also increases the risk of mental health problems such as anxiety, stress, depression and eating disorders, all of which can have a knock-on effect on our physical health.

We're just beginning to understand what serious consequences that can have. Loneliness changes the brain, taking hold of our thoughts and behaviors in ways that are likely to make us feel even more isolated. But its effects are not just psychological; they are also physical. Left unchecked, loneliness can have a physiological impact as detrimental to longevity as smoking or obesity.

Researchers at the Aarhus Sygehus University Hospital in Aarhus, Denmark ("the happiest city in the world"), tracked over 138,000 people. Men above the age of 50, and women above 60, who lived alone were particularly at risk. Despite constituting just 8% of the whole study population, these groups accounted for more than 96% of all deaths.[239]

Screaming Signal

Perhaps the biggest effect may be on the genes that control the immune system. In their first study together, Cacioppo and Cole compared gene expression in the white blood cells of two groups. In one group were six persistently lonely middle-aged adults and in the other were eight who ranked as consistently socially enfranchised.

In the lonelier people, the activity of genes responsible for inflammation was ramped right up. "The signal was screaming loud—it could not have been more clear," says Cole.

Inflammation is the body's first line of defence against injury and bacterial infection, but too much inflammation has been linked to numerous diseases, including a whole array of psychological issues, including depression, bipolar disorder, anxiety, Alzheimer's, schizophrenia, fibromyalgia and a whole host of autoimmune diseases with a strong psychological component.

But if loneliness is so bad for us, why have we evolved to feel this way? That's possibly not such a mystery. A short pang of loneliness probably helped us to survive in our evolutionary past. Social primates like us live in groups as a means of protection.

Loneliness is a potential warning symptom. Just like hunger, thirst and pain, it tells us we must do something, or suffer the consequences. Trouble is, if we cannot solve the lack, we suffer that deficiency symptom chronically. That seems to be the fate of many people today.

Summary:

- 31% of people surveyed in the US feel lonely at least once a week

- 48% of people in the UK believe we are getting lonelier

- The health impact of loneliness is equivalent to smoking 15 cigarettes a day.

- Loneliness increases the odds of early mortality by 26 percent, about the same risk as chronic obesity.

- Living alone means a 76 percent increased risk of heart disease.

- The effect of social isolation is comparable to that of high blood pressure or lack of exercize

- But perhaps the biggest effect may be on the genes that control the immune system. In the lonelier people studied, the activity of genes responsible for inflammation was ramped right up. Too much inflammation has been linked to cancer, depression, Alzheimer's disease and obesity.

How Lonely Are You?

To measure loneliness, researchers commonly use the UCLA Loneliness Scale, first developed by Daniel Russell and colleagues at the University of California, Los Angeles, in 1978. The original version is reserved for research only, in case too many people become familiar with the test and skew future results. But Russell has created the following shorter test, which is claimed to be just as accurate.

Answer the questions using a scale from 1 to 4, where 1 = never, 2 = rarely, 3 = sometimes and 4 = always, then calculate your total score.

1. How often do you feel unhappy doing so many things alone?

2. How often do you feel you have no one to talk to?

3. How often do you feel you cannot tolerate being so alone?

4. How often do you feel as if no one understands you?

5. How often do you find yourself waiting for people to call or write?

6. How often do you feel completely alone?

7. How often do you feel unable to reach out and communicate with those around you?

8. How often do you feel starved of company?

9. How often do you feel it is difficult for you to make friends?

10. How often do you feel shut out and excluded by others?

How You Scored

20 is the average score on this survey

25 or higher reflects a high level of loneliness

30 or higher reflects very high levels of loneliness

3.12 Supernoetics® and Punk Psychology®

Throughout the text, you will have noticed me referencing my science of consciousness and Being that I call Supernoetics® (*noetics/noetikos* Ancient Greek: study of mind, soul or spirit). We all know what super means: biggest, best, most complete... etc.

So you could say Supernoetics® is the best-of-ME or "ME to the max"!

It's about getting into the best possible state of mind, to make the wisest choices and get the most fulfilling outcomes, not just for yourself but for everyone around you. This isn't selfish. You may have heard of the concept of *enlightened self-interest*. It means that your world has to be good in all aspects, to enjoy the best of mental and spiritual health. You can't get there by hurting others. Indeed (scientific fact): the number one path to happiness is to serve others, not to grab what you want, as many seem to think.

Studies show that, once the basics are taken care of (food, shelter, etc.), then more and more wealth does not bring increased happiness. The only thing researchers found brought an increase in meaningful happiness was helping other people to get what they needed.[240]

Putting others first is called *prosocial* behavior. In a 2016 study, published in the journal *Emotion*, the surprising outcome was that ONLY those who were generous to others, at the exclusion of self interests, were able to report positive emotions. In turn, these increases in feelings such as happiness, joy, and enjoyment predicted increases in psychological flourishing at the end of the study.[241]

Memory Is What Makes Us What We Are... BUT

Memory is your worst enemy!

Think about it: we carry around all the hurts, conflicts, upsets and tragedies in our store of memories. This locker-full of misery is never addressed in life; it's just left to fester. We go on flinging more and more painful trash into this memory bin and then wonder why our life isn't so enjoyable.

It doesn't sound very sensible when somebody puts it like that, does it? In fact it sounds downright STUPID. But that's the basic problem with our powerful human ability to recall... we have no means (until now) of cleaning out the misery dumped in our memory locker.

The only existing technique has been to ignore things, "try to forget" and dabble in a bit of whimsical philosophy. You probably know the old joke: *we're born, life's a bitch and then we die*. All too often, that neatly sums up the experience of living.

Wouldn't it be a good idea if someone eventually figured out how to clean up the rotten-memory trash, strip it of crud and put it back in place, all shiny and harmless, useful memory that can no longer cause hurt or pain?

As an MD who has spent more than half a lifetime watching people suffer, I've always thought such a method would be a real breakthrough in relieving misery everywhere. It would be a fantastic achievement, comparable to the discovery of anesthetics, microbes, antibiotics and nutrition.

Well, not to boast: it's been done! I can prove it to you. Hundreds have already learned the truth... Memory does not have to hurt!

You don't have to lie to yourself and pretend it doesn't hurt (that's just denial).

And you don't have to sit around patiently for decades, waiting for "time to heal". Actually, here's a shock for you: time does NOT heal. It's a myth. Time just covers over the deposits of pain. It buries things but does not heal them.

We've walked boldly with individuals into the memory of events that took place over half a century previously and, within moments, found him or her bawling helplessly. Events from decades ago lose none of their power. Not one drop of the pain goes away; it's all sitting there, festering, and ready to whack you one in the dandynuts, when you are least expecting it.

In fact I have theorized at times that maybe that's actually how we die. One day, the hurt in mind finally gets to us, lots of it at once, and we can't go on living.

If that's is too fanciful for you, consider this: if left unaddressed, unpleasant, stressful memories will come out sooner or later... as disease or death. That's an established scientific fact.

Stress remains the number one killer; the Grand Emperor of all dis-ease, including cancer and heart attack.

The Double-Edged Sword

Memory has value, of course. It's learning. Memory is skill. Knowledge.

But memory is one of the deadliest tools we have in our mental armory. We couldn't manage without it—but we can never be truly happy with it!

NOT, that is, unless someone could figure out how to separate the pain from the actual memory content.

And I repeat: it's been done!

And in case you are wondering, one of the great things about this garbage-disposal operation is that memories in general become more accessible. Without the pain to obscure possibly-uncomfortable memories, recall becomes easier and broader. Your memory will improve by leaps and bounds. Sweeter Memory Is Better Memory.

I call this breakthrough Punk Psychology®. It's part of a far bigger human potential rescue package called Supernoetics®. With it, we are "working towards the purposeful re-invention of Mankind®".

Now we can not only release stress but change our emotions, thoughts and behaviors for the better.

Can you imagine the effect on our world if people just STOPPED being crazy, destructive, vicious, and hysterical? It would be like a dream... no more wars, no more murders, in fact no crime at all! That would mean no more armed police and no more armies needed to fight and kill supposed enemies!

Politicians would become sane and honest; they would govern for the people, not their own gain; government would eventually become what it is supposed to be: a system of effective management that is there to serve the individuals in society and allow them to lead the kind of life they choose! As a result of that, taxes would be something we were all more willing to pay over, since we could see the money being used how we wanted!

Divorce rates would plummet; delinquency would become a thing of the past; popular music could celebrate all the good things in life, instead of whining and moaning about loss and betrayal; mental hospitals would empty out (and a good lot of patients in regular hospitals could go home too, because stress is behind most sickness); drugs such as anti-depressants and tranquillizers could be consigned to the history books...

It all starts with the human mind. So the solutions must also start with the human mind. Can we understand ourselves fully, and correct what's not working properly? I passionately believe so and have plenty of cases and experience to back up what I say.

There are answers. Real answers. Punk Psychology® can do this!

There is far too much mystique out there, disinformation, myth and nonsense, created by under-performing researchers, who insist on confusing the mind with the brain and equate consciousness with perceptions, which are both follies of the first magnitude.

Not only are they scrabbling in the wrong direction, trying to understand the mind. They have the cheek to argue you can't go there! It's their domain of skills, they claim. Ha! We've already looked at how incompetent the so-called experts are at explaining and managing the human mind!

We don't need them. Our own existence is based in the mind and you are as entitled as anyone else to learn about yourself, to experiment, to follow threads of reasoning, and to test experience for yourself.

So Where Do We Start?

Punk Psychology® is NOT just talking, it's NOT hypnotism, it's NOT role-play, this is NOT affirmations, it's NOT EFT (which is only dressed up affirmations, anyway), it is NOT meditation or mindfulness, NOT counseling, not EMDR, yoga, mysticism, or any other modality you have likely heard of.

It's certainly NOT Freud. In fact there is 21st century science, straight out of Harvard University, which I'll come to in a moment, to back up the core technique I have evolved.

Let me start with an axiomatic principle, which I call the **Mind's Number One Algorithm**. Have you ever stopped to consider what the mind actually DOES all the time?

It is scanning the present environment for cues, which are compared with past learning and experience (memory), from which predictions about the future are made, and a course of action chosen which brings about the most enhancement.

Let's look at that in more detail... There are really four ways thinking can go wrong:

1. Faulty perception

2. Faulty memory banks

3. Faulty predictions

4. Unwise or inappropriate actions

If you are honest you will admit that, like the rest of us, you've messed up on all four counts. But if you are smart, you'll see that the number one problem is malfunctioning memory. If your databanks (to use a computer term) are telling you something different to what is true, then you can't hope to respond to your world in a meaningful and effective way. You'll mess up, either through inappropriate emotions, poor or destructive behaviors, and negative beliefs and experiences that lead you in all directions except the one most desirable?

It doesn't matter if your faulty memories have come from bad education, memes (thought viruses), hoaxes (everybody knows that... but it isn't true), or hidden pain from the subconscious mind. Without what I call *clean and useful memory* (no emotional clutter), you can't even begin to function effectively.

So, how do we clean up bad memories and emotional charges that linger to throw us off track? We are, in a sense, hypnotized by our miserable past. We need to break free; come up to the surface; regain our presence in the NOW...

Sleep Walking

The core tool in Punk Psychology® we call Hypnoetics™. Don't be disturbed by the fact that it sounds a bit like hypnotism. Hypnoetics™ is actually UN-hypnotizing people. It's taking them out of their trance, into the NOW!

That might seem a shocking idea—that people are walking around as if asleep. But it's actually not a new concept. French psychiatrist Pierre Janet (1859—1947) pioneered many extremely modern advances in the field of the mind. He even invented the term *unconscious mind* and developed amazing techniques that were later grabbed by Freud, who accidentally "forgot" to say he had stolen them from his colleague.

All that's history now and Freud has gone down the tubes, his weird sexual theories almost an historic joke; whereas Janet is literally being re-born, as scientists and psychologists in the 21st century discover his remarkable, insightful work.

Janet wrote about "somnambulism", which you probably know is a medical term that means sleepwalking. The person looks properly tuned in and present; but is not. He or she is not "here" but is working on automatic. And, as the original 19th century pioneers understood, we are all—to a degree—sleepwalking!

We function mostly normally. But we have a significant percentage of our attention units trapped elsewhere. We are in a kind of mind loop, sticking to past unpleasant events. In Supernoetics® we call these unpleasant memories *memonemes*. The more we have our attention on these issues from the past, the less attention units we have for living in the present. In other words, the more asleep or hypnotized we are!

Influential early 20th-century mystic, philosopher and spiritual teacher, Georges Gurdjieff noticed the problem too. His famous saying was: *the biggest barrier to being conscious (alert and aware) is the delusion that we are already conscious.* Most people are not. Not fully.

Our task in Punk Psychology® then, is to UN-hypnotize people and get them back to the present. It's like sending out the lifeboat, to rescue them from rough seas of the mind, and then bring them safely ashore, to relaxation, calm and insight (awareness).

Cutting The Strings That Bind Us To The Past

You can perhaps imagine that by getting our attention off many troublesome events from the past, that we become more alert, brighter, quicker at thinking and with less "baggage" in our emotional processes. In fact that's just how it feels: clean, clear, alert and efficient in mind! A spotless memory!

How do we do this? It's simple (you can learn to do it, just sign up for free at **Punk Psychology**). We guide or "pilot" the person to wherever he or she is stuck in the past and

UN-stick them! How do we know where to look? The answer is quite simple, but again quite modern: we use a biofeedback device that tells us what memories are significant and where to find the hidden, stormy memonemes. We call it GPS for the mind!

Regression therapy: isn't that old fashioned?

Nope. True, the idea has been around a long while (since 1868, when Dutch physician Andries Hoek provided the first case study of cathartic hypnotherapy in fact) but the actual modern technique we use—easy, fun and very effective—was only developed by me and a handful of colleagues in the late 20th century.

For over a quarter of a century, I have been able to produce remarkable changes, using a technique I call "make it now technique" (MINT for short). I now know I was correct in my thinking. Modern studies at Stamford and Harvard Universities have backed up my clinical experience with scientific theory. Researchers now talk about "plastic" memory. They have shown that memory is not simply a storage and retrieval system, as everyone thinks. If we want to "remember" something, we recreate the memory, on the spot, to look at. They call it reconsolidation.

Thing is, the memory is completely soft and mushy at that exact moment of creation (recall) and we can tweak it, re-fashion it, to give us better messages. We can strip out the pain, the blackness, the misdirection, the faulty thinking around it and make it nice and shiny, comfortable and clean in a jiffy!

So, far from being an old procedure, Punk Psychology® is really a modernization of a well-established (proven) concept. Hence the term "punk", something edgy, fresh, different and a bit startling!

We call it piloting because it's essentially like steering. We find a "place" in the mind! We have our detailed map and we use the mind-GPS device to know exactly where we are in a chain of events or what we call a "thread". Think of it like a riverboat pilot, knowing what to do and where to go.

Most importantly, we do not need drugs or any other chemical "solution" to improve mental function and performance. We are not trying to "solve" a difficulty, or come up with an answer or adaptation. We fully eradicate the dependence on the unpleasant emotions of the past.

Thing is, all negative emotions and unsuccessful behaviors (ineffective strategies, you might say) were installed for a reason. They worked once. But that was then! This is Now! We don't need to go back there every time an issue arises.

In piloting we don't lose our unpleasant memories altogether. We need those for learning and experience. What we don't need is the pain and misery; but that's gone!

This is an important point. If you suffer agoraphobia (fear of the outdoors and open spaces) because of being attacked in a dark alley, we want you to break out of your fear. But we want you to do it rationally, not from avoidance or denial. To recover fully, not just cope. You will be free to develop a future safety strategy for walking alone, based on what you learned. But the life-impairing fear will be gone. You will recall the events of that night, without quailing or switching on your incapacitating flight-or-fight response. Your memory of events has become helpful, instead of creating terror.

And so it goes with any kind of memory. Good to have; minus the pain.

So You Think You Know?

The Supernoetics® number one secret to a new and happy life: *the problem is not what you think it is!* Or to put it another way, where you think your problem is coming from is never correct.

There is a simple rule: when you find the real source of an issue, it vanishes. It's a kind of psychology functional magic we call Deep-IS. The surface layer, or the Simple-IS, is what appears on the outside; that's how it looks. But it cannot be true because, if it was, the problem would vanish instantly. Deep-IS is a special kind of impermanance; it's the same quality of magic at the moment of creation as at the moment of vanishment.

Zen philosophy and many sages over the ages have noticed that truth is ephemeral... Time (persistence) is a lie and only attained by altering something; in other words making it less than true. Anything which persists contains some falseness. Real truth evaporates, to become part of the infinite field of all-knowing.

Does this sound troubling and complex? Don't worry. It may be, at first sight. But you will work with this axiomatic truth throughout this book and discover for yourself that real truth does not contain persistence. Hence the difficulties we encounter only persist because there is a lie. Once you get past the lie, to the real truth (Deep-IS), the problem simply disappears. That's great. There's an old saying: "The truth will set you free". Seems that it is correct, after all.

We have a technical expression for this: *negative gains*. Getting good results by dropping out what is not wanted. No, it's not an oxymoron. It's a very real mechanism. When you find the real reason for an effect, the deeper truth, it vanishes like morning mist in the noonday sun!

Sometimes the individual forgets there even was a problem! It takes a friend to say "You're not scared of flying any more?" for the client to realize they once had a problem but it's no longer present and he or she doesn't even remember they had a difficulty!

This complete vanishment is one of the important contributions of Punk Psychology®. When it's gone, it's gone! Someone likened this to blowing up anti-personnel mines. When you've exploded one, you can ever after step on it without an explosion. Good metaphor!

Do We All End Up Identical Plastic Dolls?

Not on my watch! The truth is, by shedding unwanted strife and negativity, we come to be more our own unique selves, not more like everybody else.

In reality, the dark mechanisms of the mind are somewhat universal in character and effect. We share those. The light, free, good humored personal aspect of our thoughts and character is the part that is unique to us.

So don't worry; we are talking personal freedom and expanded awareness, not squeezing everyone into the same mould.

But without your pain and emotions, aren't you a poor shadow of a human being? That's a common misconception you will certainly come across. Again, it's misguided. Yes, stormy emotions, ridiculous beliefs and absurd destructive behaviors are common, you might even say normal, but that doesn't make these behaviors desirable.

C'mon! Road rage doesn't make you a better driver, now does it?

The idea that it is noble to suffer and we need emotional hurt and strife is, quite frankly, baloney. In Supernoetics® we call these "everybody knows it's true" follies a hoax. Hoaxing is a widespread vice we'd like to get rid of! Especially this one: that behaving badly and throwing our negative emotions all over the place is not just desirable; it's our right!

What complete and insupportable nonsense. It's peddled largely by people who cannot cope with their own irrationality and emotional overload. Getting drunk continuously or taking mind-invasive drugs is not necessary to be a creative and productive person.

Ask Michelangelo! He didn't need self-abuse to create his masterpieces, though it is generally accepted that he had some kind of *terribilitá* (Italian word for driven by personal demons of overwhelming intensity).

Helping Others

The great thing about Punk Psychology® is that you can use it to help people around you, all the time! You can also buddy up with someone and hack away at each other's lousy emotions and irrationality. That's why it's optimistic punk!

Some of us feel (or believe) we are leading very good, meaningful lives. Maybe we are not struggling, as so many people are, to find happiness, purpose and reward in life.

That doesn't mean we have no interest in the mechanics of mind and the structures of a workable philosophy of success. It just means we need to develop the expertise of helping others who are not so fortunate and may be making heavy weather of it all.

Would it not be valuable and life-changing to get a grasp of some of the key mechanics of the mind and its workings?

You could become the go-to person for your tribe or network. It really is electrifying to be able to recognize what someone is experiencing and know why it is happening to them. As you share your knowledge, people will look to you for solutions and advice.

What To Do:

Remember, **Supernoetics**® is a HUGE library of protocols, workshops, hacks and tips that can solve just about any life situation. Punk Psychology® is only a small part of the whole; but a very handy part, nonetheless.

You can look around **Punk Psychology** website as well: www.PunkPsychology.net. You can watch videos, download eBooks and pamphlets, sign up for some training to become a pilot and help change the world.

You can find detailed information in the Valuable Resources section in the back of the book.

3.13 The Pips Phenomenon

No work on holistic psychiatry and the impacts of stress could avoid this topic (even though nobody is writing or talking about it!)

I call it pipping and the individuals affected are thus "pips". I am talking about the woeful tendency of some individuals to crush or suppress others. It seems as if a small percentage of the population (less than 2% probably) seem to want to get ahead by bringing down others.

Unfortunately, these few people are difficult to spot; individuals higher in social skills and awareness can only recognize them, as their game strategy unfolds. They always seem to present a cheerful facade, often with a nervous laugh and constant smile. They appear calm, pleasant and resourceful at times.

But inside they are seething. Their "solution" to life is predicated on controlling others.

At this time I don't have a suitable name for such individuals (certainly not pipsters!) but they are the Sly Ones. Their characteristics are quite clear and the main ones can be listed as follows:

Through their appearance, words, propaganda or advertising they present themselves, their services or products as being 'so nice, so charming, so condescending and so helpful'. They may seem to be concerned about you, in politely asking probing personal questions about you, your work, your relationships, your sex life, your politics or your religion.

They are storing up ammunition, because they are highly manipulative, they engage in gossip readily but have no qualm in covertly twisting facts around, to knife someone in the back whenever, wherever and to whomever they can.

For objectives that they are too lazy or fearful to undertake themselves, they covertly manipulate and subjugate individuals above and below them on the social scale (Pips) to do their bidding and dirty work.

When confronted, they change the subject to move away from the point and are always rewriting history or changing the truth about past events to suit their current position. They will do and say anything to avoid exposure.

Their targets are any individual, families, tribes, companies or nations that they consider high on the scale and therefore a threat (e.g. +3s, +4s etc.), attempting to "pip" them and bring them down to chronic appeasement, grief and apathy (Minus 4 and Minus 5).

Their *unstated* aim is to cause ruin, discredit achievements and split up relationships. At this they can be very successful and gloat when their victims go down into the lower chronic levels of Minus 4 and 5.

Males at this level subconsciously know their fearful limitations. They can be slothful, but have a need to control and suppress women down to the -4 and -5 levels so that they can feel secure in their sexuality, (also somewhat true of males at -1 and -2).

You could never trust anyone at this level with your health, your money, your reputation, your safety, your husband, your wife, your children, your business, your company, your country, or this planet.

Grima Wormtongue, in J R R Tolkein's story *The Lord Of The Rings* was such an individual. As was Iago in Shakespeare's instructive masterpiece: *Othello*.

The victims, or **Pips,** do literally limp through life, like cripples. These are your Borderline cases. While ever they are stuck to the Sly One that is manipulating them, he or she will never be free and happy. The Sly will effectively see to that.

Borderline Personality Disorder (Emotionally Unstable) is the classic Pip characteristic; a condition characterized by rapid mood shift, impulsivity, hostility and chaotic social relationships. People with borderline personality disorder usually go from one emotional crisis to another. The wild mood swings are diagnostic: up then down, up again, then down.

For psychotherapists, Pips are a problem, because they appear to be with us and even, at times, seem to do well. But the Sly has other plans and sooner or later will bring their victim down. That reflects disastrously on you as a therapist. You will appear to have failed. You will be blamed...

Sickos. You may recognize this name from Michael Moore's jocular film title for his exposé movie about the US medical care system. "Sicko" is a pun on *Psycho*, the famous movie, of course. But by Sickos here, I mean chronically sick people. They need not be crazy (psycho), or borderline, or malingerers, or in any way wanting to be sick. But he or she has definite mental issues, as well as their physical challenges. They are definitely manifesting the "pipping" phenomenon.

I constantly warn people never to marry, or enter into a long-term relationship with, a chronically sick person. Such an individual has big personal issues and you will inevitably be drawn in. He or she is a Pip.

But a word of caution: *people are often chronically sick because no one knows how to help them.* Depression, anxiety, headaches, inflammations, metabolic disturbances, sexual difficulties, weight disorders and many other chronic conditions may be due to food allergies, chemical overload, nutritional deficiencies and other so-called lifestyle issues. Often there are multiple factors leading to ill health. The person may not really be sick at all, just burdened by toxins!

That's what this book is about. One thing is for sure: people with health issues need to clean them up, *before* deeply engaging in a relationship with others or with the whole topic of mental health and happiness.

The way back to wholeness for the individual is not to "disconnect" from the pippers. We all know Scientology made itself hated all over the world by coming up with that strategy. The thing is, disconnecting is vicious, divisive, judgmental and *totally unnecessary.*

What is really needed is that the individual recognizes that—under the pipping influence—he or she at some point decided to make themselves smaller. It is only necessary to spot that moment, then write up a full list of negative dogma that he or she bought into—and disconnect from that; dump the negative beliefs.

This is simply done. In Supernoetics®, my advanced research into mind and Being, we have a simple and effective solution. We call it the Freedom Technique, because it frees the individual from past malevolent influences (*mal* plus *volare* (to wish): Latin for evil wishing or intending evil).

Learn more about the Supernoetics® Freedom Technique on the Punk Psychology website.

3.14 The Tangled Wing

I have taken this term from the writings of Melvin Konner MD. In 1982 Melvin put out a book he called *The Tangled Wing* (Holt, Reinhart and Wilson, New York). He's a materialist, which means he misses the true nature of consciousness by a long mile. But his sensitive and straightforward discussion ranges across topics such as the roots of aggression, the basis of attachment and desire, the differences between the sexes, and the foundations of mental illness.

It is the essence of the subtitle that reveals most: *Biological Constraints On The Human Spirit*. Konner's captivating metaphor has stuck with me since I read the book: that our biology holds us down and tangles with our yearning to be spiritually free and fly away. It clips our wings, so to speak. We want higher things in mind but the nasty "creature" aspect of our nature has other ideas!

We may be adducts to the state of God but we are also mammals, brutish and violent, sometimes with a very bad attitude. It seems the two aspects of our being are irreconcilable.

From here on I depart from Konner's materialistic evolutionary view. Without agreeing with any of his deductions concerning Darwinism, I believe I can explain some or all of the nature of the conflict he highlighted.

Basically, the creature's drive is survival: reproduction, DNA, who whole nine yards of sex and spreading genes. The principal emotion of our creature self is fear. It wants to live. It is greedy with resources. It is frightened whenever there are threats. Of course living in fear leads to unruly and at times evil behavior. The creature wants to survive at all costs and pays no regard to the rights of others.

The spirit, on the other hand, cannot die (otherwise it is hardly a spirit!) So it does not know fear. The principal emotion of spirit, I believe, is LOVE. The main drive, since it is not struggling to survive, is purpose or meaning. A spirit without some purpose or meaning in its life is very much a lost soul.

This model of the two selves is not recognized in mainstream biology, psychology or psychiatry. So a great deal of confusion is generated. Depending on which aspect of human nature you focus, you will get answers that are aligned with Darwinian socialism (dominance of the strongest), or are mystical and inspiring, and speak of a higher ethical and altruistic calling.

Are we akin to Thomas Hobbes' monstrous sluggard, who renders his and the lives of others around him:

"solitary, poor, nasty, brutish, and short".

Or are we angels, as described in Shakespeare's immortal words (put into the mouth of Hamlet):

What a piece of work is a man! How noble in reason! how infinite in faculty! in form and moving, how express and admirable! in action how like an angel! in apprehension how like a god! the beauty of the world! the paragon of animals!

If you look at the mixture of cruelty and art, reason and madness, or exploitation and divinity that you find in humans, you will rightly be confused over how the two coexist. Yet they do.

But we can go further still in this explanation of our mystical or spiritual side. Here we drop off the psychology and biology Richter scale altogether.

3.15 The Complex Of Self

This section is perhaps the most crucial in the whole book. Whatever your mental challenges—or even if you consider yourself healthy and normal, with no such challenges, but are reading this book—you can understand the inner world of "Self" better, if you grasp the model I am about to share.

I call it The Complex Of Self.

In a word: *the idea that we are single Self entity or unity is false.* We only appear to be a single self. In reality we are, as one knowledgeable MD put it, a "mob". There is more than one thinking entity going to make up the psychic space that you are used to thinking of as YOU!

This is hard to grasp: when we are brought up to think wrongly; when textbooks ignore the truth; when everyday experiences that prove this model is true are simply explained away as mental weaknesses, or even disease states, then you can't expect to recognize it without some help.

Oh, it's not a new idea. The early Christian Gnostics understood this phenomenon very well: "For many spirits dwell in it [the body] and do not permit it to be pure; each of them brings to fruition its own works, and they treat it abusively by means of unseemly desires." (Valentinus, 100- 160 AD)

Basilides, teaching around 120- 140 AD, said "[Man]... preserves the appearance of a wooden horse, according to the poetic myth, embracing as he does in one body a host of such different spirits."

Life after death researcher Frederick W. Myers wrote movingly of "group souls".

In modern times, Greek-Armenian mystic George Gurdjieff (1866-1949) writes of us having many "I's" (many selves or many "Me's").

You need to start with the non-material mind model, to understand this properly. If we are all non-material thinking beings, peeping into the material domain through our eyes, listening with our ears, and generally learning, as babies, to make the physical body do what we want it to do, then you will readily see that any other non-material thought entity can do the same.

We could even have another thought entity trying to use our body to work with! That is the origin of walk-ins, possession, demons and entities (see section 6.5). This whole concept is no longer in the realm of woo-woo and weird. Modern post-material science says these things not only *could* happen but logically *predicts* that we will get these effects!

Far from being signs of mental disease or disorder, these phenomena might just be fairly normal. But the people defining "mental health" are too stupid to see that and insist—since we are a brain—the whole concept is an absurd delusion and the person is therefore sick.

You Already Know This!

All this might seem strange to you at first but actually this concept is present in our everyday language, once you know what to look for. Common expressions that represent this phenomenon include: "I'm of two minds about this," "Something tells me...," "My gut tells me...," "A little voice inside whispered to me..." "I don't know why I behaved like that. It wasn't really me..."

Some of these thought entities we share with are, in effect, multiple parts of the self ("other selves"), whereas some are present, creating an influence, but not part of self, so I would call these "non-self others". We can consider these collectively as extraneous beings or EBs, for this work.

To repeat, what we believe to be our single "self" (Me) is in fact a conglomerate of individual viewpoints, with varying degrees of penetration and expression in the individual's personality. Sometimes wholly different viewpoints may take over. But eventually the boss identity will re-assert its authority.

This is what is happening with serial killers, who slide in and out of their sadistic killer identity, but when back to their "normal" self have no recollection of what they did. If you want a little further insight into this, then read Ted Bundy's last interview, before he was executed for serial murders. You can find it online.

Of course the average person is totally unaware that his or her mind is actually divided into multiple entities, capable of acting independently. The reason is that in most people, these parts of self are so well integrated that we rarely notice the seamless join, when control shifts from one to another.

The illusion of a single mind is further enhanced by the fact that all the multiple consciousness particles are associated with the same body and thus share the same name; each one considers itself to be "I". The "I's" are most noticeable when they are in conflict with each other. We then have "mixed feelings": coexisting contrary attitudes.

A particularly brilliant model in this respect is Dick Schwartz's Internal Family Systems. He's not talking about family in the normal sense, but the family of selves within.

I use the expression "cloud consciousness" for this phenomenon.

Of course there is a kind of "executive self", one who rides over and above all, looking, thinking, sensing and above all Being, as a single-focus viewpoint. That could be called the True Self. As we progress along our spiritual pathway, shedding unwanted encumbrances and identities, we come closer and closer to our pure Self or Being.

Don't Worry. Be Happy

(words of a song by Bobby McFerrin)

If you get thoughts that are unpleasant, such as perversions, obsessions, vile desires, desperate cravings, horrible or violent ideas, compulsions or other strange effects, do not be too alarmed. Now you know, it probably isn't you. It will likely be coming from one of these "other" thought identities. (see The Hearing Voices Movement, below).

Don't let it distress and confuse you too much is the message here. Don't let supposed experts crowd you and insist you are crazy and need medication. I want to tell schizophrenics (and perfectly normal people who hear voices), don't be alarmed: there are living thinking entities out there and many of them want to communicate with you and via you

Some are angry, because you don't acknowledge their presence. Others are disappointed that you don't recognize the help they bring. Still others have unusual desires or skills, such as artistic talent, math genius and savantism.

But these extraneous entities can also contribute very bad thoughts and desires, crazy or wicked actions and baffling ideas that you somehow know are not your own ideas. I have heard many mental patients say these feelings or ideas come from "somewhere" but not within. That's correct. They are coming from some part of the greater self or "cloud consciousness" but not the real YOU!

And as you come to understand that the bizarre or obnoxious stuff is really coming from "someone else", *don't start getting judgmental.* That won't do any good. It will just drive the thought form out of communication. This whole phenomenon is really not so disturbing or frightening, if you just remain calm and acknowledge that this comes from, as I say, "someone else"!

The point is that, at some level, we all have positive intentions. That applies also to extraneous beings. They don't set out to deliberately cause mischief but their way of going about things will often seem counter-productive, strange or stupid to you. Just remember this is a separate "thought entity" with its own ideas about life.

Not Pathological

Everyone supposes that hearing voices inside your head is a sign of severe mental illness. It's one of the hallmark symptoms of schizophrenia.

But wait a minute: suppose there really are voices inside the head? Everyone assumes that the voices are unreal, or imagined—a hallucination if you like. But what if that's not true? What if the voices are REAL?

As I just explained, there truly are the voices of other parts of Self. It's something I have been working on for decades. Most of us hear them but ignore them, or it's such an ephemeral phenomenon, we just brush it off. However, certain individuals get seriously engaged with their internal voices, they hear them loud and clear, there are dialogues, arguments, agreements, conflicts...Lots of famous people have been there, done that and got the T-shirt. OK, that doesn't make it "normal" but it is "common." You may find that re-assuring.

Joan of Arc famously heard voices, which she ascribed to God speaking to her. Who is to say she was wrong?

Anthony Hopkins, the actor, tells us: "I've always had a little voice in my head, particularly when I was younger and less assured", he admitted. "While onstage, during classical theatre the voice would suddenly say, "Oh, you think you can do Shakespeare, do you?" and he added; "Recently, I was being interviewed on television and the voice inside my head said to me, "Who the hell do you think you are. You're just an actor, what the hell do you know about anything".

William Blake, the poet and painter, said: "I know that our deceased friends are more really with us than when they were apparent to our mortal part. Thirteen years ago I lost a brother, and with his spirit I converse daily and hourly in the spirit, and see him in my remembrance, in the region of my imagination. I hear his advice, and even now write from his dictate."

Edith Somerville, co-author of the hilarious *Irish Resident Magistrate* series of books, always claimed her co-author, Violet Florence Martin (writing under the name Martin Ross) continued to work with her, even after Ross had passed on. If you are a fan of the pair, you would not doubt that assertion that the two still wrote as one.

And no less a person than Mahatma Ghandi, wrote: "For me the Voice of God, of Conscience, of Truth, or the Inner Voice or 'the Still Small Voice' mean one and the same thing. I saw no form. I have never tried, for I have always believed God to be without form. But what I did hear was like a Voice from afar and yet quite near. It was as unmistakable as some human voice definitely speaking to me, and irresistible. I was not dreaming at the time I heard the Voice. The hearing of the Voice was preceded by a terrific struggle within me. Suddenly the Voice came upon me. I listened, made certain it was the Voice, and the struggle ceased. I was calm. The determination was made accordingly, the date and the hour of the fast were fixed..."[242]

I have often wondered as a compassionate physician (I hope) what would happen if we went round telling patients with this complaint, "It's OK. I believe you," instead of telling him or her they are nuts. I think it could bring about enormous relief.

There is a recognized condition called multiple personality "disorder", which even conventional psychiatrists recognize, in which a person manifests more than one identity or character. The point of this section is to show you that we all have multiple personality aspects. We are, as I said, not a single unity being or "self" at all!

3.16 Hearing Voices Movement

Perhaps you would be shocked to know how common this "voices" phenomenon is:

The published numbers vary widely, but one review of 17 existing studies across nine countries found that, on average, about 1 in 8 people surveyed reported an experience of hearing a voice that wasn't real.

Dr. Marius Romme MD PhD, a Dutch psychiatrist regarded as the founder and principal theorist for the Hearing Voices Movement, has this to say:

"In 1987, I had no idea the impact that the discovery that accepting and making sense of voices was a helpful alternative was going to have. Yet, after twenty three years of work we have built a unique and formidable movement of voice hearers and allies that has brought about a big change in the way hearing voices are regarded and has found new ways of helping people overwhelmed by their voices.

"There are many fears and misunderstandings in society and within psychiatry about hearing voices. They are generally regarded as a symptom of an illness, something that is negative, to be got rid of and consequently the content and meaning of the voice experience is rarely discussed.

"The research of Dr. Sandra Escher and myself with over 300 voice hearers has shown that over 70% of people who hear voices can point to a traumatic life event that triggered their voices; that talking about voices and what they mean is a very effective way to reduce anxiety and isolation; and that even when the voices are overwhelming and seemingly destructive they often have an important message for the hearer."[243]

A typical case would be Rachel Waddingham. She heard voices often: three men, mocking her; telling her she was stupid; urging her to kill herself. Psychiatrists diagnosed her with schizophrenia.

But Rachel Waddingham now rejects that diagnosis.

After more than a decade of taking medications and cycling in and out of mental hospitals, she has embraced a new way of thinking about her voices. She no longer tries to banish them with drugs, but accepts them as a part of herself. Waddingham now considers them a reflection of her feelings and experiences, signals that help her understand when and why she feels overwhelmed—rather than authorities whose commands she should follow.

Since going off her medications, she has been able to take on a demanding full-time job and got married.[244]

See, if only psychiatrists would get off this materialistic chemical model and actually *listen* to what patients are saying, they might learn something useful.

Charles Fernyhough, a psychology professor at Durham University in the U.K. who studies the topic, said one theory holds that the phenomenon appears to be similar to the self-talk that everyone does. It seems a certain percentage of people don't experience their internal monologues as being something that they themselves have produced, leading them to experience the voices as coming from another person.

Voice hearing "is unusual, but it's not in itself pathological," Fernyhough said.

Predictably, most of Fernyhough's colleagues do not agree. Many psychiatrists even question the patient's right to choose medication or not. They claim that people who are out of touch with reality and attempt to spurn "proper" treatment may pose a danger to themselves or others. But that pre-supposes that these people are out of touch with reality and, as you are learning, they are not at all. They may be the ones most in touch!

Notwithstanding, the pendulum is now swinging strongly away from the entrenched mechanistic view that these patients are sick and need chemical suppression of their symptoms.

Yes, it can be a heavy burden, to endure constant rattling in your skull that you are no good, stupid and a waste of space. But the best approach by far seems to be to work with these voices. If they really are the communications of independent, thinking entities, then you would expect them to get pissy and angry if nobody listens or treats THEM as idiots.

Many recovered voice hearers say that once they engage with the voices, their mental health improves—and the voices become nicer as well.

"For us, voices are a signal, they are something that tell you about your life," said Dr. Dirk Corstens, a psychiatrist and psychotherapist in Maastricht in the Netherlands and a leader in the Hearing Voices Movement. "You have to listen to [them]. Not obey, but listen."

The movement, which began in the Netherlands, has spread rapidly in the past three decades; there are now "hearing voices" support groups on all five continents, and over 180 in the U.K. alone, anchored by the Hearing Voices Network. The idea has been slower to take hold in the U.S., which has a strong medical model for treating mental illness, but is gaining momentum here, too.

There are now about 90 support groups across the U.S., according to the Hearing Voices Network USA.

Is There A Method To Make Sense Of This?

Gurdjieff was particularly insightful about this aspect of consciousness. His famous "Fourth Way" was about trying to disentangle one's True Self (the real YOU) from this net of other selves that are creating mental chatter. Gurdjieff thought you could master this phenomenon by just observing it carefully and becoming aware of what was going on. However I have found it is way beyond most people's ability to get to grips with.

I think it needs coaching, at least in the beginning stages, and I can commend the method we use in Supernoetics®, for talking to multiple identities. Our aim in doing this is to honor them and allow them to re-establish their freedom, to follow another purpose, and not feel tied or "stuck" to you! The Spiritual Rescue Technology, developed by David St Lawrence, is particularly effective in this regard and the laymen can learn to understand it and practice the method, with very little training and supervision.

In exploring these multiple selves, you will quickly learn that what you supposed were fixed thoughts, patterns or intrusive behaviors may turn out to be other parts of you, or even other thought entities that are living along with you. It's a fascinating road to self-discovery.

Most importantly, it sheds light and truth on many states of mind which are supposed to be pathological but which are only expressions of the Complex of Self model of consciousness.

3.17 We Are All Slightly Mad, Remember

To close this section, we should take a look at a phenomenon which, to a degree, makes madmen and mad women out of us all. I mean *cognitive dissonance*. What's that?

It's the mind's way of protecting itself from the truth, whenever contradictory or hard-to-integrate information comes along. Let me illustrate this with an anecdote.

The night before writing this, Vivien and I were re-watching one of our favorite British comedy shows: "*As Time Goes By*," starring Judy Dench. Dame Judy's character was a compulsive liar and fantasist. To get herself out of a tight fix she suddenly announced that her beau Lionel is a psychiatrist. He isn't.

But as the entanglement got worse and worse, someone asked to consult with him professionally. Dame Judy's character cornered him into continuing the pretense. So poor old Lionel ended up with a "patient" lying on the sofa, yakking up his guts about a flirtatious obsession with his younger secretary. Just talking about it released the man's fears and worries. He announced it is now solved and declared that Lionel was a really good psychiatrist.

Unable to contain the deception any longer, Lionel confesses that he was not really a psychiatrist at all.

"Not a psychiatrist," echoes the patient, smiling. " Oh, I see... that's very clever." And the patient is now convinced that this denial of status is a therapeutic tool and Lionel is a truly innovative psychiatrist at the top of his profession.

I mention this story in some detail because, although it's comedy fiction, it neatly summarizes the tendency we all have, to bend the "facts" to fit our own prejudices. It's something we all do and if you watch closely, a lot of comedy scripts rely on it.

And it's the basis of a great deal of supposed mental illness. For example when a man is convinced that someone is taking over his thoughts is he truly ill, or is he suffering only from cognitive dissonance?

It makes you think (or should).

Origins Of The Term

The original term *cognitive dissonance* was coined by social psychologist Leon Festinger. He and his colleagues investigated a famous case of it in some detail...

With monotonous regularity, the end of the world comes around! Despite the fact that it never happened the last time it was predicted, nor did it the time before, or the time before that... nevertheless, there is always an army of people ready to embrace such prophecies. The 2012 end of the Mayan calendar has some people in fits of anxiety... and, of course, many "spiritual" leaders got rich though offering solace for this particular end of days, supposedly foreseen long ago by a bunch of blood-thirsty savages (I have no regard for the Mayans).

One thing, however, invariably remains the same. At least since reliable historical records exist: *none of the predicted apocalypses has ever come true.*

Notwithstanding, on 20th December 1954, followers of Dorothy Martin, a housewife from Chicago, sat together and waited for the imminent deluge which would destroy the

Earth next day. But they were not afraid: before the end, they had been told, a flying saucer would land in Martin's garden and lift them all to safety.

Martin claimed to be in contact with aliens from the planet Clarion, who had chosen her as a medium for their revelations. Her true believers were well prepared for the last great journey. They had quit their jobs, left their schools, said goodbye to other family members and given away all their worldly goods. Just before midnight, according to the last instructions, they had removed all metal objects from their bodies, so as not to interfere with the flying saucer's navigational system, and waited.

In this instance, after hours of shocked and tense silence and weeping, the aliens dictated the solution to Dorothy Martin: God, moved by the sincerity of the little group, had abandoned his plan and saved the planet from destruction! This changed everything. The believers, earlier shunning the public, swarmed out and started to spread the "good news" with vigor and enthusiasm. They had "proved" to themselves that everything was alright; that God was loving and kind.

Festinger and his colleagues avidly followed the Dorothy Martin story and later published a famous study entitled "When Prophecy Fails" (1956).[245]

The fable of "The Fox and the Grapes", by Aesop, is an example of cognitive dissonance. A fox spies high-hanging grapes and wishes to eat them. When unable to reach the grapes, the fox decides the fruit is not worth eating, and he justifies his decision by claiming to himself that the grapes likely are sour, for being unripe.

We now have the expression "sour grapes", for any situation where a person rejects what he wants but can't have by convincing himself it is a worthless desire anyway. This is a way of reducing the level of dissonance and therefore being more comfortable (remember my key definition of stress in section 3.2, which is the gap between what you wanted and what you have got).

Cognitive dissonance offers the key to various social and psychological mechanisms behind religion, cults, magical thinking and various irrational behavior patterns.

And of course it is at work, deeply, within the psyche of any mentally distressed patient.

Please remember this. Have some compassion.

3.18 Engagement

The important point to make in closing this section is that we all have psychological stress factors to cope with. Life can be tough. We sometimes get hit pretty hard. There are upsets, setbacks, shocks, traumas and losses which can seem horrendous at the moment we experience them, no matter how sane and balanced we are! Experiencing these nasty events doesn't mean you are mentally ill.

In fact if you don't react in some way to these adverse situations, this precise lack of engagement could itself be a mental disease of sorts. I'm thinking of a strange syndrome calls Williams syndrome, caused by the spontaneous deletion of 26-28 genes on chromosome #7. The deletion occurs in either the egg or the sperm used to form the child with Williams syndrome. Accordingly, the deletion is present at the time of conception.

The patients manifest several disadvantages, such as developmental delays and learning challenges, but are noteworthy for their fatuous smiles and sunny personality. Nothing seems to faze them!

These preternaturally happy kids don't strike me as ill. Just under-engaged. I mean, if not reacting is a true mental disorder, then that would have to be true of meditation experts, sufis, siddhis and the like, who spend their lives trying to tune out "normal" emotional reactions to life's ups and downs.

Sometimes we react very badly, stupidly even, and over-dramatize our emotions, maybe making situations worse due to our folly or ignorance. But that doesn't make you mentally ill. Inept, maybe, but not sick. Ignorance is not a disease. It's a lack of education and learning. Let's face it, nothing in our schooling or upbringing prepares for the rough and tumble of real life.

Parents are often the worst leaders and cloud our view of what life is really like, with their own bad behaviors and raging emotions!

So... being screwed up is not a mental disorder, any more than bacteria under the fingernails is a disease!

OK, onwards to special pathology...

PART 4

HOLISTIC MECHANISMS OF DISEASE

In the fourth segment of the text, we are going to be looking at a host of possible causative factors in sickness of any kind (including mental problems) and how to prevent or eliminate them, from a holistic perspective.

These correctable factors include—but are not limited to—food allergies and intolerance, stealth pathogens, heavy metal toxicity, nutritional deficiencies, hormonal imbalances, parasites, disordered blood sugar metabolism and environmental chemical sensitivities.

But first let me establish some important principles of healing which are essential to understand the true holistic approach to medicine, including psychiatry, and the establishment of sound and thriving body and mind functionality. It is a whole new way of looking at disease and health. Without understanding these core principles, it will not be possible to fully grasp my proposed new way of approaching mental health.

The fact is, over recent decades there has been a major shift in the understanding of holism and what it really means. I took part in this era of exploration and transformation and am proud to have been one of only a handful of pioneers. We moved forward with observation and clinical acumen. There was no science at first!

We created it; we used the scientific approach, carefully weighing clinical observations and objective evidence, coupled with our reasoning skills. For example we were attacked and hounded because there was "no scientific evidence" that environmental chemicals could make a person ill. It was a fraudulent story, used to coerce deluded and gullible patients into parting with their money, was a common accusation. This, despite the fact we could, all of us, have earned far more money just doing what the other lazy or brain-dead doctors were doing. Where is the financial motive in that?

Well, it was true there no scientific support from the standard medical journals of the day. But if you turned to toxicology—a busy and rapidly-expanding discipline in the latter half of the twentieth century—there were literally tens of thousands of papers being published, all making the deleterious clinical effects of chemicals abundantly clear. Moreover, most of these papers in toxicology journals were of a far higher standard of scientific integrity than the sleazy science being peddled by the pharmaceutical, chemical and agricultural industries.

That remains true to this day.

And it also remains true there is still no official onus on the peddlers of chemical pollutants to prove that their products are safe. Instead, it is down to us, the victims, to prove that they are not safe in contact with humans. But since no-one other than the big industries have the financial clout to mount such tests, they can go on bleating "there is no scientific proof" that the current burden of environmental chemicals is harmful.

Indeed, today things are worse than ever. A new evil and dishonest climate has emerged in science. If the big industries don't like something, they suppress it. A raw example would be the matter of Gilles-Éric Séralini's 2012 paper on the disastrous effects of GMO glyphosate on a population of rats.

Seralini, a French molecular biologist, fed rats for 2 years with genetically modified corn and Monsanto's notorious herbicide RoundUp. The rats developed cancers. Up to 50% of males and 70% of females suffered premature death. Orthodoxy went into hysterical overdrive, in an attempt to discredit that paper, which was finally withdrawn by the journal (not by the authors).

They claimed, among other things, the rats (Sprague-Dawley) were the wrong sort (they were the same as those used by Monsanto in their fake 90-day "safety tests"); they said he used too few rats for the test to mean anything. But this was a toxicity test, not a carcinogen test. Using 20 rats is fine, whereas 50 are recommended for cancer studies.

Now it's possible that Seralini did not play with a straight bat. But all this is set against the background that Monsanto blustered its Roundup product through supposed public safety controls, *without even one study testing for the long-term toxicity of roundup.*

Can you imagine a test for smoking risks which had a group of subjects smoke for just 3 months and then stating it was safe to smoke for life?

That's the scale of lying here. It's unreal!

Incidentally, the tobacco industry has far from given up fighting the science showing the harm smoking does...

In a special report published in the Oct. 16, 2007, issue of the journal **Circulation**, UC Davis and UC San Francisco researchers say that after combing through secret tobacco-related documents they discovered how the industry initially worked to question scientific evidence about the harmful effects of secondhand smoke as a way to fight smoke-free regulations.

"People should understand how hard the tobacco industry has worked to undermine scientific evidence," said Tong, an assistant professor of internal medicine at the UC Davis School of Medicine and lead author of the study. "It's not just about fighting smoke-free regulations. Our analysis of the documents indicates an industry that also wants to influence the debate about how 'reduced-harm' tobacco products should be evaluated."[246]

In other words, they want to set the bar for what counts as evidence.

4.1 The Movement Towards Nature

It seems there are those who cannot accept that anything new and important can be discovered in their lifetime. Human progress is something, evidently, from the past. Yet these are exciting times to live in and be part of. It is true, we are in the throes of a medical revolution. But I can make that seem less of a cliché by pointing out that we are, in many senses, going backwards towards the Earth wisdom of our ancestors. Really, it is the 'drug revolution' that is coming to an end, at the same time that new discoveries in the realm of holistic causes and healing methods make it very opportune that this should be so.

While the drug companies are continuing to tighten their grip, using government-backed legislation to bully alternative healers and protect their monopoly, people are opting out altogether. Many are concerned about the safety of modern drugs; some are outright afraid—and not without reason.

The truth is the drug boom is over. After more than 40 years of hegemony, it has been exposed for what it is — a sham. The dream of universal health and magical cures for a vast array of ills, simply by popping a few pills, just hasn't happened. Instead, patients have become increasingly wary of drug treatment, with its frequent unpleasant side-effects and manifest dangers.

This isn't to say that drugs have no place in medicine. They can and do save lives; penicillin is one of the greatest gifts Nature has given humanity, second only to fire as an aid to our survival. But those kinds of drugs are in a tiny minority. The vast bulk of substances pushed by the profit-hungry chemical cartels are useless or worse. The problem comes with long-term medication. Even conscientious and caring doctors seem oblivious to the irony that, by definition, chronic drug treatment doesn't work. If it cured, there would be no need to go on taking it!

At best these kinds of drugs can only suppress symptoms. But at a terrible price. If the underlying destructive process of the disease isn't altered or stopped, then the body continues to deteriorate and the patient is given a false sense of security. There is the apparency that the treatment is helping, when in fact it is doing no good whatsoever. By disguising the damage, the patient may be ill served.

Then there is the vexed question of side-effects. No drug is free of this problem, though some are worse than others. It may be very hard for a patient to live with constant symptoms he or she knows are being caused by medication. This is made even more disconcerting when the doctor under-rates the unpleasantness of these symptoms, or refuses to believe in their existence, but considers the treatment approach an unqualified success.

I am minded of an exemplary study carried out in the UK; in the city of Newcastle, I believe. Three sets of questionnaires were used determine the results of a drug trial, using blood pressure control medication. The doctors were asked how it went and they ALL said it was a big success; wives and family were questioned and generally they agreed there was some benefit to the patient (not much). But when it came to the patients' replies, the vast majority said they felt *worse* on the treatment! Well, whose disease is it, anyway?

The Soil And Seed

One of the inevitable results of the overuse of drugs and their fundamental ineffectuality, is that the search for real causes is obscured.

Take a disease like tuberculosis. Leaving aside the question of the new wave of total drug resistant organisms, antibiotics have existed for several decades that can "treat" this condition and save lives, by killing the microbe that causes it (*Mycobacterium tuberculosis*). This puts firmly into the doctor's mind that TB is 'caused' by a bacterium. This was the sensation of medicine in the last century, the so-called 'germ theory of disease propounded by Louis Pasteur, who became (quite rightly) famous as his ideas gained credence.

But it isn't at all that simple. These microbes abound everywhere, but we do not all fall prey to their pathogenic potential. Why is this? Well, the reason probably varies from case to case but it is certain that there is some weakening factor at work in those who get TB. Isn't this the real cause of the disease and the microbe just an opportunist?

TB is a good example because, although often cited as one of the greatest successes of modem medicine; it isn't really. The actual reason for the drop in incidence of TB isn't science or drugs at all, but improved socio-economic factors. Poverty as it once existed is now virtually unknown in the Western world. As a result, individuals are better nourished today than ever before and have more resistance to disease.

We call this a question of susceptibility, as opposed to consideration solely of the effect of pathogens (disease-causing organisms), the 'soil and seed' theory. The germs are the seeds; but whether they grow successfully and flourish, to produce a disease, depends on the character of the soil — that is, the resistance of the patient.

This brings us to the idea of the individual in medicine. In fact, this is one of the major differences in 'philosophy' between the new and the old. My old mentor Dr Theron Randolph, coined the slightly clunky words *exogenous* and *endogenous* medicine, to describe the two opposite ends of the spectrum. Actually, exogenous and endogenous pathology would probably be better labels.

According to this view, exogeny is disease caused from without (exo-), i.e. environmentally. Endogeny is a failure from within (endo-). The second type of medicine conceives of patients only as sick people, something decrepit and malfunctioning, rather like broken-down machinery. Exogeny would see everyone as inherently healthy but for some exterior factor that is making them sick.

Modem medicine is highly endogenously orientated and its laboratory-based, reductionist, analytic, bodily-centered approach has come to dominate medicine almost entirely. Its techniques are expensive and applications complex. Without the support of Big Pharma and profit-making organizations it probably couldn't function at all. The holistic alternative I espouse, on the other hand, is simplistic, deductive and environmentally-orientated. Patients can apply it for themselves and get well easily and inexpensively.

Unfortunately, as Randolph points out, the split between these two views and the shift in emphasis entirely to endogenous therapeutics occurred before the field of holistic and environmental medicine had developed fully. If this had not been so, it is quite possible, he argues, that the endogenous approach would not have become so firmly entrenched, though this is to ignore, somewhat naively, the great influence of vested interest.

Instead, today, we have what Randolph calls a diagnostico-therapeutic gap, that is a great indifference to the actual nature and causation of disease and, instead, an almost rigid fixation on studying how to treat its end-result (symptoms). The body and its counter-role in illness is heavily subordinated to the characteristics and properties of the supposed 'pathogens'.

And by pathogens it must be said I don't just mean microbes. Today we have numerous agents cited as the real "cause" of disease, especially including genetic factors. Doctors believe that if sickness is "in your genes" you will inevitably fall sick.

Honest evaluation says otherwise and it can be easily demonstrated that change in lifestyle factors, especially nutrition, will switch off noxious genes. But the medical profession, driven by pharmaceutical interests, simply ignores that inconvenient fact.

Internal Ecology

I'd like to add my own contribution to the debate by introducing the term 'internal ecology'. The concept is very simple. We live in an age that is increasingly conscious of environmental issues. It must now be obvious to all, except those who live in unimaginable isolation, that if we go on as we are doing — polluting our world, wrecking the balance of Nature, plundering its non-renewable resources and generally making a mess of things — that life on this planet will shortly become totally untenable.

Yet we seem to be doing just as much damage to our inner world of mind and body and, so far, not nearly enough people have really become aware of the problem. We have been poisoning and pillaging just as profligately but stealing something even more precious: the ability of our remarkable body defence systems to cope with the rising tide of personal stresses and pollution.

I'm not just talking about food additives and pesticides, which is about the limit of media awareness. We have radically altered the internal balance in our bodies, through constant reckless exposure to a number of new hostile aspects of our environment. We have destroyed or altered the normal pattern of our bowel flora by constant use and some would say abuse of broad-spectrum antibiotics. Very few people in this day and age have not been given at least one course of these ubiquitous drugs; many have had staggering quantities over the years. The result has been a virtual epidemic of opportunistic infections of the Candida sort, including yeasts and molds.

This is all compounded by the poverty of modern food sources, which have undoubtedly added to the challenges our immune systems face by distorted or inadequate nourishment. This is a problem that goes deeper than mere food allergy. The question of food quality affects everybody. Agribusiness, like the pharmaceutical industry, is simply not interested in the damaging health effects it may have on its end-users. Instead it sees its own inalienable right to pervert food supplies, suppress information of the dangers, cheat, mislabel and disguise what it is doing to the population, solely on the grounds that an informed public would avoid buying their goods and thus damage profits.

Add to that the fact that we live under a virtual pall of chemical poisons that I call "the chemical blizzard", rained down on us from the atmosphere, polluting our water supplies and loaded onto our food. It is all in the bizarre belief that it is somehow beneficial for the human race; we are supposed to need these substances for our ultimate good; we are told repeatedly that none of it is harmful to health.

The fact is, nobody knows what the full long-term effect of this chemical onslaught will be, but you can be certain that our delicate and sensitive nervous systems are among the first to suffer. Some pesticides work in a similar manner to nerve gas (organophosphates), yet we are told this is no problem. But individuals are already experiencing difficulties; hence the idea of 'human canaries'. Soon we will all follow. The warning bells have never sounded more clearly than in the closing few years of the last millennium.

We live in an environment also bombarded by electromagnetic radiation that simply didn't exist a century ago. The term 'electric smog' has been coined. Radio waves, radar and microwaves permeate our planet so completely that it is not possible to find anywhere on Earth to escape exposure to this unseen and little understood 'pollution'. We cannot measure what effect it has on our tissues, long or short term, except that there is new and disturbing evidence that this 'electric smog' is far from safe.

Perhaps the real question is not 'Why are more and more people becoming ill?' but rather, 'How is it that some of us are able to remain well, despite the steadily increasing pall of toxins to which we are subjecting ourselves?' This at least would put the emphasis in the right place. We need to study the body's resources and learn how to strengthen them, before digging ever deeper into the complex detailed mechanisms of disease.

Take Action Yourself

I am not suggesting we go back to a medieval ecology. We all enjoy the benefits of science and technology. I would simply suggest that we begin to spend some of our vast industrial budgets on the development of safety precautions and better methods of production and disposal. This will mean exposing those who currently claim there is no problem, along with the politicians who will insist on putting the interests of big business above the common good of the people whom they are supposed to represent.

It seems there is little point in waiting for governments to act, or scientific integrity to come back into fashion. Instead, what we used to call *clinical ecology* has become very much a 'people's medicine'. For many years public awareness and personal action in health issues of this sort have been far ahead of medical competence or willingness to act. There is good and bad in this. It means no-one need wait for help; the principles can be applied by anyone. But unfortunately, it has resulted in a lot of what I regard as unscientific nonsense gaining common coinage, which further compounds the problem, because unsympathetic doctors can scoff. This makes it harder for practitioners like myself, who would like to build bridges with the medical establishment.

The final answer to the myths and ignorance is real knowledge and I have written this work with that in mind. With intelligence and persistence, you should be able to use it to attain relief from illnesses of the type described and for which, previously, you have had little help.

Richard Mackarness, a consultant psychiatrist and writer who virtually brought the clinical ecology revolution to medicine in the UK, once wrote to me, 'Every idea has its time. The time of clinical ecology is now!' This heartfelt statement has only become truer with the passage of years.

4.2 The Overload Model Of Symptoms and Dis-Ease

It's been wisely said that our bodies are defended from sudden death every single day. Along with all living creatures we are endowed with a number of key regulatory mechanisms. One can only be amazed that they rarely seem to break down, rather than being surprised and disconcerted when they do.

Every day, every minute, trouble is nipped in the bud before it gets started and we remain unaware of what is taking place: in other words, we feel one hundred percent OK. It is only when the defences are overworked that we actually experience any health problems at all. By the time we are aware of a symptom, any symptom, the defences have already broken down and matters are really quite serious.

We have our skin to prevent dehydration and excrete toxins; our immune system to pick off and destroy raiders; our kidneys to balance the internal acid-alkali regulation and also excrete toxins; the liver to denature toxic chemicals and render them harmless.

Our hormone glands are there to balance countless functions and make sure all works well.

The nervous system is there so we can react quickly to any threat in our environment.

The cardiovascular system rushes troops to the battle front and removes waste and dead bodies when it's all over.

The lymphatic system, which is a sub-division of the blood system, also transports refuse and toxins, keeping the tissues clean and sanitary, so to speak.

Really, we are marvelous orchestration of all these different protective systems. Because of them, we are able not merely to live, but live well, thrive and enjoy our wellness experience, even though we live in a world of dangerous pathogens and potentially deadly chemicals.

It's only when these healing mechanisms are compromised that we are at risk of falling sick, including the development of mental or emotional problems.

What could possibly cause that to happen?

Individual Variations

One of the most important understandings in biology and disease is the fact that *all individuals are different*. Body processes vary, some majorly out of tune with the rest of us. Rasputin, for example, was given a dose of cyanide big enough to kill a handful of people, yet he survived! It is usually explained by the fact he had a fondness for eating sweets, which somewhat neutralized the cyanide. His assassins finally shot him, tied him up and threw him into a freezing river.

This guy was tough as hell. The autopsy revealed that he was still alive when thrown into the water... and had almost broken free of his bonds!

In other words, Rasputin was far from "average". Yet medicine continues to make the laughable mistake of supposing everyone is "average". In fact NOBODY IS AVERAGE; *not one single human being is average.* So modern drug-based medicine is treating non-existent people!

We all vary in detail, according to our 20,000 plus genes. The effects that food, drink and chemical substances have on our bodies are extremely variable, which is why one individual can drink champagne and enjoy it, while another gets a terrible headache. Or why one human being can walk unscathed through graveyards filled with rotting piles of Plague victim corpses and yet never succumb to the disease, while others fall sick and die, quickly and easily.

I repeat: everyone is different. But modern supposedly scientific medicine ignores this simple fact. As Roger J Williams remarks in the preface to his rightly famous book *Biochemical Individuality*: "Although ancients and moderns alike have called attention to variability and individuality as factors particularly related to disease susceptibility and moderns have recognized that variability is indispensable to evolution, comparatively little research time and effort have been devoted to definitive study in physiology and biochemistry as to precisely how so-called normal individuals differ from each other. Such study necessarily involves the repeated observations on the same individuals, in contrast to a series of single observations on representative populations. No attempt to bring together the available biochemical material on normal variation has been previously made so far as I know."[247] Perhaps Sir William Osler, one the greatest physicians of all-time, used to put it more simply. Osler was fond of quoting an earlier wise British doctor, Caleb Hillier Parry of Bath (1755- 1822), "It is more important to know what kind of patient has the disease, than to know what sort of disease the patient has."[248] But it's worse than that, according to Roger J Williams: "A commonly accepted point of view in the field of biology and related disciplines—physiology, biochemistry, psychology—and in the applied fields of medicine, psychiatry, and social relations appears to be that humanity can be divided into two groups: (1) the vast majority possess attributes which are within the normal range; (2) a small minority possess attributes far enough out of line so that they should be considered deviates."

This is absurd. They are not deviates or "abnormal"; they simply differ from the majority. But medicine does not trouble itself with the outliers. For a significant number of people that is disastrous and condemns them to being failed by the system or, even worse, being hurt by supposed-safe standard treatments.

These are the people who die in the first week of chemo, whereas most patients survive the course; who turn suicidal or murderous on psychotropic drugs, such as SSRIs; who could bleed out, due to slow blood clotting control, whereas most people would make it to

ER; or who end up brain damaged, even dead, after what is, to most people, is a harmless vaccine.

4.3 The Cascade Model

It is very important to grasp that there is rarely one single cause for ill health, including mental symptoms. Even an "obvious" case, such as TB caused by the tubercle bacillus, or PTSD "caused" solely by a harrowing experience, is not that simple.

If you are healthy, balanced and well-nourished, it is most unlikely you will contract Tuberculosis. There has to be one or more contributory causes, for you to fall ill to the pathogen. Malnutrition is one of the most important predisposing condition. Populations, we now know, who are well fed, have a far lower incidence of TB.

Shock, loss or strain can predispose it too. Those grand Victorian novels of blighted love and yearning often ended with the main protagonist dying of TB (sometimes called "consumption" in those days, because the patient loses weight rapidly).

In other well-known stories, the hero or heroine was working excessively hard to make ends meet, while battling with poverty and privation. The exhaustion and overload effect was an important factor in falling sick.

Well, these Victorian authors were right, medically speaking, in that such pain and misery was often a major predisposing factor in weakening the person's immune system and he or she would suddenly worsen tragically, and die quickly.

Similarly, one traumatic event, no matter how shocking, is not really sufficient to cause a mental breakdown. Regard the number of people who survived the holocaust and years of squalor and privation in a concentration camp. Many (most of them) did not fold under the strain. Or soldiers who go to war and see their colleagues and friends blown to pieces with high explosive mines, shells and bombs. Again, the majority survive—if not totally unscathed—at least remaining functional.

The importance is to find those other predisposing factors and eliminate them. We can't change a person's past (though we can change their response to it, as you learned in section 3.12). But we can eliminate many of the contributory factors that hold the anguish in place.

[Note the word contributory. A tributary to a river means another stream flowing into it. Hence contribution or adding to...]

Take a viral illness, for instance. I rarely get colds. Or at least not usually. But when I was attacked by a virus just after a huge family problem, an emotional journey back home to the UK, excessive and tiring travel, not eating my usual foods, all of this in the middle of packing up house to move home back in California, I went down heavily with a respiratory illness. It took me a couple of weeks to shake it off.

Now the simplistic picture is: I caught a virus. That's what any doctor would say. Viruses cause illness. It's obvious, isn't it! But it's all totally mistaken. This ridiculous simplification is what renders modern medicine, including psychiatry, so ineffective.

The virus was not the cause of my respiratory illness. Stress, plus heavy emotions from many reunions, one particularly shocking surprise, plus poor foods, plus moving house and finally a virus intruder is what finally resulted in my illness. Too much body load caused my illness!

The this-plus-this-plus-this model of causation I call the "cascade principle" and it's mighty important to understand it.

The virus might have looked like the "cause" to a lazy observer, but in fact it was only the last step in a whole cascade of overload events! Each of the previous health burdens needed to be in place, before the virus could successfully gain a hold.

Incidentally, this is why, when you eradicate the microbe, sickness comes back later in some form or other. The person's general health is still weakened and at risk. So even if you kill off one bunch of pathogens, something else will come along and nail the patient.

That's why it is important to treat the whole patient; hence: (w)holistic.

4.4 Body Load

There are many factors which can overload the defenses and thus break down balance and vitality; things like chemical pollution, poor nutrition, stress factors, hidden infections, exhaustion, parasites and food allergies.

The important point is that if too many of these factors are present, the health and wellness process recovery breaks down and we enter disease-time. It may take a few months, years, or even decades, but sooner or later the body's own protective defence mechanisms will fail.

We call the accumulation of burdens the "total body load".

This puts a new perspective on sickness and disease. Instead of thinking of symptoms as the *start* of the disease process, their appearance actually marks the end of the sequence.

By the time we develop symptoms it's too late. The recovery process has run out of momentum and exhausted itself. That means we are now in serious trouble.

Sickness And The Barrel Model

The best way to grasp this is using the metaphorical barrel model. If we think of our heath status as a barrel, of fixed capacity, then symptoms can be interpreted as the overflow of this barrel.

While our body can contain the symptoms (the barrel can hold the fluid content without spilling), then we have no disease. The barrel represents your resistance to disease.

But if the barrel is filling up too fast, the body load is too great, then there is an overflow of the barrel and this represents the symptoms we experience (see diagram).

It is implicit in this model that you will be able to tolerate a definite level of each stressor and only by exceeding that do you move into overload.

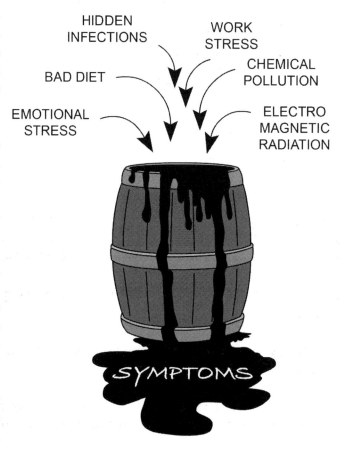

These limits may shift under different circumstances but there is always a line, drawn somewhere, which you must not cross if you want to remain well.

Factors Contributing To Overload

There are plenty of overload factors. You can probably think of a few others yourself. These are the main ones:

- Emotional Stress
- Allergies
- Chemical pollution
- Oxidative stress
- Drugs
- Parasites

- Geopathic stress
- Heavy metal toxicity (mercury, lead, etc.)
- Hidden infections
- Endocrine disorders
- Electromagnetic fields
- Fatigue
- Nutritional deficiencies
- Radioactivity
- Alcohol

The recovery process, obviously, is the reverse of this. If we shut off some of the inflow into the barrel—fix up our diet, reduce stress, start healthy living, or reduce the burden in any one of a number of ways—then we can stop the barrel from overflowing.

That means the symptoms will switch off. We will experience wellness once more. That includes a better state of mind.

It is vital for anyone suffering psychiatric or mental symptoms of any kind to stop that barrel overflowing!

The amazing thing is we don't have to have an empty barrel to have no symptoms of disease. We just need a barrel which can hold its load without spilling!

It's been a Scott-Mumby saying for nearly four decades now, that, *We don't need zero health challenges to get zero symptoms.* We just need to be able to tolerate and manage the load we have!

This can be as simple as getting rid of allergy foods, cutting back on alcohol or ensuring regular, good quality sleep. I've seen it time and time again: some small change leads to a complete reversal of the health position. Depression and anxiety lift completely; panic attacks cease; behavioral disorders calm; memory and confusion (which we often call "brain fog" or wooly brain syndrome) improve dramatically; even hallucinations and delusions vanish.

We can get rid of anything, any disease process, including psychiatric disorders, if we just reduce the body load sufficiently. Nature will help us.

Yet psychiatrists get this wrong all the time. They teach patients they are somehow busted; that they are "sick"; that they can't be cured. The only answer, doctors claim, is toxic medication (which of course only adds to the filling of the barrel).

This is an evil condemnation to a life of hell; a prison in which the pretense of medicine and healing is trapping the patient.

The Fundamental Law Of Healing

What I am sharing with you really amounts to a simple, although hugely important, Law Of Healing:

That nature will heal anything if you reduce the total body load to the point where the natural curative and restorative mechanisms can function!

Reducing total body load is how we get cures. It works every time.

So it's open to all, and anyone can become a healer and cure his or her own condition, just by applying this wisdom.

Unfortunately, as I said, modern medicine and its drugs often add to the biological burden instead of relieving it.

4.5 The Threshold Effect

Going deeper, this "barrel" model rests on another very important health principle I discovered decades ago and which is almost never talked about. I call it the threshold effect. It's very important you understand it.

When talking about body load, it is important to understand that there may be many factors stressing the body at any one time: fatigue, bad food, a virus attack, the stress of exams, jilted by a lover... It's true isn't it, that things often come in bunches like that?

Symptoms only emerge when there is too much going on for the body to easily cope, as I have explained above. Just one problem (say, lack of sleep) may not be enough to cause a symptom breakdown—healthy young kids sometimes live for days without proper sleep and they seem none the worse for it!

But when you get several effects at once, THEN the problem starts. In other words you stepped over the threshold.

The adding up of negative factors and scoring them I call the summation effect. It is usually highly unlikely that just one of the health factors, alone, could not cause a real problem. But when they all add together, that's enough to trigger damage.

It's like a health-abacus or a symptom-calculus! Say we rate the limit of tolerance at a 10 and it will take an 11 or more to cause disease (I'm just making these numbers up, you understand). A stress factor which rates a 6 is not going to harm this individual, at least not short-term.

Even when another overload factor of, say, a 3, comes along, that still only adds up to a 9. Still not enough to trigger a health crisis!

But add a third contributing stress, rated at 5 and we now have a total "score" of 14. That means symptoms are definitely going to kick in. If the encounters are far enough apart, they may not summate together to reach a 10. But if they follow rapidly one upon another, then symptoms result. And you will readily see that if all three stressors are present simultaneously, then symptoms are inevitable and immediate.

We can show this pictorially in the following diagram:

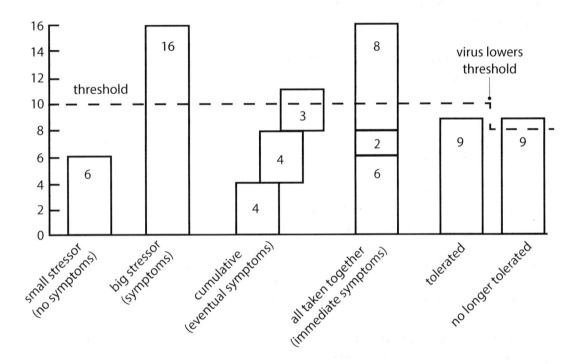

Schematic illustrating threshold values in triggering symptoms

4.6 Target Organs

There is another revealing health principle that is rarely talked about, except by doctors like me; we early pioneers of holistic medicine put in our time to fully grasp these fundamental concepts back in the 1980s. On-line health guru wannabes never mention it because they never worked with actual cases—they just Googled their "information", which is woefully lacking in depth.

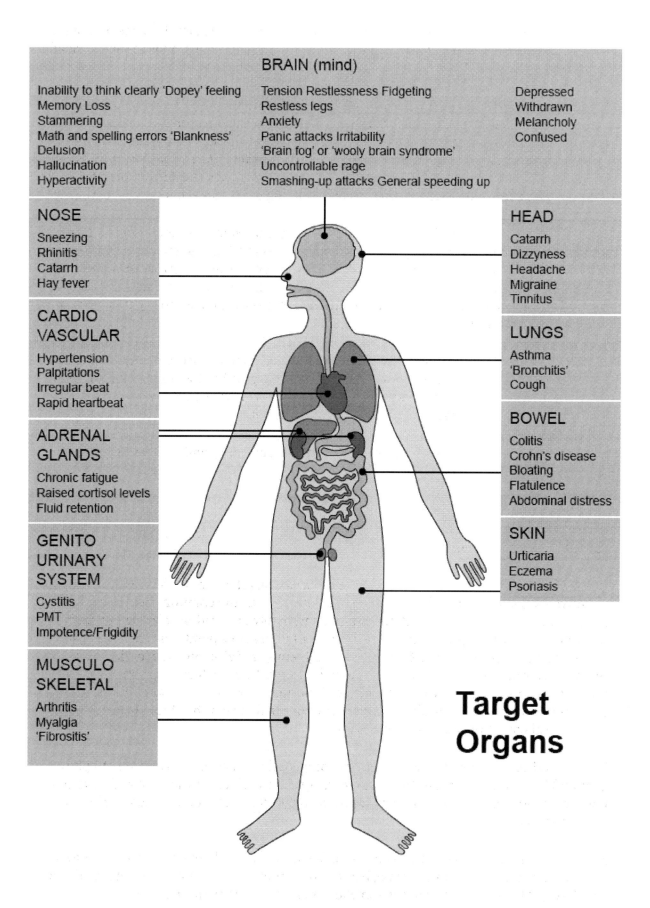

BRAIN (mind)

Inability to think clearly 'Dopey' feeling
Memory Loss
Stammering
Math and spelling errors 'Blankness'
Delusion
Hallucination
Hyperactivity

Tension Restlessness Fidgeting
Restless legs
Anxiety
Panic attacks Irritability
'Brain fog' or 'wooly brain syndrome'
Uncontrollable rage
Smashing-up attacks General speeding up

Depressed
Withdrawn
Melancholy
Confused

NOSE

Sneezing
Rhinitis
Catarrh
Hay fever

CARDIO VASCULAR

Hypertension
Palpitations
Irregular beat
Rapid heartbeat

ADRENAL GLANDS

Chronic fatigue
Raised cortisol levels
Fluid retention

GENITO URINARY SYSTEM

Cystitis
PMT
Impotence/Frigidity

MUSCULO SKELETAL

Arthritis
Myalgia
'Fibrositis'

HEAD

Catarrh
Dizzyness
Headache
Migraine
Tinnitus

LUNGS

Asthma
'Bronchitis'
Cough

BOWEL

Colitis
Crohn's disease
Bloating
Flatulence
Abdominal distress

SKIN

Urticaria
Eczema
Psoriasis

Target Organs

I'm referring to target or 'shock' organs. The concept is really very simple: some part of the body, or a particular organ (for reasons which are not clear) receives more of an overload reaction than the rest.

Whatever the environmental stressor (overload), whether it is a food allergy, a chemical, a hidden infection or some other insult to the tissues, the symptoms appear at the weak point and are referred (related) to this organ, regardless of the actual trigger. Thus you may also hear the term "end-organ failure". Here's the thing: *the symptoms experienced will depend largely on the function of this organ and whether it is excited (stirred up) or depressed (slowed down)*. The symptoms have nothing to do with whatever the stressor is!

Dairy allergy, for instance, is not associated with any particular symptoms (except lactose intolerance, which affects mainly the gut). In one patient with a true milk allergy, the skin may be attacked (rashes); in another, the lungs (asthma and wheezing); a third patient may have aching painful joints (arthritis); while a fourth is intolerably depressed until dairy is removed from his or her diet. Same allergen: the symptoms vary, according to which part of the body breaks down first.

Incidentally, this tells us why sometimes even just one hand or just one joint is affected. That's the first point to feel the impact. In time it may spread to the other hand and then the rest of the body. And, of course, it may eventually spread to the brain and nervous system, where it creates havoc with feelings and perceptions.

On the previous page is a chart of some of the main target organs and the typical symptoms one may encounter.

4.7 Brain Allergy

Of the utmost importance to this text is the brain as a target organ. Undoubtedly our most sensitive tissues are those of the delicate machinery inside the cranium. Even if you work in the non-material mind model, the brain is intimately involved in relaying our highest functions and thought processes can easily be disrupted at this point. The resultant disturbance can be as mild as forgetfulness or as frightening as full-blown dementia. Probably the most common symptom of all is 'woolly brain syndrome' which is surprisingly common; so much so that many people consider it normal to be foggy and forgetful. It is only when they try an exclusion diet or a similar unburdening step that they realize it was a pathological condition, because it clears up!

Food allergies, nutritional deficiencies, environmental chemical sensitivity, stealth pathogens and heavy metal burdens (lead and mercury are notorious for this) can and do mimic many diverse conditions, such as depression, anxiety, violent outbursts, hallucinations and schizophrenia.

Most effects are not strictly classified with a diagnostic label, therefore doctors tend to be dismissive of the patient and assume, because their presenting complaint is not found in a standard textbook, that he or she is somehow making the symptoms up.

In fact one of the strongest characteristics of food allergy induced symptoms is that they are subjective (highly personalized), protean (changeable) and come and go with no apparent pattern. Symptoms shift over time... gut one week, headaches a month later, then depression, then aching joints. Underperforming doctors are quick to diagnose the patient as weak or inadequate and refer him or her to a psychiatrist. "It's all in your mind," the unlucky patient is likely to be told, and ends up on disruptive chemical medications which virtually block any chance of recovery.

Here are some of the many symptoms I have encountered over the years, that can be attributed to brain excitation and suppression, from any of the causes in the previous paragraphs:

Mental Malfunctions

- inability to think clearly
- memory loss
- 'dopey' feeling
- stammering (attacks)
- terrible thoughts on waking
- insomnia
- maths and spelling errors
- mispronouncing words
- blankness
- delusion
- crabby on waking
- hallucination
- difficulty waking up
- desire to injure self
- convulsions
- light-headedness
- twitching

Stimulated, Overactive

- silliness
- anxiety
- intoxication
- panic attacks
- hyperactivity
- irritability
- uncontrollable rage
- tenseness
- restlessness
- smashing-up-attacks
- fidgeting
- general speeding up
- restless legs

Depressed, Underactive

- 'brain fag'
- depression
- feeling withdrawn
- lack of confidence
- melancholy
- low mood
- unreal or depersonalized feeling
- confused
- tearful

Quite a list, as you will readily agree.

The Master Indicator

There is one amazingly valuable red flag system I have, which can put you on the path to recovery virtually instantly.

It starts with one killer question: **do you ever have symptom free days?** In other words, do you experience abrupt changes from feeling well to unwell and back again? This is the master health indicator. Why do I say that? *Because if you can ever have a symptom-free day, you are NOT sick.* Think about it: you are not suffering from a degenerative process, nothing is broken or missing, your organs are all working reasonably well, you don't have a hidden infection, it isn't cancer, hardening of the arteries, diabetes, dementia or any other crippling and permanent condition.

Same idea with blood pressure, incidentally. If you ever come in with a normal reading, even just once, you do not have hypertension!

The good days tell you how you can feel when at your best. This is your real state of health!

I have a great saying to complement this: **if you can have one day without symptoms, every day can be without symptoms.** In other words something is doing it to you on certain days (overload!) and it is not that you are weak or "busted" as the doctors would have you believe.

Mold Allergy and Bipolar

Let me finish with a bizarre case of bipolar I was able to solve, where mold sensitivity (allergy, not toxicity) was causing big problems.

The patient was a very intelligent, prosperous, pleasant and dapper man in his fifties. His wife, I remember, spoke as if she had a delicious plum in her mouth!

He came to see me with bipolar disorder. Sometimes he would get quiet manic; mostly he went into inexplicable depressions. We found some food allergies, neutralized them and gave him a diet, avoiding the most troublesome foods. How much simpler than a complicated regimen of toxic drugs, such as SSRIs.

Some time later, he reappeared and needed a re-assessment and adjustment to his low-dose antidote remedy. Again, I was satisfied with the outcome. When he appeared a third time, the following year, the penny dropped! It was always the same time of year. A fresh appraisal of his history told me that he tended to get sick every summer. Up until then, his depression was quite manageable. But—come late-July every year—he was off the rails again. It was a recurring pattern.

I happen to know that in the UK where this took place, the mold Cladosporium went into maximum sporing late July every year, peaking about midday. It was regular as clock-work.

Cladosporium is one of the most common colonizers of dead plants and soil. This is the mold that is frequently found on uncleaned refrigerators, foodstuffs, window frames, straw, houses with poor ventilation and in low damp areas. This mold has also been isolated from fuel tanks, face creams, paints and textiles. It is the primary source of mold allergy.

I tested this man for allergy to Cladosporium and his reaction was fierce. Once neutralized, he felt much better. Taking the low-dose desensitizing antidote he recovered rapidly and was able to avoid the need for psychiatric monitoring or any kind of psychotropic drug. He was well when I left England in 1997 and I hope he still is.

4.8 General Adaptation Syndrome

While we are here, gaining understanding on important general principles, let's take a second look at Hans Selye's General Adaptation Syndrome (it appeared first in section 2.7). It's a whole model of stress and its progress.

Hans Selye, a Viennese by birth who moved to Canada and practiced medicine in his adopted country, began with the observation that many people, ill from different causes, had similar symptoms. These were general symptoms, which seemed common to all afflictions, such as pallor, fatigue, loss of appetite, vague pains and a coated tongue. Selye, still a medical student, likened this to the 'syndrome of being ill' and he couldn't' understand why his teachers didn't pay more attention to these symptoms: they were obviously important, since everybody got them, no matter what the illness!

Instead, his teachers got bogged down in specific and unusual symptoms, that seemed to represent nothing in particular, despite the fancy labels they liked to use for these syndromes.

Selye eventually pursued his interest, to the point of describing a mechanism of stress and adaptation that seems to be universal. It is not just applicable to humans but to all life: any organism, any stress – from an amoeba crawling into tainted water to a busy executive having a tough time at board meetings. The stages of 'adaptation' to outside stress he called the General Adaptation Syndrome, or GAS for short.

Briefly, as I said before, Phase One is the first encounter, when the body reacts and alarm signals herald the onset of some adversity (a stressor). Selye called this the Alarm Phase. If the individual takes steps to eliminate the stressor, symptoms will go away.

But if the individual does not desist and instead keeps doing whatever it is, eventually he or she might learn to tolerate the stressor and find it doesn't worry him or her too much for a time. We call this Adaptation Stage Phase Two.

This stage could last years or even decades. But all the while the individual is "coping" he or she may be paying a hidden price: resistance is being ground down. One day, overload goes UP and he or she starts being sick.

This is Stage Three and Selye called it Mal-Adaptation.

We can illustrate this with an example from an allergy doctors' experience: If an individual, as a child, is allergic to milk, he or she will experience unpleasant symptoms when ingesting it, such as mood changes, colic, rashes, hyperactivity, recurring ear infections, or whatever (Alarm Stage).

If the parents insist that the child must continue to drink milk 'because it is good for you', not knowing that is the cause of the condition affecting the youngster, the child may get used it and learn to tolerate it. The rash or other symptoms may even clear up. Doctors often say that a patient can 'outgrow' an allergy this way. He or she is now Adapted to the milk allergen (Stage Two).

As the years go by, little of note may be observed; perhaps just the occasional bout of illness or digestive disorder, probably made worse at examination times and other periods of stress. But gradually the clock is running down. That individual's intolerance of milk is slowly wearing out the body's resistance. Trouble will inevitably follow.

Either because of aging, or at a specific trigger, the milk allergy will return and symptoms start up all over again. This time it could be asthma, eczema, depression, anxiety, panic attacks, headache, or any one of dozens of conditions. The patient may be quite unwell and yet never suspect milk – because he or she has always drunk it and has never (apparently) had any previous trouble when ingesting milk.

In fact patients often become addicted to their allergy food and may find that avoiding it for any period results in unpleasant withdrawal symptoms. This encourages further ingestion of the food; the patient may even feel it "does me good," since it tends to relieve the symptoms. At this stage eating the food 'masks' unwanted symptoms; it keeps them at bay. Providing he or she eats the food regularly, ill effects are kept at a minimum. This is what we mean by a hidden or masked allergy.

One other example might serve, and that is smoking. Those who smoke will doubtless remember that their first attempt was accompanied by unpleasant consequences: headache, dizziness and nauseas are not uncommon (stage one). But by persisting, the would-be smoker gets used to tobacco and the symptoms are no longer experienced (stage two). Finally, as the addiction takes hold, the individual will find that unpleasant symptoms come on with a vengeance when going too long without a 'fix' for the nicotine craving. This is phase three and one of the hardest of all addictions to break.

Incidentally, readers of this book will learn that tobacco smoking has a well-known association with schizophrenia. Well now you understand enough to know that schizophrenia patients should never EVER smoke!

Potts and Kalita On Smoking

It would be a grave disservice to the reader, patients (and family) not to *really* emphasize the dangers of smoking in the psychiatric context. For that, I call upon the work of pioneer clinical ecologists William H. Philpott MD and Dwight K. Kalita.

This is not about lung cancer and the usual recognized risk factors of smoking. This is about state of mind. In their seminal book *Brain Allergies* (Keats, New Canaan, CT. 1980), the authors quote two highly instructive cases of profound psychological disturbance due to the act of smoking.

Case one was a 25-year-old schizophrenic man who verbalized his delusions after smoking a cigarette. He was also excessively hungry and thirsty (likely low blood sugar). His fasting blood glucose was mostly normal (around 100 mg/ml) but on certain days this soared to 200 – 300 mg/ml.

It turned out that on the days his blood sugar test was ridiculously high, he had been sneaking a cigarette.

As a test he was asked to smoke several cigarettes over the space of 30 minutes. In response his fasting blood sugar shot up from 75 mg/ml (normal) to over 200 mg/ml. Most noteworthy he was symptom-free speaking normally before the test but after smoking for 30 minutes was rambling and delusional, compulsively verbalizing his delusions.

The second case was a 3-packs-a-day male, age 24 years. He went 24 hours without smoking, prior to a smoking test. His fasting blood sugar was 80 mg/ml (again, normal). Yet after smoking just one cigarette, he was sweating and too weak to stand. After 30 minutes, his blood sugar level had plunged to 30 mg/ml, a state of profound and dangerous hypoglycemia.

Such cases make it clear that maladaptive reactions to tobacco can have profound physiological effects. Philpott and Kalita go on to remark: it has been observed clinically that petrochemical hydrocarbons, such as exhaust fumes, perfumes and gas stoves or heating units are equally potent sources in producing disordered carbohydrate metabolism and erratic blood sugar levels.[249]

(see also section 5.8 on hypoglycemia to learn the profound mental disturbances that can be caused by changes in blood sugar)

Up To Date Observations on Schizophrenia and Smoking

Orthodoxy, at least, has noticed that schizophrenic patients are often addicted to tobacco. At least they have got as far as debating whether or not smoking causes or aggravates the delusional condition, or whether the patient is simply "self-medicating" because it makes him or her feel better.

Apparently the idea of banning smoking in psychiatric hospitals has not yet occurred to them. It's effect is still "uncertain". But here's where an understanding of the general laws of health would shed light. Once the third phase of GAS is understood, one can assume it likely that *anything which relieves symptoms is actually causing them.*

It's no different than heroin addiction. No-one really wants to take very expensive powders or risky IV shots! The addict takes his or her fix for one simple reason: it relieves the horrible symptoms of withdrawal. That doesn't make heroin healthy or attractive, does it? Everyone knows that heroin is causing the unpleasant symptoms the user is trying to escape.

It has been found that nicotine increases release of dopamine, so it is hypothesized that smoking helps correct dopamine deficiency in the prefrontal cortex and will thus relieve negative symptoms. ... But this ducks one major mistake: there is no proof whatever that dopamine deficiency (or any other "chemical imbalance") is the cause of schizophrenia!

Altogether the GAS model is a most satisfying theory. It is simple and easy to understand. It explains a great many observations that would otherwise remain puzzling. It is very much in accord with the idea of body load and target organs. Patients should understand it and use it to avoid making obvious and avoidable mistakes in interpreting their condition.

Signs Of Danger

Finally, Selye published a list of warning signs that patients should look for when they are under stress and about to become maladapted to foods and other stressors. It is remarkably similar to the lists that food allergy doctors have arrived at, traveling via a different route. I reproduce them here and have bolded the ones which seem specially relevant to this work:

- **General irritability, hyper-excitation or depression**
- Pounding of the heart
- Dryness of the throat and mouth
- **Impulsive behavior, emotional instability**
- **The overpowering urge to cry or run and hide**
- Inability to concentrate

- **Feeling of unreality, weakness or dizziness**
- **Predilection to become fatigued and loss of joie do vivre**
- **'Floating anxiety' – afraid but not knowing what causes the fear**
- **Emotional tension and alertness, feelings of being 'keyed up'**
- **Trembling, nervous tics**
- Tendency to be easily startled by small sounds, etc.
- High-pitched, nervous laughter
- Stuttering and other speech difficulties which are frequently stress-induced
- Bruxism, or grinding of the teeth
- **Insomnia, usually a consequence of being 'keyed up'**
- Hypermotility (technically known as hyperkinesis), the inability to relax
- Sweating
- The frequent need to urinate
- Disturbed gastrointestinal function – diarrhea, indigestion, queasiness in the stomach and sometimes even vomiting, irritable bowel
- Migraine headaches
- Premenstrual tension or missed menstrual cycles
- Pain in the neck or lower back
- Loss of or excessive appetite
- Increased smoking
- **Increased use of legally prescribed drugs, such as tranquilizers or amphetamines**
- **Alcohol and drug addiction**
- Nightmares
- **Neurotic behavior**
- **Psychoses**
- Accident proneness

Altogether this is a most satisfying theory. It is simple and easy to understand. It explains a great many observations that would otherwise remain puzzling. It underpins addictions and explains withdrawal symptoms. Patients should understand it and use it to avoid making obvious and avoidable mistakes in interpreting their condition.

4.9 The Assemblage Point Model

I now come to an energy medicine model which is "Western", in the sense that it is not from Asia, but rather from the North American Native Tradition. I feel sure it will greatly appeal to many readers who have not encountered it. And for the detailed description which follows, I am indebted to my friend Jon Whale, director of Electronic Gem Therapy Ltd., Axminster, Devon, UK, who could fairly be described as the world's number one scientific expert on this topic.

I'm talking about the human "Assemblage Point".

I dealt with it in my classic text *Medicine Beyond*. But this present work would be woefully inadequate without it and I make no apology for leaning on my other writings in this respect. I simply have to get this text into the hands of my readers, as soon as possible.

Like many practitioners, I had never heard of this model, until it was published in the journal *Positive Health*, in the October 1996 issue entitled: *Core Energy Surgery for the Electromagnetic Body*. They have since reported that this article was the most outstandingly popular and ever-in-demand article their journal has ever published[7].

I was intrigued and spotted that the author, Jon Whale lived in Arnside, Cumbria (England), only a few miles from my own home at that time, near Lake Windermere. I could not resist visiting him and spent a very fascinating half day learning a whole raft of new ideas, not confined to explanations of the Assemblage Point, but including the scientific principle of electronic gem therapy.

I learned to move the assemblage point to a healthier position, as Jon taught me, and it remains a fascinating model of health, much more realistic and rewarding for me than the chakra system.

I must here caution the reader that the description of this process given by Carlos Castaneda in his book *The Fire from Within* is not only unhelpful but definitely misleading. I have reason to believe that what he describes is a special variant of the technique used by shaman Tom 'Two Bears' Wilson (on whom he may have modeled Don Juan, the sorcerer). This was an atypical version because Castaneda himself was in bad shape!

In any case there continues real doubt about what Castaneda's sources were; he was certainly good at hiding them. Indeed there are many who consider his whole evocation of shamanism a fraud. The years before his death hardly add to his image; in the words of Mick Brown, 'Rather than dying the immaculate death of the sorcerer, it's suggested that the sorcerer's apprentice died a frail, paranoid and angry old man lashing out at the world with lawsuits'[8].

Over the years 1996 and 1997 Jon Whale published two more comprehensive articles in *Positive Health*, detailing the medical symptomatology and dangers of unhealthy Assemblage Point locations 3-part series and the methods for correction. The following year Jon received a litigious restraining Fax from Carlos Castaneda's offices. It stated that only

REAL SECRETS TO TRANSFORMING MENTAL HEALTH

Castaneda had the rights to the medical applications of the Assemblage Point. The irony is that Carlos Castaneda failed to provide his readers with any methods or details on how to correct an unhealthy or detrimentally located Assemblage Point.

In fact Castaneda had no such rights. He was far from the discoverer. He was just an arrogant opportunist; a plagiarist, if you like.

Meeting Swiftdeer

A decade previously (September 1988) Jon Whale had met with a well-known North American Indian Shaman called Harley "SwiftDeer" Reagan. SwiftDeer employed large specimens of machined and polished quartz crystals within his Shamanic work and teachings. At that meeting Jon Whale showed SwiftDeer one of his early prototype electronic gem therapy instruments. SwiftDeer said that he was all in favor of combining electronics with crystals and gem stones for the purpose of increasing their healing power. See my book *Medicine Beyond* for the fulfillment of this promising combination.

SwiftDeer also explained the human Assemblage Point and demonstrated how he used a large rose quartz crystal to shift it to the center of the chest. This was a ritualistic practice used at important events, such as before entering a native Indian 'Sweat Lodge' ceremony.

All those present at the meeting had their Assemblage Points moved, followed by a 'Sweat Lodge' ceremony. This event was for Jon and other people present a profound experience, each person experiencing the living proof that their Assemblage Point was a life giving reality.

Incidentally, SwiftDeer—a real life shaman, not a fictional character—was far from complimentary about Carlos Castaneda's books, intimating to Jon Whale that it was important to research, record and publish the different Assemblage Point locations relating to medical health problems; he as good as charged Jon with this important task.

SwiftDeer used a 'The Sliding Shift' method to shift the Assemblage Point described by Jon Whale below, as opposed to the back slapping method described by Castaneda. Jon Whale taught this technique directly to me, along with the other methods he had developed. It is neither a version of chakras nor meridians but the similarities are startling. Again we are talking of a universal life energy flowing in and around the body. But in this shamanic model there is a definite vortex coming in at the chest, an actual assemblage of energy flows (assemblage: gathering together).

Let me give here the "seven rules" which govern this model:

THE SEVEN RULES

1. At the physical, emotional, atomic and quantum level, a human being is an independent oscillating energy field. All oscillating energy fields, by virtue of the fact that they are oscillating, must have an epicenter or vortex of the rotation. The epicenter of the human energy field is called the Assemblage Point.

2. The location and entry angle of the Assemblage Point with respect to the physical body dictates the shape and distribution of the human energy field.

3. The shape and distribution of the human energy field are directly proportional to the biological energy and activity of the organs and glands in the physical body, also to the quality of the emotional energy.

4. The biological activity of the organs and glands determines the position of the Assemblage Point, and thus the shape and distribution of biological energy throughout the physical body.

5. The location and entry angle of the Assemblage Point has a direct influence over the biological activity of all the organs and glands including the brain and these have a direct influence on the location of the Assemblage Point.

6. The location and entry angle of the Assemblage Point regulates how we feel and behave. Disease also dictates the Assemblage Point location and entry angle.

7. The way we feel and the manner in which we behave; our state of health or disease—particularly mental health—is reflected in the location and entry angle of our Assemblage Point.

How It Works

Our Assemblage Point location fixes in a healthy, stationary, near-central position at around the age of seven if we are brought up in a stable home environment and positively identify with good parents. The Assemblage Point has a critical relationship with our embryonic life force. A stable location near the center of the chest is essential for good mental and physical health.

But an unstable and displaced Assemblage Point is likely if we had a consistently negative relationship with our parents, a troubled background or having a displaced upbringing. Genetic reasons or disease can similarly produce abnormal and unstable Assemblage Points.

Sufferers of an involuntary Assemblage Point shift downwards experience that 'something' deep inside them has changed. Although they can remember how they behaved and felt before the incident, returning to their former energetic and happy self is impossible for them. That indescribable 'something' deep inside all of us that can suddenly shift following an adversity, changing our whole perception of reality and our physical health, is the location and entry angle of our Assemblage Point.

Gross misalignment of the Assemblage Point location is present in many diseases such as: depression, bipolar syndrome, paranoia, schizophrenia, drug and alcohol addiction, epilepsy, senile dementia, coma, Parkinsonism, toxicity, leukemia, cancer, AIDS, myalgic encephalomyelitis (ME or fibromyalgia), multiple sclerosis, and many others. Many of these conditions are accompanied by compromised pathology of the patient's hematology and biochemistry.

In other words, it is a vital model in any consideration of holistic psychiatry!

The diagram below should make the basics clear. Above center is over-stimulation, below center is depression; to the (patient's) right means anxiety/tension states (extrovert psychosis), to the left means hallucination and delusions (introvert psychosis). With this in mind, it is possible to tell, from the position of the assemblage point, all which is important about a person's energy state.

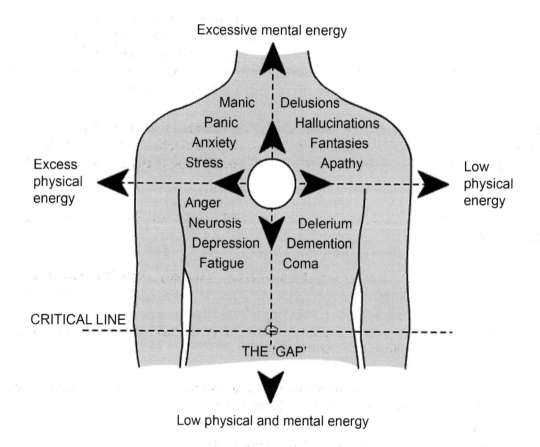

Note: The location for an average healthy woman is 2 – 3 inches higher than that of an average healthy man.

Locations higher than the optimum are accompanied by symptoms of too much energy: hyperactivity, anxiety, panic, insomnia and so on, along with hyper liver/adrenal activity. Attention deficit hyper activity disorder (ADHD) in children is now very common and is an example of this.

Lowered locations are accompanied with hypoactivity: the depressive illness spectrum and hypo liver/adrenal/thyroid activity.

The bipolar disorder spectrum or manic depression is accompanied by an oscillating Assemblage Point location, which switches between a high manic location and a low depressive position on the right side of the chest.

Interestingly, with the schizophrenic spectrum there may be several Assemblage Point locations, as also happens with the epilepsy spectrum.

Dangerous Drop

If the Assemblage Point drops beyond a certain distance for example, with chronic fatigue, down to or below the liver area, despite what medications or therapies are employed, it is very difficult for the individual to recover their former health and state of being. Their Assemblage Point is most unlikely to return unaided to its previous healthy location. Literally the biological energy levels are too low, so preventing recovery.

Raising the Assemblage Point location and angle upwards, closer to the center of the chest, is an essential intervention in such cases. Unfortunately, accepted orthodox medical diagnostic and management procedures do not take the patient's Assemblage Point location into consideration.

States that can drop the assemblage point below "the gap" and into the danger zone include the following:

1. Serious accident, bereavement, disease, fever, tragedy, chronic stress or depression.

2. Distressed or oppressed childhood, rape or sexual assault, violent intimidation, kidnapping, abduction, enslavement.

3. Self laceration, mutilation or poisoning, attempted suicide, substance and drug indulgence, drug overdose, mental institution.

4. Mugging, robbery, burglary, fraud, identity theft.

5. Genocide, war, terrorism, homicide, torture, post military combat trauma, imprisonment.

6. Physical or psychological intimidation, interrogation, brainwashing.

7. Betrayal, financial or legal intimidation, blackmail, malicious divorce, bankruptcy, redundancy, home repossession, arrest, prosecution[9].

Under any of these circumstances many people can undergo a significant and seemingly permanent lowering of mood or even a personality change. They may also develop physical symptoms and illness. This may eventually lead to more serious disease. Any of these incident types can and do cause an involuntary shift of the Assemblage Point to a dangerous dropped location.

Locating The Assemblage Point

Finding the precise location and entry angle of the average, healthy, balanced person is a very quick and simple affair. The following is a description of one the numerous methods used to locate the Assemblage Point. You can find detailed and clear graphics of how to do this on Jon Whale's website (check for the link in the Valuable Resources section at the back of the book): The person should stand upright, looking ahead at the horizon. The investigator should stand facing the person's right-hand body side.

1. Form your left hand into a shallow cup shape. Use it to 'feel' for the person's Assemblage Point at the back around the area between the shoulder blades.

2. Form the fingers and thumb of your right hand into a tight, concentrated point, like a 'bird's beak'. Use the fingertips of the right hand to 'feel' for the cluster of energy lines entering the person's chest.

3. Hold both of your arms wide apart. Hold your left hand behind the person and your right hand in front. Standing relaxed, be keenly aware of your physical feelings and your weight on the floor. It helps to close your eyes or look away. Moving both hands in a slow circular motion, slowly bring your hands towards the back and towards the chest, feeling for the maximum energy disturbance or potential in the fingertips of your right hand and in the palm of your left hand. Allow the person's energy lines to control your arm muscles.

4. The difference in energy potential along the collection of energy lines of the Assemblage Point is easy to distinguish, being concentrated and stronger closer to the chest. When your cupped left hand and right hand pointed fingers are lined up with the person's cluster of energy lines, you will experience an 'energy surge'. This will pass along your arms and through your chest between your shoulders.

5. Bring your hands together, feeling for the maximum power and connection with the person. Allow your hands to touch the person's back and chest at the points of maximum energy connection.

6. Move your right-hand fingers back and forth across the energy lines of the Assemblage Point. Most subjects will feel a 'pulling' sensation deep inside their chest. Use small, adhesive labels to mark the front and rear position.

The location of a woman's Assemblage Point is generally, but not always, several centimeters higher than that of a man. Broadly speaking, a woman's vibrational rate, her behavior, the way she feels and her view of the world are quite different to a man. Therefore, female and male locations tend to be different.

At the location of the Assemblage Point, the skin is less resilient and more painful to the touch. The skin may occasionally be blemished or marked in some way, sometimes by a small diameter reddish spot. Touching or pushing the spot with a fingertip will cause the skin to redden more than skin elsewhere on the chest. The spot is tender, sore or uncomfortable.

Pushing it causes the person a feeling of slight unease. The feeling passes deep into the chest, often right through to the shoulder blade or the place of exit at the rear. Any sensitive person touching the precise location of a person's Assemblage point will feel an exchange of energy. It will feel like a faint or weak electric shock and often has a vibrating quality to it[10].

Shifting The Assemblage Point

Obviously all this new knowledge would be of little value, unless some means were known that could shift the Assemblage Point back to the central healthy position. But in fact it's surprisingly easy! I learned to do it in less than an hour. The procedure takes mere minutes.

Those with the requisite skill, such as Tom Two-Bears Wilson, can probably correct it with a well-placed whack on the person's back! The way Jon taught me to do it was to use a crystal rod (as an attractor) and just "bump" or drag it to the desired location. It's easier to describe than do, but it is certainly not difficult. Anyone with enough life energy in them should be able to do it for another individual.

Doing it for yourself would be near impossible, I think.

There are a number of methods of doing it. The following is the one I learned from Jon and is good for beginners. You will need a heavy chunk of quartz crystal, about 200 grams (7 – 8 ounces), a length of at least 18 centimeters (6 inches) and a thickness of 3 cm or more (1½ inches). Most large towns and cities will have shops that support the sale of crystals.

The crystal must have a ground and polished dome at one end and must have a well-defined point at the opposite end. It should be as clear as possible. The point should have at least three perfect triangles among its six facets and it must be energetic and dynamically "alive" (the crystal should be washed in running water after each use, to keep it energetically clean).

Check its power: hold the crystal with your right hand and direct the point at the palm of your left hand. You should feel a breeze of cool, tingling energy penetrating the skin of your left hand, where the crystal is pointing. If it's "dead", switch for another one which isn't. The crystal is a crucial tool.

Just don't drop it on a hard floor!

Here's the procedure:

Having found the Assemblage Point, front and back (previous section), you now know the start position. Your intention is to literally drag or shove it to the center ideal location. Done right, you can get this shift in one go. If not, repeat the procedure. You'll see an immediate change in the patient's body and energies. When Jon first showed this to me, an MS patient of his, who could barely walk, was instantly able to walk normally!

1. Mark the Assemblage Point position, front and back, with a felt tip marker or small self-adhesive labels.

2. Instruct the subject to stand upright and look straight ahead, not at you.

3. Position yourself to the left-hand side of the patient's body. Holding the crystal in your left hand, place the smooth, domed end on the precise location of the subject's Assemblage Point, where it enters the chest.

4. Place your right hand over the exit point on the rear of the chest, ready to slide it to the desired location.

5. Have the subject take three deep breaths, exhaling slowly over several seconds. Make sure they really are deep and if not ask for three more, to really expand the lungs and chest cavity.

6. On the third inspiration, instruct the patient to hold their breath and squeeze their perineal sphincters (anus and genital area). At the same time instruct him or her to half swallow, which closes the throat, and then hold that moment.

7. With the retained breath and closed body exits, pressure will build up and this "loosens" (for want of a better word) the person's energy field. It becomes detached from the body. Act swiftly and firmly, executing the next step...

8. Using the quartz crystal as a kind of handle, slide your subject's Assemblage Point to the center of the chest. At the same moment, drag the rear location to its correct position, between the shoulder blades, using your right hand. The di-

rection of movement is critical: you must sweep up, across and DOWN onto the desired position.

9. Twist the crystal a half turn and remove it from the chest. At the same time tap the person's head with the palm of your right hand and instruct him or her to resume normal breathing.

10. If you fluffed it or the patient is nervous and fails at keeping still or holding their breath, start again with locating where the Assemblage Point has now moved to and its new angle and repeat the procedure, beginning from this new position.

Obviously, you should instruct your subject beforehand what to do and what to expect. Then these verbal instructions while doing the procedure are merely reminders.

Confirming the shift: - Once done, you will need to orient the subject to the new location. Have them feel it and notice that the spot may be tender. He or she may have reduced or vanished symptoms, as a direct result of the shift of Assemblage Point.

For comprehensive information and instructions on locating and correcting the location and entry angle of the Assemblage Point, please refer to Jon Whale's EBooks and paperbacks. You can find more information in the Valuable Resources section at the back of the book.

His books *The Naked Spirit* or *The Catalyst Of Power* are both extremely insightful and innovative books, in my view. If you like brilliant and novel ideas, you will also enjoy learning about Jon's electronic biologic energy devices. I feature one called the Stellar Delux (former Caduceus Lux) in Chapter 22 of my *Medicine Beyond*.

Now The Science

So far, this might sound like just another esoteric model, about right for a level of New Age whimsy. But Jon Whale is an electronic design engineer and speaks a mathematical and scientific language I find agreeable and convincing. Alongside his scientific work in electronic engineering, he also practiced and studied Eastern mystical disciplines and philosophies relating to the control and manipulation of the body's 'Life Force' energy (*prana* or *Ch'i*, Chapter 11).

Jon states that the oscillating human field has an epicenter of rotation, which is called the Assemblage Point. This does not fit with the Chinese or Indian view but does provide a familiar system structure supported by quantum physics. The Assemblage Point then is a cluster of strong energy lines or strings running through the center of the field. Where these clusters of energy lines cross in the center of the chest, they form a toroidal (donut-shaped) energy structure. Close to the body they have an average diameter of about 1.0 centimeter or less. These lines pass through the chest and out of the back not unlike the Earth's magnetic North and South Pole.

Where the cluster of lines enters the physical body, they induce a tender or very sensitive area of skin when pressed or touched. This tenderness can be quite uncomfortable and can penetrate through to the back.

There is an energy potential both along the length of the lines (front to back) and across their diameter. The energy potential is strongest close to the body where the lines are closest together. Further away from the body the energy lines diverge or spread out and the energy potential spreads with them.

For a healthy person, infrared digital thermometers and infrared image scanners will show a slightly lower reading of approximately 0.2 degrees centigrade at the precise location where these lines enter the chest, compared to the immediate surrounding skin. This is due to a dip in the energy field of 2 - 5% and this is clearly seen as a colder area in the frontal thermogenic body image. Whale Medical Inc. sells a device which will enable you to easily map the body's temperature.

This measurable physical effect is a major finding and confirms the reality of the Assemblage Point. Locating and experiencing these Assemblage Point phenomena provide clear personal proof that in addition to our physical body, we all have an energy body.

The Assemblage Point is not part of the physical body. Although it has serious beneficial medical applications, like the acupuncture meridians, chakras and nadis, it is an integral component, the epicenter of, the energy body that surrounds and saturates the physical body and is almost entirely a spiritual matter.

In other words, it's an intensely personal thing and directly connected to the 'life force' of the individual.

Moving the assemblage point on an individual who is in some psychic and mental stress becomes a vital aspect of treatment. It does not exclude other healing modalities. But it does markedly enhance the effect of any adjunct therapy.

Definitely something to learn, if you are a Western health practitioner.

PART 5

TREATABLE CAUSES
OF MENTAL DISEASE

Now we come to the nub of this book (nub: *the crux or central point of a matter* - Oxford Dictionaries) Simply stated: 99% of individuals are not "mentally ill" or "psychiatric patients", but are suffering from correctable physical ailments, imbalances or disorders (often multiple), which leads to the feeling of not being well or sound in mind.

5.1 Inflammation

Central to almost all these conditions is the element of brain dysfunction, most often to due to an inflammatory process in the brain itself, or secondary to widespread inflammation in the body as a whole. More and more research is backing up this important new understanding. For example, the orthodox view of depression is that people who are depressed have a deficiency in monoamine neurotransmitters in the body, which leads to low levels of neurotransmitters like serotonin and norephinephrine in the brain. There is no actual evidence to back up this hypothesis, but it sticks as a belief system and psychiatrists don't question it.

How could they? If this model is wrong, it makes a nonsense of the powerful and destructive chemicals they prescribe to "correct" this deficiency.

The truth, as I reported earlier in this text, is that there is now abundant evidence supporting the idea that some forms of depression may be linked to ongoing low-grade inflammation in the body. Consider a study published in *The Journal of Clinical Psychiatry*, which examined data from 14,275 people using the Patient Health Questionnaire (PHQ-9) to screen for depression and had blood samples drawn. They found that people who had depression had 46% higher levels of C-reactive protein (CRP), a marker of inflammatory disease, in their blood samples.[250]

Note these markers are indicators of body-wide inflammation and not specific to the brain. In other words, clinical depression may only be a side effect of a more general process going on within the body—and one which is correctable without psychiatric drugs.

Brain-specific inflammatory markers, on the other hand, may be associated with suicidal tendencies. According to a 2017 study, patients with major depressive disorder (MDD) who were experiencing suicidal thoughts had increased brain levels of a marker of microglial activation, a sign of inflammation.[251]

Let's start with an understanding of the mechanisms of inflammation. As the name suggests, it's a condition characterized by heat and pain, like fire. In fact the four marked conditions that are present are heat, redness, swelling and pain. These define a state of inflammation. In most instances there is also loss of function; for example an inflamed joint hurts when moved even slightly, so the person tends to hold it still.

The important point to grasp is that inflammation is a very powerful defense mechanism. Without it we wouldn't last more than a few days. It's a way of blocking infectious pathogens, sealing them off so that they cannot spread widely throughout the body. Without it, that simple whitlow beside a fingernail could end up killing you.

Better to have a swollen, hot and painful finger for a few days than have those microbes rampaging throughout your bloodstream!

A dental abscess is very severe and pain is the prominent feature. But that too, no matter how miserable to endure, is an important safety mechanism, that keeps the bacterial invasion confined to the tooth root and jaw bone. There are many cases where the bacteria do finally escape and spread around the body—a condition called septicemia—and it's highly fatal. So never ignore toothache or any other flare up of infection! You can no longer rely on antibiotics to save you.

The problem we have is not this wise and very efficient phenomenon of rapid inflammatory response to a real threat. We call that *acute inflammation* (acute is a medical expression meaning quick, urgent, and right now).

The trouble comes when the inflammatory process won't stop. It just goes on and on, eventually for years. We call this *chronic inflammation* (chronic, as in "through time").

It can be caused by an unresolved infection that simply cannot be got rid of. The important thing to understand is that almost anything which shouldn't be going on in the body (called an "insult") will lead eventually to chronic inflammation.

Insults are many and varied: food allergies, stealth pathogens, parasites, heavy metal poisons (mercury, lead, etc.), pesticides and pollutants, radiation, to name just a few. The number one insult we face is bad food. Not just inadequate diet but inflammatory foods: refined carbohydrates, sugar, color additives, trans-fats, MSG, xenoestrogens, anti-nutrients and hormone disruptors.

Second to that are the abundant chemicals we face in our food, water and the air we breathe. There are something like 70,000 chemicals currently in commercial production and none of them have been tested adequately for human safety. There is what I call a "chemical blizzard" going on out there. Poison falls from the skies; we breathe it and swallow it, whether we choose to or not.

This is not the place for a diatribe about socio-political issues with Big Ag and Big Food (agricultural methods are designed for maximum profits, not for food quality. Similarly the food industry is not interested in human health, only in profits).

The point to make is that chronic inflammation *from any source* is able to damage individual organs in our body and cause them to dysfunction. That includes the brain and nervous system.

Any and all psychiatric disorders can be caused by, worsened by or prolonged by inflammation, somewhere or anywhere within the body. The idea that mental problems could be caused or enhanced by generalized inflammation goes back at least as far as the early 20th century.

Reducing Dietary Inflammation

I reported earlier on new science (2017) showing that dietary changes and anti-inflammatory supplementation with fish oils (omega-3s) was robustly shown to reduce the symptoms of inflammation, compared to controls.

When people with severe depression followed the Mediterranean diet, they experienced a significant reduction in symptom severity that lasted up to 6 months.

Tooth Abscesses and Psychiatric Illness

Here's a strange story, which has something important to teach us, including the mistakes that were made!

Right at the start of the 20th century, American psychiatrist Henry Cotton began removing decaying teeth from his patients in hopes of curing their mental disorders. We all know we feel lousy in mind, when driven crazy by toothache. But this was certainly a leap into the dark!

It's not clear what success rates Cotton had but he certainly started a fad.

Bret Stetka, an editorial director at Medscape, tells us that Cotton was director of the New Jersey State Hospital for the Insane and was acting on a theory proposed by influential Johns Hopkins psychiatrist Adolf Meyer, under whom Cotton had studied, that psychiatric illness is the result of chronic infection. Meyer's idea started with observations that patients with high fevers sometimes experience delusions and hallucinations.[252]

If tooth extraction didn't work, Cotton moved on to more invasive excisions: tonsils, testicles, ovaries and, in some cases, colons. That, I think, was going too far. His mortality rate was around 45%, which is horrifically high.

Undeterred, in 1921 Cotton published a well-received book on the theory called *The Defective Delinquent and Insane: the Relation of Focal Infections to Their Causation, Treatment and Prevention*. A few years later The New York Times wrote, "eminent physicians and surgeons testified that the New Jersey State Hospital for the Insane was the most progressive institution in the world for the care of the insane, and that the newer method of treating the insane by the removal of focal infection placed the institution in a unique position with respect to hospitals for the mentally ill."

Eventually Cotton opened a hugely successful private practice, catering to the New Jersey elite. Following his death in 1933, interest in Cotton's cures waned. But today we are returning to the concept, if not to the brutal and extravagant surgery (one presumes his patients had little choice).

Symptoms Of Mental And Physical Illness Can Overlap

In 2014 Turhan Canli, an associate professor of psychology and radiology at Stony Brook University, published a paper in the journal *Biology of Mood and Anxiety Disorders* asserting that depression should be thought of as an infectious disease.[253]

"Depressed patients act physically sick," says Canli. "They're tired, they lose their appetite, they don't want to get out of bed." This is remarkably close to Hans Selye's suggestion of the syndrome of "being sick" (see section 4.8).

Canli points to the fact that Western medicine tends to focus on the psychological symptoms of depression, while in many non-Western cultures, patients who would qualify for a depression diagnosis report primarily physical symptoms, in part because of the stigmatization of mental illness.

"The idea that depression is caused simply by changes in serotonin is not panning out. We need to think about other possible causes and treatments for psychiatric disorders," says Canli. We've looked in full into that in section 1.4.

Canli points to how certain infections of the brain—perhaps most notably *Toxoplasma gondii*—can result in emotional disturbances that mimic psychiatric conditions. He also notes that numerous pathogens have been associated with mental illnesses, including Borna disease virus, Epstein-Barr and certain strains of herpes, including varicella zoster, the virus that causes chickenpox and shingles.

An important Danish study published in *JAMA Psychiatry* in 2013 looked at the medical records of over 3 million people and found that any history of hospitalization for infection was associated with a 62 percent increased risk of later developing a mood disorder, including depression and bipolar disorder.[254]

Canli believes that pathogens acting directly on the brain may result in psychiatric symptoms, but also that autoimmune activity—or the body's immune system attacking itself—triggered by infection may also contribute.

You will notice my important speculation that schizophrenia is a kind of auto-immune disease of the brain. I think I'm right. This Danish study also reported that a past history of an autoimmune disorder increases the risk of a future mood disorder by 45 percent.

Antibodies Provide A Clue

The idea that there could be a relationship between the immune system and brain disease isn't new. Autoantibodies were reported in schizophrenia patients in the 1930s. Subsequent work has detected antibodies to various neurotransmitter receptors in the brains of psychiatric patients, while a number of brain disorders, including multiple sclerosis, are known to involve abnormal immune system activity. Researchers at the University of Virginia recently identified a previously undiscovered network of vessels directly connecting the brain with the immune system; the authors concluded that an interplay between the two could significantly contribute to certain neurological and psychiatric conditions.

Multiple studies have linked depression with elevated markers of inflammation, including two analyses from 2010 and 2012 that collectively reviewed data from 53 studies, as well as several postmortem studies. A large body of related research confirms that auto-immune and inflammatory activity in the brain is linked with psychiatric symptoms.

Now a new study (2017) has shown that lupus (an autoimmune disease) almost doubles the risk of a certain type of dementia (1.97 times, in fact).[255]

Once again, I repeat the maxim that association doesn't prove causation.

But it might be the price we have to pay for our powerful, even over-reactive, immune systems. The good news is that lowering allergies (hypoallergenic diet) and quenching inflammation—all part of this text—can have a calming effect on most autoimmune diseases.

Dr. Roger McIntyre, a professor of psychiatry and pharmacology at the University of Toronto, implicates inflammation in general, not exclusively inflammation caused by infection or direct effects of infection itself, as a major contributor to mental maladies. "It's unlikely that most people with a mental illness have it as a result of infection," he says, "but it would be reasonable to hypothesize that a subpopulation of people with depression or bipolar disorder or schizophrenia ended up that way because an infection activated their immune-inflammatory system."

McIntyre says that infection, particularly in the womb, could work in concert with genetics, psychosocial factors and our diet and microbiome to influence immune and inflammatory activity and, in turn, our risk of psychiatric disease.[256]

In other words, McIntyre is saying what I am saying. Physical factors are the real cause of mental disorder, not some twisted state of mind.

5.2 Post-Vaccination Syndrome

This too is a strong player and often overlooked, in the search for causes of mental ill health. Someone has to think of it, for it to be diagnosed.

Not to put too fine a point on thigns, vaccines have been linked to decline in mental health and social interaction; some are even speculating this could be a cause of increase in mass school shootings. It makes sense, since the most heavily vaccinated demographic are children and youths.

Let's consider a recently published study in the journal *Brain, Behavior, and Immunity* titled "Low-Grade Inflammation Decreases Emotion Recognition – Evidence from the Vaccination Model of Inflammation". It clearly links low-grade inflammation to a decrease in mental health and human social interaction. [257]

One of the well-known sources of low-grade inflammation is the grumpy and disturbed immune system after it has been whacked with vaccines. Obviously the more vaccinations a child receives, the worse the inflammatory disturbance, up to and including loss of cognitive function and control (such as autism).

The study, authored by a team of researchers from the University of Birmingham in the UK and headed by Leonie J.T. Baltcr, called attention to the already well-established fact that systemic inflammation can disturb mind function. Depression, indeed, in mainly an inflammatory disease, not a mental process at all (as described in section 2.1).

To test out the effects of post-vaccination syndrome on mind function, the team decided to use the typhoid vaccine because, according to their research, this particular vaccination induces inflammation, without apparently causing their participants to suffer from sickness, fever, or mood change.

This is important, of course, because discomfort and sickness are factors that could also account for temporary cognitive dysfunction and social impairment.

Results

About 6h30m after injection in each condition, participants completed the Reading the Mind in the Eyes Test (RMET), a validated test for assessing how well the mental states of others can be inferred through observation of the eyes region of the face.

According to Balter, when deciding on the health of their participants, she and her team had decided to exclude any individual who had had a previous history of a suspected vaccine-related allergy, a food allergy or intolerance, an inflammatory, cardiovascular, neurological, mental health or immune related disorder, smokers, a visual impairment (unless corrected to normal), or anyone on medication seven days prior to the test.

That cuts the field down a lot but I consider that very prudent and such a decision puts this study in a class of its own, from the point of view of integrity. From over four decades of clinical work, I know that food allergies and other immune reactions produce profound cognitive impairment (section 4.7).

In summary, typhoid vaccination elicited a transient low-grade inflammatory response in healthy young men and decreased performance on the Reading the Mind in the Eyes Test, tested in a double-blinded placebo-controlled crossover design.

The importance of this test, showing a reduced ability to tell what other are thinking, is that it is a strong pointer to the possibility of autism (ASD is nothing so much as an inability to respond to others)

Hereby the current study provided direct empirical evidence for a link between heightened inflammation, caused by vaccinations, and lower ability to infer mental states of others. The study to be of great significance, because it could also demonstrate a link between vaccinations and depression. That could explain why U.S. News recently reported that between 2013 and 2016, the diagnosis of depression had risen by 33 percent in the U.S. alone.

In other words, the drive for mass vaccination (to generate more profits) could be a major contributing factor to what has become an "epidemic" of depression.

Nice business model, by the way: drive for mass vaccinations (make lots of money); make people sick and depressed; sell lots of antidepressants to the victims you just made sick (make lots MORE money). That's Big Pharma all over!

Missing Link

Many of us are worried, not to say convinced, that vaccinations are certainly the origin of autism. Mass vaccinations means more autism. Bad news.

This study could be one of the missing links that proves the connection. After all, if the typhoid vaccination can cause a lowered ability in facial recognition, a recognized symptom of autism, then perhaps other vaccinations can cause similar problems.

However, the Balter study was not purely about autism; their study was mainly about depression. It's therefore a bit weird that the researchers had decided not to include women in their study because, in general, depression affects a higher number of women than men. [I have not written to Leonie Balter, asking what the thinking was behind that]

Referred to as sickness syndrome, models of inflammatory depression are characterized by symptoms that could be designed to reallocate energy resources for recovery.

Those symptoms include loss of appetite, lack of social interest, irritability, slowed thinking, low libido, increased sleep, anhedonia (lack of pleasure or enjoyment), and lethargy.

Depression was likely an short-term adaptive response in human history of acute infectious stressors but has been rendered disabling in a landscape such as we live in today, of chronic, unrelenting assaults on response systems.

Vaccinations and Depression

Balter and her team were not the only researchers to have examined the link between the typhoid vaccination and depression.

In 2009, Neil A. Harrison et. al., wrote a paper titled Neural Origins of Human Sickness in Interoceptive Responses to Inflammation, which was published in Biological Psychiatry.

Harrison's team also used the typhoid vaccination as their vaccination of choice. They wrote:

Inflammation is associated with psychological, emotional, and behavioral disturbance, known as sickness behavior.

Inflammatory cytokines are implicated in coordinating this central motivational reorientation accompanying peripheral immunologic responses to pathogens.

Studies in rodents suggest an afferent interoceptive neural mechanism, although comparable data in humans are lacking.

For their study, Harrison and his team also chose to vaccinate male participants, however, unlike Balter and her team, Harrison's team asked their participants to complete a Profile of Mood State questionnaire, at the two and three-hour baseline. Their results were as follows:

Typhoid but not placebo injection produced a robust inflammatory response indexed by increased circulating interleukin-6 accompanied by a significant increase in fatigue, confusion, and impaired concentration at 3 hours.

Performance of the Stroop task under inflammation activated brain regions encoding representations of internal bodily state.

Spatial and temporal characteristics of this response are consistent with interoceptive information flow via afferent autonomic fibers.

During performance of this task, activity within interoceptive brain regions also predicted individual differences in inflammation-associated but not placebo-associated fatigue and confusion. Maintenance of cognitive performance, despite inflammation-associated fatigue, led to recruitment of additional prefrontal cortical regions. (emphasis added)

They concluded:

These findings suggest that peripheral infection selectively influences central nervous system function to generate core symptoms of sickness and reorient basic motivational states.

Once again, we can see that post-vaccination these participants became increasingly confused and lacked concentration.

On-Board Inflammagens

In 2015, psychiatrist Kelly Brogan, M.D., published a paper tilted Psychobiology of Vaccination Effects: Bidirectional Relevance of Depression.[258]

In her abstract, Brogan stated that:

> Emerging research on inflammation-mediated processes that underpin depressive syndromes reveals a possible link warranting greater exploration.

Because of its often insidious onset and varied presentation, depression as a sequel-ae of pharmaceutical interventions can be difficult to assess.

This review explores the available literature considering the relevance of pre-existing depression to vaccination response as well as the association of vaccination with adverse psychiatric events/depression and the mechanistic plausibility of that association.

As we all know, many of the vaccinations that our children receive contain trace amounts of toxic metals, such as Thiomersol (US spelling failure: Thimerosal) which contains mercury and aluminum.

The CDC (Centers for Disease Control and Prevention) has stated that these are added to the vaccinations as either adjuvants or preservatives. Adjuvants are added to the vaccine to help the vaccine be more effective, and preservatives are added to the vaccine to help the vaccine remain unchanged.

However, in some recipients, these adjuvants and preservatives can cause serious adverse reactions. The CDC seems to be arguing we have to make this stuff nasty, otherwise there is no immune response.

The trouble is, these toxic heavy metals are not gotten rid of when no longer needed. So they are bound to produce a long-term inflammatory response and that, as we all know, is dangerous indeed. Inflammatory depression might be among the least of the problems. Brain damage, autoimmune disease, diabetes, vascular inflammation and cancer are likely results too.

In other words, it's like having on-board inflammagens you cannot expel.

Evidence exists that shows that organic mercury (notably ethylmercury) can act as a mitochondrial toxin in brain astrocytes. Thiomersol (US: Thimerosal) has also been found to promote overflow of the excitotoxic chemical, glutamate, in the prefrontal cortex causing "behavioral, neurochemical, and neuropathological abnormalities"and "lasting neurobehavioral impairments and neurochemical alterations in the brain" in animal studies.

It's important to be aware that a toxicological assessment of injected quantities has never been carried out. But due to the absence of liver-based detoxification mechanisms and the gut barrier, direct injection of heavy metals can be presumed to have a significantly greater potential toxicity compared with oral delivery.

As mercury was phased out of most vaccines 10 years ago as a precautionary step, aluminum replaced it as a primary vaccine adjuvant, and it is now present in 18 vaccines in the current pediatric schedule—hepatitis B (HepB); diphtheria, tetanus, and pertussis (DTaP); hepatitis A (HepA); hacmophilus influenza type B (Hib); and pneumococcal conjugate vaccine (PCV).

But it's laughable to pretend that aluminium (aluminum) is safe. On what grounds? Not science...

A recent study stated, "Aluminum in adjuvant form carries a risk for autoimmunity, long-term brain inflammation, and associated neurological complications, and thus, may have profound and widespread, adverse health consequences." [259]

In other words, watch out. Any vaccines could contain any combination of serious toxic adjuvants and be a part of mental impairment, including difficulty relating, mood swings, cognitive dysfunction and ultimately, dementia.

Testing For Inflammation

It is possible to put a figure on how-much inflammation is going on. To do that we measure blood levels of what are called inflammatory cytokines.

An inexpensive C-reactive protein (high-sensitivity) blood test (CRP-hs) can help reveal if you suffer from systemic inflammation. If your CRP-hs level is over 1.3 (mg/L), this is an indication that you have an inflammatory event occurring in your body. Those with elevated CRP-hs levels (and who suffer from a disease associated with chronic inflammation) should consider using a supplement protocol and/or prescription drugs known to suppress elevated pro-inflammatory cytokines (see below).

Other tests for inflammation are expensive but definitely reveal more information. The principle ones are Tumor Necrosis Factor-alpha (TNF-a), Interleukin-6 (IL-6), Interleukin 1 beta (IL-1(b) and Leukotriene B(4) (LTB(4).

The cost of these cytokine tests can be outrageously expensive. You'll need to make an arrangement with your doctor and/or your insurance company. I have links in the **Valuable Resources** section at the back of the book that might be helpful.

Generalized Quietening of Inflammation

There is no question that finding and eliminating specific causes of inflammation, such as stealth pathogens, food allergies, inhalants, chemical sensitivity and toxic metal overload is the prime approach, but understanding how to quench or dampen down the body's inflammatory response is crucial knowledge.

There are a number of anti-inflammatory "tools" that can be brought to bear but these are unlikely to be entirely successful, unless the cause is found a disposed of.

Omega-3s. These essential fatty acids (EFAs) have a quenching effect on inflammation. The body can synthesize most of the fats it needs from the diet. However, two essential fatty acids, linoleic and alpha-linolenic, cannot be synthesized in the body and must be obtained from food. These basic fats are used to build specialized fats called omega-3 and omega-6 fatty acids.

Put simply, omega-3s are good and the omega-6s are pro-inflammatory. The trouble is, our typical diet of civilization contains a huge excess of omega-6 fatty acids and very little omega-3s.

Hence the diseases of civilization—also the diseases of aging—diabetes, arthritis, dementia, etc. It's no coincidence that the incidence of these diseases has soared, since our diets have deteriorated under the onslaught of manufactured foods and turning away from fresh whole foods.

Everyone should supplement omega-3 EFAs, particularly eicosapentaenoic acid (EPA) and docosahexaenoic acid (DHA). Plant sources include borage, oil of evening primrose and flax seeds. Fish oils and krill have been popular but, as the oceans get more and more polluted, there is a concern over purity. Surprisingly, the richest source of all is grass-fed beef. That might be surprising at first but, if you think about it, cattle do a good job of turning grass into nice, rich fatty milk. They can do the same with essential fatty acids!

The ideal dose is around 3 grams daily for an adult.

Bromelain-Papain mixes (example: Wobenzym)

Inflammation throughout the body produces pro-inflammatory cytokines and other aggravating substances. These can affect the brain, as well as any other organ or tissues, as we have seen. Any legitimate way of lowering the presence of these pro-inflammatory substances is good. We can digest them away!

Digestive enzymes make a fine neutraceutical, used intelligently. Large doses may even benefit cancer, but that's another story.

Simple, natural digestive substances can be obtained from plant sources, notably bromelain from pineapple and papain from papaya. Vegetarians can find mixtures of these two enzymes. Better by far, if you are not vegetarian or vegan, is animal based proteolytic (protein digesting) enzymes.

In fact the very best product in this field is a German formulation: Wobenzym®. It contains the following: pancreatin, papain, bromelain, trypsin, and chymotrypsin. Each one of these is a protease, which simply means that they break down proteins. You can buy it online from many sources (make sure it is authentic, not a cheap knock-off).

Of course Wobenzym® is not the only effective formula. A good test for checking if an enzyme product is working is to put a tablet on the back of your tongue. If it doesn't start to sting or smart quite quickly (due to digesting your tongue), don't rely on it!

Moderate Exercise

Gentle exercise can be anti-inflammatory and very helpful. Quiet, gentle walks are highly recommended for all acutely distressed individuals, preferably in relaxing, easy-on-the-mind surroundings, such as by the ocean shore (see also the section on forest bathing 2.4).

This is definitely NOT a case where more is better. Extreme and damaging workouts, such as the Crossfit cult, marathons, etc. are contraindicated. Vigorous exercize, in fact, is quite *pro*-inflammatory.

However, I feel I should refer the reader to an important series of studies relating physical fitness and brain health.

In fact, compelling evidence shows that physical exercise helps build a brain that not only resists shrinkage through aging, but increases cognitive abilities and creativity. Researchers at Stanford University found that walking can increase creativity up to 60 percent. This applies to mild or moderate exercize.[260]

Even more importantly, we now know that exercise promotes a process known as neurogenesis, i.e., the brain's ability to adapt and grow new brain cells, regardless of age. Exercise also promotes mental health by normalizing insulin resistance and boosting natural "feel good" hormones and neurotransmitters associated with mood control, including endorphins, serotonin, dopamine, glutamate and GABA.

Most recently, Canadian researchers found high-intensity workouts helped boost memory by improving hippocampal function—a finding they say could prove to be an important prevention strategy against Alzheimer's disease, the most serious and deadly form of dementia.

The hippocampus is an important memory processing part of the brain. I say processing because there is no suggestion that memory is stored there. Indeed, memory is non-material, whatever the mechanistic dinosaurs want to preach.[261]

A recent scientific review from Australia's National Institute of Complementary Medicine (NICM) at Western Sydney University and the Division of Psychology and Mental Health at the University of Manchester in the U.K. shows that aerobic activity can improve your memory and overall brain health as you age.[262]

According to Joseph Firth, PhD, study author and research fellow at Australia's National Institute of Complementary Medicine: "Our data showed that, rather than actually increasing the size of the hippocampus per se, the main 'brain benefits' are due to aerobic exercise slowing down the deterioration in brain size. In other words, exercise can be seen as a maintenance program for the brain."

This is all good news for older citizens, who may be worrying about dementia. Stay active is the message!

Supplements Against Inflammation

The reader will have realized from comments throughout this text that omega-3s (fish oils, krill oil, or plant-based sources of alpha-linolenic acid (flaxseed oil, canola, soy, perilla, and walnut oils) are the star anti-inflammatories. Take 3-4 grams daily.

But there are other players to bear in mind.

DHEA, an important hormone precursor (see below), has anti-inflammatory properties. I would suggest a dose of 50-100mg daily for men. Women should take substantially less, because it will cause greasy skin and possibly spots.

Curcumin (from the spice turmeric) is currently enjoying huge popularity and being extensively clinically tested as an anti-inflammatory. Mounting evidence from studies shows that curcumin modulates numerous molecular targets and exerts antioxidant, anti-inflammatory and neuroprotective activities.

Abnormal microglial cell activation, oxidative stress, and neuronal death are associated with the progression of the Alzheimer's disease. Curcumin has been found to inhibit this. So it's a good bet for most disturbances of mood and cognition.

Unfortunately, curcumin taken orally is poorly absorbed and rapidly metabolized and eliminated. Therefore, the potential of curcumin as a therapeutic agent is limited.

Some curcumin supplements have added piperine, to increase the bioavailability of curcumin. This is not a good idea. Piperine interferes with detox pathways and those need to be kept open and flourishing for all patients with mental health issues.

Trials suggest that curcumin is quite harmless, up to about 12 grams.[263]

Typical doses would be around 2 – 3 grams daily. According to the European Food Safety Authority Panel, the acceptable daily curcumin dosage is 3 mg/kg bodyweight.

Research studies have used between 0.5 g and 7.5 g curcumin per day, divided into three or four even doses.

There's a great article in LE Magazine (January 2002) that breaks down anti-inflammatory supplements. I'll place the article information in the **Valuable Resources** section in the back of the book.

5.3 Food Allergies

There is no question that the number one cause of systemic inflammation in our bodies is food: unwise foods, such as manufactured junk, or specific food allergens. These are sometimes referred to as "inflammatory foods" or "pro-inflammatory foods". But that's a major mis-representation of the truth, as I shall reveal: *there are NO foods that are anti-inflammatory, or pro-inflammatory in all individuals.*

Such generalizations are erroneous and may cause failure of treatment and confusion.

The truth is: everyone is different and each person has to work out which foods inflame his or her body. THEY WILL BE UNIQUE FOODS. There are no universal inflammatory foods, applicable to all.

Incidentally, "organic" or "GMO-free" labels have nothing to do with this. Whereas junk foods are universally bad for us, I am calling attention to the fact that some foods that, even in the organic wholefood form, may make an individual severely ill, in body, mind or both. These are true food allergies (or intolerance), a reaction to the pure food, not manufactured substitutes.

This is a good starting place. Let's take a look at what I consider probably the number one and number two causes of mental disorder: food allergies and inhalant allergies, particularly chemical susceptibility and mold toxicity.

5.4 Not All In The Mind: Food Allergies and Intolerance

I chose the heading for this subsection carefully. "Not All in the Mind" was originally the title of a seminal book by a British psychiatrist called Richard Mackarness, published in 1976. He was tired of encountering patients who had been referred to him because "there was nothing wrong" and the patient had been told "It's all in your mind," "You need to see a psychiatrist", etc.

Doctors were coming up with negatives on the labs and thus assumed the patient was faking their problems. But the doctors were failing to test for the number one health phenomenon that disturbs brain function. In fact the vast majority of cases had food allergies and intolerance to foods and that was the main reason for the patient being ill!

I almost invariably advize a patient with a significant number of mental symptoms—whether benign (like lethargy and "brain fog") or severe (like violence, depersonalization, hallucinations and depression)—to start by trying to identify any food allergies and intolerances. If you haven't yet looked at the inventory of likely symptoms, do so first and see how you score (appendix). The point is that you may find many other symptoms that will suggest food allergy, not merely mental problems.

Some symptoms are real give-away for food reactions:
- Bloating and flatulence
- Food binges
- Food cravings

- Overweight, underweight or wildly fluctuating weight (gain a few pounds in a day)
- Symptoms actually come on while eating
- Symptoms after food (falling asleep, chills, sudden rapid heartbeat, after a meal)
- Feeling unwell when going for hours without food (food addiction)
- Feeling tired, crabby or very lethargic on waking

The last may seem strange: most everybody wakes up feeling bad, don't they? No, but it is common; that's because very many people are suffering the addiction effects of food allergy. Common doesn't mean normal, however.

Think about this: by the time we wake in the morning, we may not have eaten for 10- 14 hours; that's more than enough time to set up withdrawal symptoms. With breakfast, we get our first "fix" of wheat, sugar, caffeine, or whatever is the trigger food and the symptoms start to clear right away. You don't believe me? Wait until you have followed the exclusion diet instruction in this section and you'll see the truth of what I say. Even the most incorrigible morning bear-head gets a pleasant surprise.

A Good Place To Start

This is not to say that everything mental is just a food allergy. But diet adjustments are a great place to start because there is usually some kind of beneficial result and they are relatively easy to do. If you can feel much better just avoiding, say, milk or wheat, that is far easier than battling against multiple environmental shocks and stressors. The reason is simple if you understand the overload principle: avoiding one stressor, especially if it is an important one, may free your body defences up enough so that it can cope with the rest, without your help!

Even if you feel no better after eliminating certain foods, that doesn't mean that you don't have food allergies, but it may mean that you have co-existent environmental allergies and intolerance.

The secret of successful identification of food allergies is to give up sufficient foods to be able to feel well, then to re-introduce these foods one at a time, so that detecting a reaction is relatively easy. We call this elimination and challenge dieting. It rarely works to give up just one food at a time because anyone who is ill is almost certain to have more than one allergy. If it was simply one major allergen, the person would have spotted it eventually, as indeed some lucky people do.

Pediatrician Dr Doris Rapp MD, author of "Is This Your Child?" and several other books, coined an instructive term: the "eight nails in the shoe trap". Doris points out that if you have eight nails sticking out in your shoe, and then pull just one of these nails, you will still not be comfortable – because of the other seven. It can be the same with multiple allergies. You have to work at it just that little bit harder.

It is important to remember that I am talking here of a trial diet, an experimental procedure we call an "elimination diet" or "exclusion diet". You do not need to stay on a tough diet long-term; indeed you are specifically cautioned not to do so, otherwise you run into other problems. The purpose of the strict diet is to isolate the culprits. Once you know these, you can eat most anything else. This means you shift into a maintenance diet, solely avoiding the offending foods, something you stay on for months or years. Almost anyone who feels much better by avoiding one or two foods has the will power to continue; the rewards are high!

Let me outline my 3-tier elimination dieting plans. You can get full details from my self-help book Diet Wise (www.DietWiseBook.com), where I discuss things like medication, organic foods, GMOs and the like.

You must also stop smoking if you are serious about getting well. I have indicated the strong connection between smoking and severe mental disturbance in section 4.8.

Let's start with the easiest level diet as an entry.

An easy elimination diet (14-21 days)

It is logical to start by eliminating only the common likely food allergies. This leaves plenty of foods to eat and you should not find this diet too onerous. It is especially suitable for a child and consists basically of fresh meat, fish, fruit and vegetables, with juice and water to drink. We call it the 'Stone-Age' or 'Caveman' diet. I used this diet from the 1970s onwards and it nicely pre-dates the current fashion of paleo-eating.

Foods You Are Allowed To Eat:

- Any meat (not processed or smoked)
- Any vegetables (fresh or frozen, not tinned)
- Any fruit, except the citrus family (lemon etc.)
- Any fish (not processed or smoked)
- Quinoa (grain substitute)
- All fresh unsweetened fruit juices, except citrus
- Herb teas (careful: some contain citrus peel)
- Spring water, preferably bottled in glass
- Fresh whole herbs
- Salt and pepper to taste

Foods You Are Not Allowed To Eat:

- No stimulant drinks – no tea, coffee, alcohol

- No sugar, honey, additives or sweeteners

- No grains: absolutely no wheat, corn, rye, rice, barley, oats or millet. That means no bread, cakes, muffins, biscuits, granola, pastry, flour or farina

- No milk or dairy produce: no skimmed milk, cream, butter, margarines or spreads, not even goat's milk

- **No manufactured food**: nothing from tins, packets, bottles or jars. If somebody labeled it, they likely added sneaky ingredients to it.

Here are some important points to keep in mind:

It is vital to understand that you must not cheat on this or any other exclusion diet. This is not a slimming diet, where you can nibble a piece of chocolate cake and still lose weight. Remember that it takes several days for food to clear your bowel and eating it as little as twice a week will prevent you clearing it from your system. If you do slip up, you will need to extend the avoidance period for several more days. Later on, when the detective work is complete, the occasional indiscretion won't matter. In the meantime, follow the instructions exactly.

Don't forget about food addictions; they are real. It is quite likely that you will get withdrawal symptoms during the first few days. This is good news because it means you have given up something important. Usually the effects are mild and amount to nothing more than feeling irritable, tired, or perhaps having a headache, but be warned: it could put you in bed for a couple of days. I have seen wheat "cold turkey" that was just as grim as narcotics.

Please also note that it is possible to be allergic even to the allowed foods - they are chosen simply because reaction to them is less common. If you are in this unlucky minority, you might even feel worse on this diet, but at least it proves you have a food allergy. In that case, try eliminating, also, the foods you are eating more of (potato is a common offender) and see if you then begin to improve. If not, you should switch to the Eight Foods Diet, or a fast as described below.

While on the elimination diet, try to avoid hanging on to a few favorite foods and eating only those. You must eat with variety, otherwise you will risk creating reactions to the foods you are eating repeatedly. It is senseless to go on with old habits. The whole point of exclusion dieting is to make you change what you are doing - it could be making you ill.

Don't worry about special recipes or substitutes at this stage. By the time you have fried, baked, steamed and grilled everything once, the first ten days will almost have passed! If in the long term it transpires that you need to keep off a food, then you can begin searching for an alternative.

Patients usually ask: What about my vitamin and mineral supplements while on an elimination diet, do I need to take those? The answer is NO. Most vitamin and mineral tablets contain hidden food ingredients, such as corn starch. Even those that say "allergy-free" formulas are sometimes misleading. They may not be made up with common allergens, such as wheat, corn or soya derivatives; but nevertheless, vegetable ingredients are present, such as rice polishings and potato starch. To call these allergy "safe", or even hypoallergenic, is in my view dishonest.

Don't take the risk, you won't come to any harm without supplements for a short period. *This leads on to another major Scott-Mumby Rule:*

The biggest and commonest health hazard by far today is not what you are lacking that you should be eating, but what you are already eating that you shouldn't! In other words, giving up allergens, toxic or overload items has far more dramatic results in terms of health recovery than supplementing stuff you are deficient in.

How Did You Get On?

If you felt a whole lot better, skip to the section on food challenge testing:

DO NOT, simply because you do not improve or feel any different, make the erroneous assumption that you could not then be allergic to milk, wheat or other banned foods. Remember the eight nails in the shoe? This would be a serious mistake which could bar your road to recovery.

You can, in any case, carry out useful challenge tests, taking a note of what happens when you re-introduce a food. Careful! You do not want to hammer a pointed nail back in that shoe!

The Eight Foods Diet (7-14 Days)

Not as severe as a fast but tougher than the previous regime, is what can be called the Few Foods Diet; I prefer to use an 8-food plan. Obviously it is more likely to succeed than the previous plan, since you are giving up more foods. Any determined adult could cope with it, but on no account should you subject a child to this diet without his, or her, full and voluntary cooperation. It could produce a severe emotional trauma otherwise (factually, there is rarely a problem—most children don't want to be ill and will assist you, providing they understand what you are trying to do.)

The basic idea is to produce one or two relatively safe foods for each different category we eat. Everyday foods are avoided since these include the common allergens. Thus we would choose fruits such as mango and papaya, not apple and banana; flesh such as duck and rabbit, not beef and pork; quail and ostrich, not chicken... you get the idea? The diet below contains my suggestions. You can vary it somewhat according to what is available to you locally.

The Few Foods Diet

Meat, protein:	rabbit, venison
Fowl:	ostrich or quail
Fruit:	persimmon, kiwi fruit
Vegetables:	spinach, turnip
Starch:	buckwheat, quinoa

In addition to the stipulated foods, you are allowed salt to taste but not pepper, spring water but not herb teas or juices. Even herbs and pepper must be challenged correctly on introduction. Note that neither of the suggested starch foods are in the grains family.

The main problem with such a restricted plan is boredom. However there is enough variety here for adequate nourishment over the suggested period of seven to ten days, providing you eat a balance of all eight foods. Exotic fruits can be expensive, but you won't need to eat them for long and, in any case, few people would deny that feeling well is worth any expense.

The chances are that, on a diet like this, you will feel well within a week, but for some conditions, such as depression, eczema and arthritis, you will need to allow a little longer. Be prepared to go the full ten days before deciding that it isn't working.

A variation of this diet is the exotic food diet. Don't worry how many foods you can round up to eat, choose as many as you can find; just make sure they are all unusual, you personally have never eaten them and they are not related to any common food category. The book Diet Wise gives you further useful information, like food families (foods that are somewhat related in character): www.DietWiseBook.com

The Fast (5-7 Days)

Although a fast is the ultimate approach in tracking down hidden food allergies, I don't recommend it lightly. It is quick (fast!), inexpensive and an absolute yes-no statement on whether your illness really is caused by food allergy. Although it can be tough at first, by the morning of the fifth day, you can expect to feel wonderful! That's why fasting is popular as a religious exercise and why sometimes people with a severe attack of gastro-enteritis, who expel almost all the food content of the bowel by diarrhea and vomiting, are suddenly "cured" of some other health condition.

The real problem is that sometimes it can then be difficult to get back on to any safe foods. Everything is unmasked at once and the patient seems to react to everything he or she tries to eat. This can cause great distress.

Undertake a fast only if you are very determined or you still suspect food allergy and the other two approaches have failed.

Fasting is emphatically not suitable for certain categories of patient:

- Pregnant women
- Children
- Diabetics
- Epileptics
- Anyone seriously weakened or debilitated by chronic illness
- Anyone who has been subject to severe emotional disturbance (especially those prone to violent outbursts, or those who have tried to commit suicide)

The fast itself is simple enough—just don't eat for four or five days. You must stop smoking. Drink only bottled spring water. The whole point is to empty your bowels entirely of foodstuffs. Thus, if you have any tendency to constipation, take Epsom salts to begin with. If in doubt try an enema! Otherwise the effort may be wasted.

It may help to do what I call a grape-day step-down. This means eating grapes only for a day, as an easy-in step towards fasting.

Special note: A variation, which I call the 'half fast', is to eat only two foods, such as lamb and pears. This means taking a gamble that neither lamb nor pears are allergenic, and it is not as sure-fire as the fast proper. It is permissible to carry this out for seven days, but on no account go on for longer than this.

Food Challenge Testing

As soon as you feel well on any of these elimination regimes, you can begin testing, although you must not do so before the four day unmasking period has elapsed. Allow longer if you have been constipated.

Of course, you may never improve on an elimination diet. The problem may be something else, not a food. In that case, when three weeks (maximum) have elapsed on the simple elimination diet, two weeks on the Eight Foods Diet, or seven days on a fast, then you must begin re-introducing foods. This is vital. It is not enough to feel well on a very restricted diet; we want to know why? What are the culprits? These are the foods you must avoid long-term, not all those which are banned at the beginning.

Even if you don't feel well, as already pointed out, this does not prove you have no allergies amongst the foods you gave up. Test the foods as you re-introduce them, anyway - you may be in for a surprise

My recommended procedure is as follows, except for those coming off a fast:

Eat a substantial helping of the food, preferably on its own for the first exposure. Lunch is the ideal meal for this.

Choose only whole, single foods, not mixtures and recipes. Try to get supplies that have not been chemically treated in any way.

Wait several hours to see if there is an immediate reaction, and if not, eat some more of the food along with a typical ordinary evening meal.

You may eat a third, or fourth, portion if you want, to be sure.

Take your resting pulse (sit still for two minutes) before, and several times during the first 90 minutes alter the first exposure to the food. A rise of ten or more beats in the resting pulse is a fairly reliable sign of an allergy. However no change in the pulse does not mean the food is safe, unless symptoms are absent also.

Alkali Salts

If you do experience an unpleasant reaction, take Epsom salts. That clears the food from your bowel as fast as possible. Also, alkali salts (a mixture of two parts sodium bicarbonate to one part potassium bicarbonate: one teaspoonful in a few ounces of lukewarm water) should help. Discontinue further tests until symptoms have abated once more. This is very important, as you cannot properly test when symptoms are already present; you are looking for foods which trigger symptoms.

Using the above approach, you should be able to reliably test one food a day, minimum. Go rapidly if all is well, because the longer you stay off a food, the more the allergy (if there is one) will tend to die down and you may miss it.

Occasionally, patients experience a 'build up' which causes confusion and sometimes failure. Suspect this if you felt better on an exclusion diet, but you gradually became ill again when re-introducing foods, and can't really say why. Perhaps there were no noticeable reactions.

In that case, eliminate all the foods you have re-introduced until your symptoms clear again, then re-introduce them more slowly. This time, eat the foods steadily, several times a day for three to four days before making up your mind. It is unlikely that one will slip the net with this approach.

Once you have accepted a food as safe, of course you must then stop eating it so frequently, otherwise it may become an allergy. Eat it once a day at most - only every four days when you have enough 'safe' foods to accomplish this.

Psychiatric Patients

Some care needs to be taken when the patient has pronounced mental problems, that is to say severe enough to have been admitted to a psychiatric ward or hospital. Food reactions can be so violent as to precipitate mania and psychotic delusion; this sometimes has to be seen to be believed.

Equally serious, is the possibility that the patient may try to injure him or her self, or even try to commit suicide, when challenged in this way.

Never leave such a patient unattended, even if the response appears mild at first.

I hope to see the day when, once again, environmental control units can survive and flourish. This is a set up where very sick people can be admitted under professional medical care, with skilled doctors and trained nurses in attendance full time, breathing only pure air and drinking pure water, and then fasted for five days before challenges. Unfortunately, the economic set up today makes it impossible today for such units to survive.

Special Instructions For Those Coming Off A Fast

Begin only with exotic foods which you don't normally eat; do not be tempted to grab for that coffee or cake! The last thing you want to happen is to get a reaction when beginning to re-introduce foods – it will mean you cannot carry on adding foods until the symptoms settle down once again.

Instead, for the first few days, you want to build up a minimum range of 'safe' foods that you can fall back on. Papaya, rabbit, artichoke and dogfish are the kind of thing to aim for - do the best you can with what is available according to your resources.

The other important point is that you cannot afford the luxury of bringing in one new food a day: you need to go faster than this. When avoided even for as little as two weeks, a cyclical food allergy can die down and you may miss the proof of allergy you are looking for. Quicker means testing two or even three foods a day when coming off a fast. Pay particular attention to the pulse rate before and after each test meal and keep notes. It is important to grasp that some symptom, even if not very striking, usually occurs within the first 60 minutes of eating an allergy food and it may be subtle, only blowing up into full force hours later. You need to be alert to this, or you will miss items and fail to improve without understanding why.

If the worst happens and you are ill by the end of the day and can't say why, condemn all that day's new foods.

The build-up of foods is cumulative: that is, you start with Food A. If it is OK then the next meal is Food A + Food B, then A + B + C and so on.

An example table of foods tests might be:

Days 1- 4   no food

Day 5

- breakfast - poached salmon
- lunch - mango (plus salmon)
- dinner - steamed spinach (plus salmon and mango)

Day 6

- breakfast - baked pheasant, quail or partridge + day 5
- lunch - kiwi fruit + pheasant + day 5
- dinner - steamed marrow or zucchini (courgette), kiwi and/or pheasant + day 5

Day 7

- breakfast -lamb chop (plus any of the above) + days 5,6
- lunch - baked potato (do not eat the skin) + lamb + days 5,6
- dinner - banana + days 5,6 etc...

Grape not allowed on day 5 if you used a grape-day step-down. Best to leave it a week or 10 days.

All proven safe foods are kept up after an allergic reaction. Therefore, if Food F causes a reaction, while you are waiting for it to clear up, you can go on eating foods A-E, until symptoms clear.

Within a few days, you should have plenty to eat, albeit monotonous. From then on, you can proceed as for those on elimination diets if you wish.

Your Personal Exclusion Program

An elimination diet is not a punishment and not a "cure". It's simply an experimental, fact-finding exercise. *You do not need to remain on an exclusion diet for long; indeed, you should not.*

Whichever program you chose, once you have carried out the challenge tests you will have a list of items you do not tolerate well. You must now avoid these, if you are serious about your health. You have, in effect, designed your own personal diet plan for health. Use it as something you return to in times of trouble or stress, a safe platform.

There should be no rush to try and re-introduce any of these bandit items, if at all. Design your living and eating plan without them, long-term. However the good news is that allergies do settle down, sometimes quite rapidly, especially if you pay attention to everything else I have explained in this book. If you develop and practice a newer safer ecological lifestyle, you may have surprisingly little further trouble. You may feel better than you have felt in years. Many patients act emotionally and energetically younger, free of worries and cares; so much so that friends and relatives often comment. I noticed this over thirty years ago and that is one of the reasons I now find myself pioneering holistic alternatives to psychiatry.

A Food Diary

It is a good idea to keep a food diary during your experiments with food. Write down everything you eat at each meal, or between meals, and also mark in any symptoms which you experience, with the time of onset in relation to meals. It is often possible to spot a pattern which recurs time and time again but which is not evident when relying only on short-term memory.

Warning: a food diary does tend to make you very conscious of food, which is probably a good thing in the short term. However, taking the long view, try to avoid the exercise making you too introverted about feelings and symptoms, otherwise it can start becoming an obsession. Many allergy patients become so consumed by anxiety about what they are eating that they cannot eat or socialize normally. Food allergy investigations, as described here, are merely a tool not an end and should not become a way of life, otherwise family and friends will feel excluded and that in turn leads to rejection.

Many "amateur" gung-ho food allergy books actually tend to create this major social incompetence, because the authors do not have sufficient experience to be aware of the dangers (and likely because they too are obsessive). Make no mistake, food allergy restrictions can ruin relationships and break up marriages, if it is taken to extreme, as many know to their cost. I do not automatically take the patient's side but sympathize with both points of view (because ultimately I see this as in the patient's broader interests).

Eating can become a psychological burden on the patient and intolerable nuisance to family and friends, if you go too far. True health does not mean isolation from society, it means full social wellbeing included in the deal.

The food diary is merely a tool and should be discontinued as soon as practicable.

5.5 Chemical Intolerance (Environmental Illness Syndrome)

We come now to one of our BIG topics, albeit it a highly controversial one: the question of "chemical allergy" or intolerance. I am not talking here merely about chemical pollution in the atmosphere but contact with substances common in the home and that release fumes which we breathe on a daily basis.

Some of this chemical exposure is deliberate and part of our modern living style: cosmetics, detergents, aerosols and even medical drugs are all intentional chemical exposures. I particularly object to the concept of spoofily-named "air fresheners", when all they do is add more chemicals to the air, in an attempt to disguise existing contaminants. It is rather like taking dirty trench water to wash away stains --- "Not logical", as Mr Spock (Leonard Nimoy, not the pediatrician) would have said.

It is surprising to most people to learn that indoor chemical pollution is often many times the allowed safety limits allowed at work. A 5-year-study carried out by the US Environmental Protection Agency (EPA) found that peak concentrations of 20 toxic compounds monitored were 200-500 times higher inside some homes than those outdoors. Formaldehyde and toluene (from paints and varnish) are good examples of dangerous indoor pollutants. Formaldehyde, given off by many home substances, from PVC to particle board, is a known carcinogen. Toluene, released by fresh paint, dissolves brain tissue and causes permanent brain damage. There is a move to ban it in industry as a health hazard but homes have no such protective legislation. In the di-isocyanate form (tdi= toluene di-isocyanate), released by wet varnish, it is notorious for sensitizing people to allergens. Significant exposure to this latter chemical has been the start of a descent into Allergy Hell for many individuals.

Human Canaries

Increasing numbers of people simply cannot accommodate the everyday load of ambient chemicals and it begins to undermine their health in many unsuspected ways. In my radical 1986 book *Allergies: What Everyone Should Know* (London, Unwins) I introduced the term "human canaries". The phrase seems to have caught on. This likens chemically sensitive people to the canaries taken down mines in olden days. If the bird fell dead it meant that the air was dangerous and was a warning to humans to get out fast. It seems to me that we have many human canaries today but few people are heeding the warnings.

Are you a canary? You can download a free questionnaire (the link is in the **Valuable Resources** section at the back of the book).

Chemical sensitivity is with us, big time. A 1999 survey reporting the prevalence of people with sensitivities to chemicals found approximately 12% of the population had problems.[264]

No wonder.

Something like 6 million new chemicals have been manufactured since the 1960s, when the chemical boom got under way worldwide. Of these, upwards of 100,000 are in production at any one time. In just the 25 years between 1970 and 1995, the volume of synthetic organic chemicals produced tripled, from about 50 million tons to approximately 150 million tons. And today it is much more, according to Lynn R. Goldman, Dean of the George Washington University School of Public Health.[265]

We call these synthetic substances xenobiotics (foreign to life). This is not an idle word: it implies that our bodies do not know how to deal with these substances. Nature did not endow us with the necessary enzyme equipment to safely detox them because they are not naturally occurring compounds. This increases their danger considerably.

In my view it is unarguable that we will all go under if we don't soon start to reduce the total chemical load in our environment. This is not merely green politics but an out and out survival issue. There is dirty work afoot and that, of course, means Big Business dollars getting in on the act and perverting truth. We are told we need most of this chemical junk, that pesticides save lives and help grow more crops, which we need to feed the planet, and so on. I am not in the agribusiness, I'm a doctor. My take on this is very simple and very blunt:

The word "pesticide" is a con trick. Plant and animal physiology does not recognize human value judgments, such as "useful" and "nuisance" life forms. The correct word is *biocide*, which means that it *kills any life*, not just pests.

Moreover, the idea of "responsible" or "controlled use" of toxic substances and talk of "reducing" usage levels is meaningless and dishonest: chemicals in the environment persist. *Last year's out put is added to that of the year before, to this year's, next year's and so on. It's cumulative.*

There are already enough xenobiotic substances in our environment, working their way through the water table and eco-system to keep us all ill for decades, even if output was curtailed tomorrow, a pretty unlikely event in any case.

Now that's said, let's get back to chemical sensitivity:

The arguments I have heard against this phenomenon are frankly absurd:

Many otherwise sound clinicians refuse to accept that small traces of chemical substances can make an individual ill. Yet the toxicologists, who have very precise and quantitative scientific techniques, know it and have written tens of thousands of papers on what I have termed "low grade poisoning" – susceptible individuals who feel the ill effects at doses that are supposed to be safe in normal circumstances.

The explanation lies in the statistical tool known as a bell curve (because it is shaped like a bell). Individual reactions vary from those who can tolerate very little of a stressor, to those who seem hardly fazed at all, even by large exposures. In the middle lies the majority. But the majority sensitivity is NOT the defining condition. It is wholly inaccurate to consider only the middle response on this curve.

Further confusion may stem from the fact that it may be long-term exposure which causes the trouble, as the chemical accumulates in the tissues (especially the brain). Exposure levels that are allegedly safe don't count if you are storing the toxin.

Small simple molecules don't command an antibody response, is another ridiculous assertion. We all know that people can be highly sensitized to nickel: that's just one unique atom! You can't get simpler than that. But experts should know also about haptens. These are small molecules which plug in to an antigen-antibody pair and excite a reaction which might not otherwise have happened.

Overload

The key to chemical intolerance of this type is the matter of individual biological variation. It is no good measuring averages or the mean when it comes down to the fact that most people are not at all average and some individuals are very far from average. Is it right to condemn and ignore individuals who are extremely poorly tolerant, or accusing them of making it up, when we know (for sure) that there are individuals equally far from average in the opposite direction, who can tolerate very large exposures apparently without harm? An enlightened and compassionate medical science must include everyone and not dismiss those who don't fit the reductionist demographic formula.

Dr Theron Randolph, who first pioneered chemical susceptibility in a massive seminal book *Human Ecology and Susceptibility to the Chemical Environment*, points to this major difference between conventional medicine and the allergy/ecology approach: the one is for the mass, the other is for the individual. He called these two approaches endogenous and exogenous medicine. It is worth tabulating the key differences.

ENDOGENOUS MEDICINE	EXOGENOUS MEDICINE
Treats the average	Treats the individual
Blames the patient	Blames exterior causes
Symptom-oriented	Cause-oriented
Sees averages	Sees uniqueness
Over-rides nature in the cure	Seeks to enlist nature in curing
Treatment adds burden	Treatment by reducing burden

The point is that, sooner or later, everyone reaches their threshold limit and from then on, symptoms escalate. It matters not whether we call it susceptibility or overload; the result is the same.

When to suspect chemical intolerance and overload.

Suspect chemical intolerance or overloading when you develop the following signs:

- Symptoms worse in closed spaces (shopping malls, long car journeys)
- Symptoms worse on week days (chemicals at work)
- Symptoms better on holiday (fresh air!)
- Worse in an urban environment
- Gasoline or gloss paint gives you a headache
- Acute sense of smell to chemicals
- Lost sense of smell or it comes and goes
- You get a "lift" or liking for certain chemical odors
- Intolerant of synthetic fabrics (sneezing, skin rash, irritation)
- Others similarly ill in the home or workplace
- Illness began after moving to present location or current employment

Does the idea of a "lift" or buzz from chemicals sound crazy? Why should it? Think about glue and solvent sniffers. They do it on purpose – but just because they are too stupid to realize the dangers that doesn't mean it is not pleasurable brain stimulation.

Note that with exposure at work symptoms may not begin till Tuesday or Wednesday, as the cumulative effect builds up. Similarly, symptoms may not clear by Saturday morning but could linger through till later. Yet you may get the worst reaction on Monday and Tuesday, as your body is challenged by chemicals which have gassed out over the weekend.

Why Would Someone Develop Chemical Intolerance?

I have learned of at least five reasons a person becomes chemically sensitive. Others may come to light in time:

- Chronic over-exposure (as in the workplace)
- Sudden massive over-exposure (as in a contamination incident)
- Metabolic (enzyme) deficiency
- Overload
- Candida (so-called)

Once intolerance to one chemical substance is established, it tends to multiply rapidly, with more and more substances causing problems. We call this the "spreading effect".

Scott-Mumby's Rule Of The Nose: I have a maxim, based on decades of experience, which is that if there is enough substance present to cause an odor, there is enough to cause symptoms. Some chemical substances, of course have no odor.

There are many other chemical contacts, of course: plastics, urban atmospheric pollution, perfumes and cosmetics, cleaners, solvents, aerosol sprays, paints and food additives, to name but a few. Most of these are derived, ultimately, from petroleum and the whole group we call "hydrocarbons" from their chemical structure. Interestingly, all petroleum (and coal) products originated as pine trees in carboniferous forests millions of years ago. Yet we find pine and its terpene derivatives today are quite potent allergens! Is there a connection?

Chemicals At Work And School

Don't forget the work environment as a source of chemical exposure. In some trades there are specific hazards and the monitoring of these exposures since the Health and Safety at Work Act of 1974 has come under the control of the Environmental Safety Officer (ESO) in the Environmental Medical Advisory Service (EMAS). However, to pretend this system is working efficiently and protecting workers properly is to be foolish and gullible in the extreme. Only a very small percentage of workers - those employed in larger factories and offices - effectively come under this sort of umbrella.

Although the Act supposedly covers all offices, factories and places of work, in actual fact it is impossible to monitor the countless small businesses that this represents. Only if the individual worker complains is any action likely to be taken in the event of a hazard and many workers are reluctant to report breaches of the codes for fear of losing their jobs, either as retribution or indirectly because the works are closed down due to not being able to afford all the safety procedures required.

It may be obvious to you that you are working with major chemical toxins. Elaborate precautions and safety instructions would tell you that. However, many chemical allergens at work are much more insidious and difficult to detect unless you consider the possibility. Problems can come from photocopier fluids, solvents, aerosol, powerful cleaning agents and detergents (common where contract cleaners are employed), air purifiers and, last but not least, the fabric of the building and its furnishings (formaldehyde particularly). If your office has that new 'plastic' smell, this could be a problem. Air conditioning often makes matters far worse by circulating indoor pollution.

Sick Building (Tight Building) Syndrome

This problem can be so bad that we have begun to pinpoint what is called the Sick Building Syndrome. It is, in and of itself, a new kind of psychological health issue. Some modern buildings have such a high internal accumulation of these obnoxious substances, that almost everyone feels ill to some degree. Headaches, sore eyes and runny nose, fatigue and inability to concentrate are almost the norm. The effect on work efficiency is disastrous and absenteeism runs sky-high.

Contaminants, like pollutants from motor vehicle exhaust, plumbing vents and building exhausts (bathrooms and kitchens) can enter the building from outside through poorly located air intake vents, windows and other openings. Combustion byproducts can enter a building from a nearby garage. Radon, formaldehyde, asbestos, dust and lead paint can also enter through poorly located air intake vents and other openings.

The most common contaminant of indoor air includes volatile organic compounds (VOCs), especially formaldehyde, which is almost ubiquitous. Other VOCs include adhesives, upholstery, carpeting, copy machines, manufactured wood products, pesticides, cleaning agents, etc. Environmental tobacco smoke, respirable particulate matter, combustion byproducts from stove, fireplace and unvented space heater also increase the chemical contamination. Synthetic fragrances in personal care products or in cleaning and maintenance products also contribute to the contamination (so-called "air fresheners" are a joke, which simply add to the chemical burden).[266]

In order to have an acceptable indoor air quality with a minimum energy consumption, The American Society of Heating, Refrigeration and Air-Conditioning Engineers recommends a minimum outdoor-to-indoor air flow rate of 15 cubic feet per minute per person (cfm)/person to avoid the problems related to inadequate ventilation. The standards are 20 cfm/person in office spaces and 60 cfm/person in smoking lounges. Poor design and construction of buildings with too many offices crammed in a building (to increase the salable area) has also been blamed for inadequate ventilation.

Other factors that have been blamed for sick building syndrome are electro-smog, unpleasant acoustics, fluorescent lighting and inefficient ergonomics.

The solution, if changing the place of work is not an option, is to try to take control of the immediate personal environment. Chemicals should be removed from the office or workroom, air filters fitted or upgraded, and personal substances, such as perfumes, after-shave and hair spray, banned (a good idea anyway).

Even a small desktop air filter can make a big difference. But the more powerful HEPA type (high efficiency particulate air), can remove 99.97% of particles down to about 3 microns in size.

See section **Improving Air Quality** below.

Since it is costing industry money in lost man-hours, you may be sure (especially if you are cynical, like me) that a lot of money is now being spent on researching this problem.

In the meantime, the answer is simple. Open the windows! The problem is made far worse by the modem craze for energy efficiency. For allergy sufferers at least, draughts are good news. They help to circulate air and keep down internal pollution. This applies in the home also - double glazing and draught-proofing may be disastrous to those who suffer within the home environment.

The list below gives pointers towards chemical overload in the work environment.

- The presence of any known hazards (eg. Toluene diisocyanate, formaldehyde)
- You feel better at weekends
- Symptoms clear up on holidays
- Co-workers affected ('sick' or 'tight' building syndrome)
- Reaction started when you started your present employment
- Worst on Monday and Tuesday
- You have an unusually keen sense of smell
- You have lost your sense of smell
- Chemical odors seem to give you a lift or "high"

Nowadays, thanks to the pioneer work of my great mentor Theron Randolph, and his successors, such as William Rea MD and Sherry Rogers MD, we recognize the widespread and diverse manifestations of chemical sensitivity. We call this phenomenon Environmental Illness Syndrome, or EI for short.

You will sometimes hear the expression "chemical allergy" but this attracts criticism. I have introduced a better concept: low-grade poisoning. The fact is that almost all chemicals are toxic and when inhaled over long periods, even in small quantities, can produce cumulative overload and symptoms. But some individuals are more susceptible than others, and react at levels most of us can tolerate. Some unlucky patients are exquisitely sensitive and react adversely to even the smallest traces of certain substances. We can label them chemically hypersensitive. Often there are complex reactions intermixed and the term multiple chemical sensitivity has come into common use.

Such susceptibility produces reactions which are easily confused with true inhalant allergens. Sometimes, of course, the two coexist within the same individual. Always bear in mind the possibility of chemical sensitivity when investigating symptoms due to apparently airborne triggers.

Universal Reactors

"Allergic to the twentieth century!" screamed the derisory newspaper headlines as these stories began to emerge a few decades ago. Universal reactors suffer from what has sometimes been called 'total allergy syndrome'. While this did give some insight into the origin of the problem it was grossly overstated and was the cause of much confusion and misinformation about real allergies.

There are persons who have a very tough time from a wide variety of foods and environmental excitants, and they find it difficult to share our ordinary way of life. Sometimes the sheer number of triggers can seem endless and baffling. Even clinical ecologists have tended to use the term *universal reactors* for such people, without stopping to think what this means.

Nobody can be sensitive to everything, so the term has no meaning. But it can seem that way. Gulf War Syndrome can have this aspect at its most extreme. Looking beyond the official vacant denials, it may be said that the jury is still out over whether the latter is caused primarily by poisons or by vaccination overwhelm of the immune system. My own view is that, as always, it will turn out to be a combination of such factors.

What is actually being described is a condition in which most of the immediate substances in view seem to cause symptoms. In other words, allergics trying to find a safe diet and encountering only foods that cause symptoms may well in despair get the idea that they are allergic to 'everything.'

Others are alarmed about chemicals in the environment: they wear masks, panic at the sight of a felt-tip pen, claim they react to yesterdays aftershave on visitors and would rather starve than eat food that might have been sprayed with pesticides. There is something irrational about the beliefs of patients who reach this level of anxiety about chemicals. Many such 'chemical victims' have lost sight of, or are unaware of, the irony that the foods they allow themselves to eat contain high levels of some of the toxic chemicals they claim to react badly to. Many foods are highly toxic in nature, especially when eaten raw. Common carrots, for example, have a toxin (caratotoxin) that is classed with organophosphates (nerve gas). Falcarinol is a natural pesticide found in carrots An even more potent toxin in carrots is cicutoxin. Clinically, cicutoxin causes grand mal siezures and eventually death in its victims. OK, not such a threat to humans in the quantities found. But red beans? If these are not cooked properly, the toxins they contain can put you in hospital.

Isolationism

There could be, in the environmental view of disease, the germ of fanaticism; the foundation of the (erroneous) notion that all one has to do to enjoy good health is to isolate oneself from the outside world. It is a tempting notion on the surface and I have seen many examples of people trying to cope with their problems in this way. But their 'victory' has come at such a cost.

Health in its fullest sense means well-being of body, mind and spirit. This cannot really be achieved by severing all practical contact with other human beings. I am talking about holistic medicine and that means the whole self. To fixate on the body at the expense of the mind and spirit is a sad slight to the totality of our humanity.

If this isn't reason enough, there is a very sound technical reason why extreme avoidance is wrong. It means the patient will unmask large numbers of food and chemical allergies simultaneously. It can then become extremely difficult to find a way back without having to pass through many reactions while readapting to the environment. This can actually fuel the impression that you react to everything.

The Way Out

Urgent reduction of body load is needed. This applies also to psychological burdens: counseling or Supernoetics® piloting (section 3.12) may be called for. If life difficulties have not been to blame for precipitating the condition (as is usual), the individual will certainly have crept into a psychologically negative space and needs bringing back to a balanced center.

All means of reducing body load are legitimate. A holiday, however fearful to contemplate, can be soul-saving in the event. Sometimes just such a simple measure can break what has hitherto been a vicious circle. Exotic foods are better than starvation. Malnutrition will only add to the body's problems.

Some kind of low-dose desensitization can be very helpful. The best general program I know lies with a rotation diet and neutralizing drops, in accordance with Miller's method.

The environmental control unit (ECU) approach may be the answer, where available. This is a facility where the patient can rest while on a 5-day fast, breathing only filtered air and drinking pure water. Foods are then returned to the diet, after careful challenge testing, followed by screening chemicals. It is a laborious approach but highly accurate.

Unfortunately, insurance companies today have squeezed every last ECU unit out of business. They don't want cures. We may have to wait years or decades before this important healing approach can once again become financially viable for the individual.

Cleaning Up Your Chemical Environment

It makes good sense to clear your environment of as many unnecessary chemicals as possible. This will reduce your overall environmental burden. We choose the home for this because it is something you can control to a great extent. You can't do much about what is beyond your doors and windows (except move if you are down-wind from a factory or such) but, unless you have a particularly unsympathetic and selfish family, you should be able to effect enough changes indoors to produce a worthwhile improvement. Some substances you will be able to replace with safer substitutes. Many you will be able to dispense with altogether. Some you will need and no substitutes can be found. The answer is to recognize the danger, use them as infrequently as possible, preferably get someone else to carry out the task involved and store these substances outside the house, for instance in the garage

I usually get patients to comb the whole house, room by room, cupboard by cupboard and shelf by shelf, listing all the chemicals found. Sometimes, the list itself is a shock and this is salutary. To pinpoint all potential trouble, I get them to supplement what can be seen with what can be smelled. Most chemical allergics have a very sensitive sense of smell; others have none and will need to enlist the help of someone else - I call this a nose survey: if you can smell it, it can make you ill. That is, if there is enough to cause an odor, there is enough to cause symptoms.

The list of some potential chemical allergens shown below will help you search out trouble. Store, replace or throw out as much as possible of what you find. There are nearly always safer or less reactive alternatives.

- Aerosol sprays of all kinds
- Air fresheners
- Tap water
- Cavity wall insulation
- Cleaning materials
- Cooking utensils
- Fabrics
- Flues
- Garages, integral - Petrol fumes
- Gas
- Heating

- Cosmetics
- Paints
- Toothpaste

Don't forget car and upholstery are potential hazards. Nowadays, most are treated with complex stain-repellent and preservative chemicals. You may not want to throw out your nice new carpet or sofa but at least if you can diagnose that's where the trouble is coming from, you will feel less distressed. Things will probably improve in time. However, for an unlucky few, the truth is simple, if bleak - they will never be well until the luxury wall-to-wall hazard is disposed of!

Organic Foods

It pays to avoid food additives and eat only wholefoods. It makes no sense going to the trouble of cleaning up your personal local environment, if you let in foodstuffs that are loaded with poisons.

Dr. Sherry Rogers emphasizes eating whole foods uncontaminated with pesticides and drinking unchlorinated, unfluoridated water that is as uncontaminated with agricultural runoff where possible. "The sick body cannot rally if it is busy detoxifying pesticides and other chemicals." Tests show that pollutants from plastics are "a million times higher than any other pollutants."

Plastic bottles, so beloved of spring water suppliers and soda manufacturers, give off significant levels of phthalates which can migrate into the food, water, and milk causing hormone disruptions in all the endocrine systems, nervous tissue, and the immune system, causing a plurality of confusing symptoms and combinations of symptoms.

Science for Toxic Times

According to a July 2012 study of 400 primary care patients (published by Claudia Miller, an environmental health expert at the University of Texas School of Medicine in San Antonio, and her colleagues in the popular family practice journal Annals of Family Medicine), 22 percent of individuals with chronic health issues suffer from some degree of chemical intolerance. That's more than one in five — and, says Miller, they are vulnerable to chemicals, or what she calls TILT (toxicant-induced loss of tolerance), if life happens to toss them too much toxic exposure.[267]

"The fact that chemical intolerance is so prevalent, yet unrecognized, is important for primary care physicians," says physician David Katerndahl, Miller's colleague and lead author on the study. "On the one hand, simple therapeutic approaches (avoiding chemicals) may be quite effective, while on the other hand, conventional treatments (allergy shots, immune suppressants) may fail. This means that we must change our clinical paradigm with these patients."

The 2012 study is based on an inventory of 50 questions called the QEESI (the Quick Environmental Exposure and Sensitivity Inventory, available for free at familymed.uthscsa.edu/qeesi.pdf). The QEESI isolates sensitivities to common triggers, such as diesel, paint thinner, foods and products like fabric softener. It is very effective at culling the one in five individuals who are vulnerable to severe TILT, and it has been validated in Sweden, Denmark, Japan and the United States.

Some patient's lives were devastated by chemical sensitivity. "In the study, I was astounded to find that over 6 percent of people visiting a primary care clinic for any kind of chronic health condition were greatly affected by TILT, based on their symptoms and chemical and other intolerance scores from the QEESI. By greatly affected, I mean that they had chronic health symptoms that were severe, and they scored high on sensitivities to common chemicals, foods and medications," says Miller. "Another 15.8 percent were moderately affected, with scores that were still well above average."

Like Dr Miller, I would like to see the QEESI survey form administered frequently, if not always, in the primary care situation. Have you been "tilted"?

It's unique to our age.

5.6 Airborne Allergens

Environmental triggers can include both airborne particles, such as dust, pollen and mold spores, and of course, chemical pollution, though the two problems are often inextricably bound together.

This section is to look at airborne allergens, not necessarily chemical overload.

Suspect environmental allergies if your symptoms change as you re-locate in different places or at different times. If you are well at home but feel bad at work, an environmental allergen or chemical pollutant in your work environment may be to blame. Perhaps you are better on holiday (away from home); that would suggest an environmental factor, but be careful – you may eat differently on vacation, where normal habits do not apply!

Classic summer symptoms are a sign of a reaction to airborne allergens, such as pollen and mold. But some individuals are worse in winter. On hearing this I immediately suspect indoor pollution; in winter time we close our doors and windows, turn up the furnace and suffer from combustion fumes. Indoor chemical pollution can rise to many times the levels that would be permitted by safety regulations at work! Lack of fresh air also raises humidity, which allows house dust mite and molds to flourish.

What Do We Mean By Airborne Allergies?

Environmental or inhalant (breathed in) allergies are quite common. Indeed, for half a century they were the only kind to be recognized. Inhaled allergens can include such diverse substances as pollens, house-dust mite, feathers, mold, fur and fabrics. The one thing these substances all have in common is that they are light enough to float in air and so be breathed in. Thus the target area is often the nasal and respiratory passages. However I discovered early on, by challenging sensitive individuals, that even a dust or mold allergy can induce strong and unwelcome mental reactions, such as altered perception or inappropriate changes of mood.

It is vital in the investigation of any mentally disturbed patient that inhalant allergens are borne in mind.

We can classify inhalant allergies into two main categories:

- Seasonal (specific times of the year) and

- Non-seasonal (sometimes known as perennial or all-year-round)

Seasonal triggers are due to pollens and mold spores. 20% of the US population is affected by seasonal allergies, that is, up 35 million sufferers. Non-seasonal triggers include dust, mold and chemicals.

Molds

No review of airborne allergens capable of causing profound mental disturbance could possibly be considered comprehensive without reference to the effects of molds.

Unfortunately, mold allergies are very common. Drug reactions to antibiotics, such as penicillin, are actually mold allergies. Most exposures, however come from mold spores floating in the air. Molds are rather like an all-year-round pollen, only absent during hard frost or when the ground is covered with snow.

Some indoor molds, notably *Stachybotrys chatarum*—the toxic black mold—can be very dangerous. Stachybotrys causes lung bleeding in infants. It may even be a cause of sudden infant death syndrome. It is recognized as a contributor to sick building syndrome.

Stachybotrys has been implicated in a variety of a variety of mental symptoms in adults, including memory loss, disorientation, confusion, difficulty in focusing and personality changes. All psychiatrists and mental health workers should be aware of its ominous potential.

Suspect mold allergy if…you are bad on damp, humid days
- better in cold weather

- have cravings for bread, alcohol or yeast foods
- damp, musty buildings make you ill
- you have a skin mold (athlete's foot, Tinea versicolor, ringworm)

Ringworm, of course, is not a worm! It is a mold which grows outwards from the center and thus has a circular shape, with an active (growing) outer ring. This and other skin fungus growths are called Tinea. There is a phenomenon which I identified over 30 years ago and which I called "the moldy patient". It denotes an individual who seems to be a natural growing place for a mold and a "yeast garden".

The above symptoms point to such an individual

The science is becoming clear: a 2007 study published in *The American Journal of Public Health* reported a link between mold and depression. In this study led by Brown University epidemiologist, Edmond Shenassa, the team actually set out to disprove the association between mold and depression reported in several studies out of the United Kingdom (one of my bitches with so-called science is that they set out to prove something or other—shouldn't they just set out to find what the truth actually is?).

In fact they achieved the opposite and established a clear link between the two. The main outcome for the study was depressive symptoms, measured by an index based on the presence of 4 symptoms of depression (sleep disturbance, decreased interest in activities, low self-esteem, and decreased appetite) during the 2 weeks prior to the assessment.[268]

Any symptom can be caused by mold. Stuffy nose is obvious. But the most overlooked symptoms are mental ones. These can be extremely bizarre and frightening. In medieval times people would sometimes eat rye bread infected with poisonous ergot mold (*Claviceps pupurea* and its LSD-like mycotoxin). Ingestion resulted in an intense burning of the skin (St Anthony's fire) and wild, violent and irrational movements (St Vitus' dance). It has even been suggested that the outbreak of hysteria and hallucination in Salem, Massachussetts, in 1692, attributed to witchcraft, could have been an outbreak of rye mold poisoning. If so, lives were tragically lost due to ignorance of this malady.

Mold toxicity can manifest with so many different and diverse symptoms, that it is frequently misdiagnosed. It is likely that some cases of chronic fatigue, fibromyalgia, mast cell activation disorder, histamine intolerance, irritable bowel and leaky gut, multiple sclerosis and post treatment Lyme syndrome, which do not respond to treatment, are due to a chronic inflammatory response caused by toxic mold.

Unfortunately mold toxicity is not on the radar of many practitioners, and thus they do not include it as part of the differential diagnosis.

I have seen patients acting very strangely on mold challenge tests. One woman shook uncontrollably, from head to toe. Another patient cried for hours, though he explained that he felt fine and definitely not sad or anguished.

Psychology Today gives the following list of likely symptoms (note, as with all lists like this, none of these symptoms are mold-specific. They are in fact mainly OVERLOAD symptoms):

1. Fatigue
2. Weakness
3. Aches
4. Muscle Cramps
5. Unusual Pain
6. Ice Pick Pain
7. Headache
8. Light Sensitivity
9. Red Eyes
10. Blurred Vision
11. Tearing
12. Sinus Problems
13. Cough
14. Shortness of Breath
15. Abdominal Pain
16. Diarrhea
17. Joint Pain
18. Morning Stiffness
19. Memory Issues
20. Focus/Concentration Issues
21. Word Recollection Issues
22. Decreased Learning of New Knowledge
23. Confusion
24. Disorientation
25. Skin Sensitivity
26. Mood Swings
27. Appetite Swings
28. Sweats (especially night sweats)
29. Temperature Regulation or Dysregulation Problems
30. Excessive Thirst
31. Increased Urination
32. Static Shocks

33. Numbness

34. Tingling

35. Vertigo

36. Metallic Taste

37. Tremors[269]

Reducing Mold Exposure

Consider mold problems if no other obvious cause of organic illness is found and your house is low-lying in a damp valley. Older houses are especially suspect, particularly those with a condensation problem. Sometimes it is possible to see the mold growing on the walls and carpets!

If there is any doubt, order mold growth plates to be exposed around the home and see what grows on the plates after this collection.

You will need professional advice to be sure of getting rid of the damp. It may entail major structural repairs. If the problem is too extensive, you should consider moving, if you value your health. In the meantime, a dehumidifier should help to reduce the damp.

Clean mold wherever you find it, using a dilution of chlorine bleach to four parts of water. Do not soak fabrics and soft furnishings in this process. Moisture is the enemy. Remove all moldy fabrics, once contaminated.

Once again, dieting has considerable value in reducing cumulative overload. Certain foods are actually fungus or molds (mushrooms and cheese). Yeast products are similar and often cross-react. A suitable diet for a mold-sensitive individual would of course avoid these and also foods containing yeast and fermentation products:

- alcoholic and fermented drinks
- bread (except unleavened)
- vinegar
- sauces
- malt and malted foods
- yeasted cakes
- coffee and chocolate (fermented during processing)
- B-vitamin products (unless stated yeast-free)
- over-ripe and moldy food
- carton-packed and bottled fruit juices also contain significant amounts of yeast, but not when freshly squeezed

Remember that house plants encourage molds which grow in the damp soil. You may need to get rid of them.

Improving Air Quality

If you suffer psychological problems, or any other symptoms, caused by airborne particulates or chemicals, it makes sense to try and improve the quality of the air you breathe. There is nothing to be done about urban pollution, or summer allergens, apart from keeping your doors and windows closed. But there are a number of air purification devices on the market which may help you to produce a *clean local environment*, whether in your bedroom or at the office. Bedroom is especially valuable, because we spend about one third of our lives there!

Some people will find the equipment below very useful, enabling restful nights and symptom-free days, perhaps for the first time; others will benefit only little and find trying to tackle inhalant particles and gases not worth the trouble. People vary and there are no hard-and-fast rules. A little experimentation is recommended. Good manufacturers and suppliers will often lend you equipment on an approval basis, so you have a chance to try it first.

It isn't realistic to expect to achieve an environment that is 100-per-cent controlled, except in an environmental control unit (ECU).

Face Masks:

There are situations where a multiple sensitive person may want to wear a protective mask, for example when cleaning in a damp and dusty enclosed space. However it is not a good idea to get into the habit of using artificial aids on a semi-permanent basis. Often this means little more than psychological dependence that may not have any relation to scientific removal of impurities. Patients who squeal and hold a handkerchief over their face every time someone takes the top off a felt tip pen are inviting ridicule, moreover (my point entirely) there are far better ways of conquering your problem than this.

If you need to use a mask, be aware of the different types and their limitations:

- Lightweight, cotton surgical masks strain out particles such as pollen, dust and smoke. People sensitive to wheat and flours who work in the catering industry may need one of these. They are not completely effective against particles.

- For chemical vapors you may need an activated-charcoal filter mask. There are many simple versions of this design which, in its full form, is the gas-mask worn by troops in combat. Suppliers claim these are effective against benzene, ozone, diesel fumes, lead salts, hydrocarbons, nitrous oxide and sulphur dioxide. Most people would probably benefit from one of these masks when encountering smog.

Air filters:

If you can't face the expense of major household filtered air purification, consider a small, mobile system. Standards are variable and if possible you should try out a model before buying. Beware of settling for a unit that seems inexpensive but is inadequate to the task; check volume air turnover and compare this to the size of the room you are trying to maintain pure. Aim for at least four changes of air per hour.

The best units combine chemical purification (activated carbon) with particulate removal of varying standards (see next 3 sections).

Avoid units with the deplorable addition of scents and 'fresh air' perfumes; this adds chemical pollution.

There are portable models for the car that plug into the car's cigarette lighter socket. Used properly these may assure that you arrive in a refreshed state after a long drive, instead of semi-drugged with traffic fumes!

Activated carbon filters:

These are fairly effective at absorbing cooking and food smells, cigarette and tobacco odors, perfumes, diesel and petrol fumes, smog, ozone and animal smells. They are less effective against pollen, smoke, mildew, chlorine, fish odors and some noxious gases. Unfortunately, they perform poorly against two dangerous indoor chemicals, carbon monoxide and formaldehyde.

Electrostatic air cleaners:

A fan draws in particles and these are then given an electric charge that causes them to stick onto a screen or plate. Manufacturers claim they remove 90 percent of particles. In fact performance falls off very rapidly and within days the unit may be less than 50 percent effective. This type of purifier also needs constant cleaning and maintenance.

Another problem is that charged particles that 'escape' the screen or plate will stick on walls and furniture. There can be considerable build up, which causes discoloration. This type of filter may also produce ozone, a highly toxic gas that causes headaches in susceptible people.

Not really recommended.

High efficiency particulate air (HEPA) filters:

These are 95% efficient for particles down to about 0.1 micron in size (see Table 1), and 99.7% efficient down to 3 microns, according to the US National Bureau of Standards. Predictably they are also quite expensive. They are sometimes called absolute filters and are used to maintain sterile air in hospital operating theatres and burns units.

HEPA filters work particularly well against important sensitizing allergens such as pollens, molds, yeasts, fungi and bacteria. They are also effective against viruses, which means they may help to cut down on colds and other infections.

When combined with an activated carbon filter, these devices can produce very good quality air in a limited space.

Do not fall for ad wordings such as products that claim to be "HEPA-type", "HEPA-like", "HEPA-style" or "99% HEPA". None of these are of value to a real pollution sufferer.

Ionisers:

It has been observed that people often feel better and more zestful when they are near mountain streams or beside the sea. At least one possible cause for this is the presence of excess negatively charged ions in these places.

The earth is positively charged and so attracts these ions, yet they tend to be diminished in buildings such as homes and offices. In fact, for comparison, the average negative ion concretion near a waterfall is 50,000 per cubic centimeter, in mountain air 5,000 and in the countryside 1500 or so; yet in a modern office, this figure can fall to as low as 50 per cubic cm.

What happens to the ions in buildings? They are electrically precipitated by particles in the air, notably dust, cigarette smoke and fabrics such as synthetic carpet fibers. Modern closed ventilation systems and of course the ubiquitous office computer make the problems many times worse, because of the static build-ups they create.

The atmosphere in ionised spaces is generally cleaner and 'feels fresher' because there is an increased rate of precipitation of particulates, thus reducing cigarette smoke clouds and circulating dust. The potential benefits for sensitive patients seem obvious.

Additionally, ionisers may remove harmful bacteria from the air. Since droplet spread from exhaled breath is a potent method of cross-infection, this may mean less illness. ioniser trials in a Swiss bank reputedly showed a dramatic fall in absenteeism due to coughs, colds and other infective complaints.

Given the "feel good" factor, it seems a good idea to try and supplement your environment with negatively changed ions. Studies are poor to date but one 'double-blind' trial carried out by an insurance company in the UK using ionisers showed a remarkable 78 percent drop in the incidence of headaches and other minor symptoms.

At least one of my patients did a blind controlled trial study with an ioniser. His wife would switch it on only on certain nights, without telling him which. It didn't take long for them to realize that on the nights when the machine was switched on he had angina-like symptoms and felt quite ill. Indeed at one point he felt ready for hospital. So the effects are not always necessary beneficial.

Thus, a note of caution must be sounded amongst the enthusiastic claims that manufacturers make. Mains–operated ionisers generate adverse electromagnetic fields pulsating at 50 to 60 Hertz. Some individuals will be highly sensitive to these fields.

Some machines will produce ozone levels that exceed guidelines in small, non-ventilated areas. One study showed that ozone can react with other constituents, namely cleaning agents to increase pollutants in the air, such as formaldehyde.[270] As with so many environmental considerations, individual experimentation is called for. But please be very careful.

5.7 Candida and Yeasts

Related to the mold phenomenon—and in some people's minds the same thing—is the problem of so-called Candida and yeasts.

Around 40 years ago now, Orian Truss MD, a holistically-inclined psychiatrist from Alabama, set the clinical ecology world alight with his revelation of the role of Candida in profound psychologically disturbed states. In a series of articles published in *The Journal Of Orthomolecular Psychiatry* he labeled Candida as "the missing diagnosis" and set about establishing the foundation of his hypothesis that it was a potent cause of mental illness.[271]

Of course every endeavor has been made to discredit his observations, his hypothesis and his treatment methods. But the concept has survived all criticisms and hostility and is now firmly established in the public's mind.

My late friend, William Crook MD, took up the banner and launched what was a virtual crusade, with his book titled *The Yeast Connection*, which ironically outsold Truss's own book *The Missing Diagnosis*.

I myself made a considerable addition to the debate by pointing out that *Candida albicans*, per se, was not a likely candidate for the syndrome created by Truss and Crook. I do not dismiss the diagnosis, or the patients' experiences; I have merely pointed out that there are several (better) candidates for the role of arch-villain!

Read on if your mind is open to it!

Intestinal Fermentation Syndrome

The fact is there are health gains to be made by following an anti-Candida program, taking antifungal drugs and excluding sugar and yeast foods from one's diet. Yet Truss's idea is no more than a theory.

If there is one valid complaint that members of the medical profession have against clinical ecologists, it is their tardiness in backing up ideas with research. It has been more than 35 years now since Truss's innovative papers; ample time to carry out detailed studies that would validate his claims. Yet they are singularly lacking. A catalogue of startling recoveries does not constitute scientific study. We may be getting the right results for the wrong reason.

Here's something you may not know... Despite a degree of 'brand identification', Truss was in fact far from being the first investigator in this field. His ideas were anticipated almost 70 years earlier by a man called Turner, who presented a paper on what he called 'intestinal germ carbohydrate fermentation'.[272]

In 1931 Hurst was in his footsteps, writing about 'intestinal carbohydrate dyspepsia'. In the 1930s and 1940s this dyspepsia was being treated with *Lactobacillus acidophilus*, B vitamin supplements and a low-starch diet (remarkably like modern anti-Candida treatment except that legumes are no longer banned, as they were at that time).

Others wrote about "autointoxication":

'The control of man's diet is readily accomplished, but mastery over his intestinal bacterial flora is not...the innumerable examples of autointoxication that one sees in his daily walks in life is proof thereof. They are the cases that present...malaise, total lack of ambition so that every effort in life is a burden, mental depression often bordering upon melancholia, frequent attacks of indefinite abdominal pains due to flatulency, sudden attacks of acute diarrhea alternating with periods of constipation...A battle royal must be fought and when this first great struggle ends in victory for the Bacillus bulgaricus it must be kept on the field of battle forever at guard...'[273]

A wild flamboyant English surgeon called Sir William Arbuthnot Lane (1856-1943) got into the act. He viewed the colon as a simple 'sewage system'. Within this 'cesspool', as Lane called it, the normal intestinal bacterial flora was said to be altered and a migration of bacteria toward the small intestine would encourage an even greater absorption of intestinal toxins. The symptoms, as usual, were far and wide, although they were most notable in the gastrointestinal and mental realms – dyspepsia, abdominal pain, constipation alternating with bouts of diarrhea and malaise, but also notable psychological symptoms: melancholia, incapacity for prolonged mental or physical exertion, insomnia and neuroses.

The catch-all diagnosis for all of these symptoms - a cluster of modern day co-morbid disorders: irritable bowel syndrome, chronic fatigue, myalgic encephalomyelitis, fibromyalgia, anxiety and depressive disorders – were cast as neurasthenia, and Lane was convinced that neurasthenia was almost always a matter of colonic toxemia. Not entirely wrong, as we shall see in the next section, but the strategy was pretty grim: beyond lifestyle interventions and internal disinfectants for mild or early-stage colonic stasis, a chronic state, in Lane's view, this condition could only be resolved by surgery, typically a colectomy or complete colon bypass (so-called short circuit).

I should point out the Lane's mortality rate was appalling: 16%. One is reminded once more of the pioneering madness (that may be an oxymoron) of 20th century American psychiatrist Henry Cotton in New York (section 1.4). His surgical mortality rate was said to be as high as 45%. That's practically murder![274]

Medical literature has tried to define the patient-type who suffers with this unhappy syndrome. A major text on gastroenterology in 1976 described victims as 'Essentially unhappy people... any suggested panacea or therapeutic straw is grasped... no regime is too severe and no program too difficult... with the tenacity of the faithful, they grope their way from one practitioner to the next in the search for a permanently successful remedy.' This disparaging description shows a lamentable weakness on the part of doctors for blaming any patient they cannot help.

The 'problem patient' attitude was probably what sank the condition in the 1950s. At that time, the psychosomatic theory of disease was enjoying a great revival. The tendency was to dismiss all patients with vague, ill-defined symptoms as psychiatric cases. Unlike today, there were no physical findings to disprove the psychiatric label and so it stuck. It's still with us, to a large degree.

On-Board Brewery

So the idea of a yeast-like organism that lives on starches and sugars and causes bowel disturbance is far from new. It seems to enjoy a vogue in medical circles every few decades and then lapses out of sight once again. The reason is probably that, as in the 1980s, some doctors become convinced they know what causes the syndrome, but then can't seem to find a workable proof that affords a satisfactory explanation. This casts doubt on the basis of the theory. So it is today with Truss's 'Candida'.

The success of antifungal drugs may have fed a myth. In some cases, anti-Candida therapeutic agents such as Nystatin seem to work only in very high doses (10 to 100 times the usual dose). This has led to the speculation that it may be helping by some other mechanism than just that of eradicating the yeast micro-organism; possibly by blocking bowel permeability, which would heal so-called leaky gut (see section 5.6 if you are not familiar with this term).

One thing is certain, there is virtually no correlation between Candida in the stool sample and the existence of the 'yeast syndrome'. Indeed, *Candida albicans* is rarely identified in specimens, despite its known very wide occurrence, in and on the human body. This lack of correlation is disappointing but hardly surprising, especially if we are looking for the wrong culprit.

It is true: treatment directed towards this type of organism can be highly effective in selected individuals, so clearly a real phenomenon exists. But that doesn't prove that Candida is to blame.

Incidentally, just as Candida isn't the only contender for the role of pathogen, ordinary ethyl alcohol is not the only product of fermentation we seem to be dealing with. Many other products can be derived from the breakdown of sugars and starches, including short-chain fatty acids such as acetate, proprionate, succinate and butyrate, and other alcohols such as iso-propanol, butanol and 2,3 – butylenes glycol.

All of these substances are capable of producing severe psychological changes, from inebriation to depression, and so must be excluded in any comprehensive investigation into physical illness posing as a psychiatric disorder.

Further, if detoxification pathways are blocked due to overload, other unwanted metabolites are produced, such as epoxides (carcinogenic), aldehydes and even chloral hydrate, ingredient of the classic 'Mickey Finn'. Typically this chemical produces a tired and 'spacey' feeling. Here is at least part of the reason these patients can't take alcoholic drinks. Naturally, these by-products too have a bad effect on the patient; most are quite toxic.

Note: The Mickey Finn is most likely named after the manager and bartender of the Lone Star Saloon and Palm Garden Restaurant, in Chicago, which operated from 1896 to 1903. He poisoned his customers with the intention of incapacitating them and subsequently robbing them.

The Human Microbiome and Dysbiosis

A better idea than the Candida model, and calling forth a ton of meaningful up-to-date science, is the problem of disturbed intestinal flora. We called it dysbiosis. We pioneers thought of leaky gut, among other things (see next section). The emerging picture is far, far bigger. It is also of absolutely pivotal interest in the field of holistic psychiatry.

I'm talking about the make up of the human microbiome.

The dinosaur medical view is that what you eat has no effect on how you feel; the brain is not affected at all by foods or digestion. Nothing that happens down there in the damp and dark of the intestines has any effect on our emotions, thoughts or wellbeing. Wrong! The modern, scientific view, is that the gut *dominates* our mental and physical health.

It's interesting to look at the history of this aspect of medicine. It's a concept that has been round a l-o-n-g time... Hippocrates (circa 400 BC) wrote, "All diseases begin in the gut."

Not just bodily diseases but diseases of the mind too. French psychiatrist Phillipe Pinel (1745- 1826), known as the father of modern psychiatry stated, "The primary seat of insanity is the region of the stomach and intestines."

"So early as Hippocrates, the abdominal viscera were regarded as the principal seats of disease in mania and melancholia. This doctrine has been, at various times, forgotten and revived from that period to the present moment, according as circumstances have occurred to influence the minds of the medical practitioners and as the opinions of the metaphysical or physical pathologists have prevailed."

David Uwins, MD, Physician to the City of London Dispensary, 1818

By the beginning of the 20th century, microbes were considered to be directly (and indirectly via the by-products released) involved in various diagnoses of the day, such as melancholic outlook, malaise, neurasthenia, and what were known as 'the neuroses'. Preliminary reports suggested that the administration of beneficial microbes could be helpful in cases of depression and dietary alterations, especially macronutrients, were part of mainstream discussions concerning ways to manipulate intestinal microbiome for health.

For example, manipulating dietary protein and carbohydrate in animals could induce changes in behavior with associated changes in the intestinal flora (see 5.5 which is Yeasts or intestinal fermentation syndrome). The behavioral changes were attributed to a combination of both direct macronutrient influences on mood, and the indirect ability of foods to shift the production of mood-altering microbial byproducts.

Physicians of the day also thought (quite correctly) that the nervous system and its moods could influence the microbiome:

"Disturbing the sympathetic and autonomic nervous centers as to result in disturbance of the digestive apparatus, such disturbance may lead to the development of an excess of certain bacteria...we need not even assume it is always the same bacterium which gives rise to symptoms like those of melancholia. Various antibodies and various metabolic by-products called out by the presence of bacterial enzymes, may be the particular poisons causing the 'cough' known as melancholia."

Robert T. Morris, MD, 1919

In fact, some of the scientific findings during what the authors of the *Journal of Clinical Pharmacology and Neuroscience* called the 'bacterio-mania' of the early 20th century were to become groundbreaking. However, the science of what was called "intestinal toxemia" was rudimentary, and largely speculative; risky intestinal surgeries were performed to "rid" the body of its toxic reservoir, and as that journal article remarked, it was all very premature: the lucrative 'microbial product' cart was placed before the proverbial horse.[275]

This first wave of serious interest in bowel flora, as it's sometimes called, and the effect on mental health spanned from approximately 1900–1930, and left a legacy of unnecessary surgeries, useless products and unwarranted fears concerning frequency of what constituted normal bowel movements.

It has resurfaced today, with renewed interest and, hopefully this time, some real answers to some important conundrums. So buckle up for an amazing ride!

The Second Brain

Today we know that there is a vast deal of neurological tissue in the intestines, known as the enteric nervous system (ENS), which has been christened the "second brain". Consider:

The ENS is a large and independent network of neurons, with accompanying neurotransmitters, and special proteins we know are responsible for communications, "thinking," "remembering," and even "learning". The esophagus, stomach, small and large intestines are lined with sheaths of tissue containing some 100 million neurons: more than in either the spinal cord or the peripheral nervous system! This large body of neurones releases the same neurotransmitters that exist in the brain and are influenced by these neurotransmitters.

In fact, enteric neurons secrete an intimidating array of over 30 neurotransmitters. For example, 95% of the body's serotonin is found in the gut, not in the brain! Serotonin has a reputation with the layman as the "happy hormone" but it's far from that simple. Serotonin is actually pro-inflammatory, meaning it's big trouble. Too much of it will set your brain on fire!

Which is why SSRI drugs (like Prozac), which prevent the safe re-cycling of serotonin, are so hazardous: the result is that the brain is awash with serotonin and way overstimulated and the individual just may run out on a crazed mass shooting spree.

It's interesting to note too—a kind of confirmation—that the other side-effects of SSRI drugs is to cause gastro-intestinal symptoms. Irritable bowel syndrome is known to arise, at least in part, from too much serotonin in our guts, and could perhaps be regarded as a "mental illness" of the second brain.

Another major gut neurotransmitter is acetylcholine. In general, neurons that secrete acetylcholine are excitatory, stimulating smooth muscle contraction, increases in intestinal secretions, release of enteric hormones and dilation of blood vessels.

But there's also noradrenaline or norepinephrine as the Americans call it, glutamine, gamma-aminobutyric acid and encephalins, plus endorphins and weird stuff you don't need to know about, such as cocaine and amphetamine regulated transcript (CART).

It's quite a list! Note that last enzyme: cocaine and amphetamine related. You can just sense it spells trouble... and it does!

We have a lot to learn about our "second brain", the ENS. But it's beyond question that it is capable of giving rise to unwanted psychiatric symptoms, even the major ones, such as depression, anxiety, hyperactivity in kids and even schizophrenic manifestations.

Some of the most intriguing work has been done on autism. For decades, doctors, parents, and researchers have noted that about three-quarters of people with autism also have some gastrointestinal abnormality, like digestive issues, food allergies, or gluten sensitivity.

What's been found so far is that a common microbiome species called *Bacteroides fragilis*, is present in lesser quantities in some (not all) children with autism.

Restoration of B. fragilis from humans to mice with symptoms similar to autism, improved their behavior: the mice became less anxious, communicated more with other mice, and showed less repetitive behavior.

It's been speculated that a chemical called 4-ethylphenylsulphate, or 4EPS, which seems to be produced by gut bacteria, may be to blame. They found that mice with symptoms of autism have blood levels of 4EPS more than 40 times higher than other mice. What's more, when healthy animals were injected with the compound, they developed autism-like symptoms.[276]

Control Of Digestion

It's actually a two-way traffic. Stress and anxiety can hinder the immune system and over time lead to rampant overgrowth and dysbiosis in the gut, signaled clearly by digestive disturbances. Most people under stress make matters worse by binge eating junk food to try to increase dopamine levels and elevate mood, and in doing so further imbalance the gut microbiome.

Many of the expressions in our language pay tribute to the fact that we notice our thoughts and moods affect the gut: "my stomach turned over" (fright), "I felt I had been punched in the stomach" (shock), "I felt sick to my stomach" (anger, disappointment) and ""I had a gut feeling that..." (apprehension).

The "real" brain and nervous system exert a profound influence on all aspects of digestive processes, namely motility, molecular ion transport associated with secretion and absorption, and gastrointestinal blood flow. But the ENS too has an enormous array of functions, as reflected in its magnitude and complexity.

So the ENS is best seen as the 3rd component of the autonomic nervous system, along with the sympathetic and parasympathetic nervous systems.

The ENS regulates all aspects of gut function, from breaking down food (enzyme secretion), absorbing nutrients, and expelling of waste, to the mechanical mixing and rhythmic muscle contractions that move everything on down the line.

"The system is way too complicated to have evolved only to make sure things move out of your colon," says Emeran Mayer, professor of physiology, psychiatry and biobehavioral sciences at the David Geffen School of Medicine at the University of California, Los Angeles (UCLA). For example, scientists were shocked to learn that about 90 percent of the fibers in the primary visceral nerve, the vagus, carry information from the gut to the brain and not the other way around.[277]

According to Mayer, psychiatrists are going to have to expand to take into account the second brain in addition to the one atop the shoulders. How times change! It makes old Philipe Pinel seem pretty clever.

The truth which has emerged is that depression, stress, anxiety and autism, among numerous other psychological conditions are all proposed to be at least partially sensitive to manipulation of the gut microbiome. Studies have suggested that a variety of less obvious conditions are influenced by the microbiome, including obesity, functional gastrointestinal (GI) disorders, chronic fatigue syndrome and inflammatory illnesses. All of these disorders are known to have an important central nervous system component.[278]

So now we have a new specialty: neurogastroenterology.

What Is Dysbiosis?

Holistically-oriented websites are pretty liberal with the term "dysbiosis". But it is important to note that it has no absolute definition; it's just a concept. There has been no research that shows unequivocally what an "unhealthy" gut microbiome is. There is too much variability among "normal" individuals in the composition of the microbiome, superimposed on variation in genetic and epigenetic susceptibilities to disease and dietary and environmental exposures.

Thousands, probably millions, of microbial species inhabit human populations and the distribution of microbes across hosts vary greatly, providing challenges to statistical descriptions of human microbiome data. Moreover, there is little consensus in the literature regarding what species are most likely to have therapeutic properties, and it may be the case that a balance of organisms, supported by a specific diet, provides the most benefit for any particular health condition.

Trials of single or a few species may not represent an adequate approach to manipulating an individual's microbiome.

All I know for sure is that changing what you eat dramatically alters the balance of bowel flora *within hours*. I'm not even the first to publish that: it goes back to 1910![279]

Psychobiotics

So now we have psychobiotics! Gut microbiomes may have a significant impact on mood and cognition, which is leading experts towards a new frontier in neuroscience (I've been there for decades... yawn). Studies have shown that increase in the amount of good bacteria in the gut can curb inflammation and cortisol level, reduces symptoms of depression and anxiety, lowers stress reactivity, improves memory and even lessens neuroticism and social anxiety. This shows that, probably the beneficial gut bacteria or probiotics function mechanistically as delivery vehicles for neuroactive compounds.

Thus, a psychobiotic is a live organism which, when ingested in adequate amounts, produces a health benefit in patients suffering from psychiatric illness. Study of this novel class of probiotics may open up the possibility of rearrangement of intestinal microbiota for effective management of various psychiatric disorders.[280]

Studies

Human studies remain limited but intriguing.

Animal studies, however, consistently report that behavior and the function of the nervous system are modulated by gut microbiome. Disrupting the gut microbiome in mice with antibiotics is associated with altered brain-derived neurotrophic factor in the hippocampus and amygdala, which increases anxiety states (measured as an increase in mouse exploratory behavior).

What about probiotics? Bifidobacterium longum NCC3001 normalized anxiety in mice with a deliberately-induced low-grade inflammation. Note that a strong calming influence is also mediated by the vagus nerve. Interference with the function of this nerve will have negative effects.

Chronic administration of Lactobacillus rhamnosus str. JB1 also increased exploratory behaviour and this effect was associated with brain region–specific changes in the γ-aminobutyric acid (GABA) system.

All this is very technical sounding; just take it in one breath: altered bowel microbiome in animal studies shows it is very important for psychological and behavioral stability.

And despite the relative lack of human studies, the science is definitely hotting up. A search of PubMed in January 2017 yielded almost 400 results from a search limited to reviews of "brain microbiome." Searching for "depression microbiome" alone yielded more than 100 reviews, and "anxiety microbiome" and "autism microbiome" yielded slightly fewer.[281]

That's a far cry, remember, from saying that swallowing your yoghurt or a daily dose of probiotics would normalize brain function or alter major psychiatric disorders or change human behavior. Actually, at least one study reported that taking probiotics actually reduced cognitive reactivity and induced a sad mood. It's not the effect we would want but it does prove these changes are possible.

So, while adjusting the balance of bowel flora clearly has a lot to offer in the domain of holistic psychiatry, simply and solely taking probotics does not seem the way to go. It just doesn't have the powerful impact of reducing inflammation that allergen elimination does.

Yet case–control studies comparing gut microbiota of patients with psychiatric disorders to healthy controls show that there are significant alterations in the balance of Firmicutes, Actinobacteria and Bacteroidetes and with a loss of richness and diversity, in patients with clinical depression.

Changing The Microbiome For The Better

I have already hinted that, rather than taking probiotics, altering what we eat is a very fast way to change the microbial pattern in our gut; in fact it can take place within hours, not weeks.

What can be done?

Sarah Campbell-McBride has been ploughing her furrow, describing a resurrected old diet called the GAPS diet (gut and psychology syndrome diet as she calls it). It's based on a very out of date concept, the Specific Carbohydrate Diet or SCD, invented by American pediatrician Sidney Valentine Haas in the first half of the 20th century. Dr. Haas and his colleagues spent many years researching the effects of diet on celiac disease and other digestive disorders. The results of this research were published in a comprehensive medical textbook "The Management of Celiac Disease", written by Dr. Sidney V. Haas and Merrill P. Haas in 1951.

When celiac disease was defined as a gluten intolerance or gluten enteropathy, the SCD was forgotten as outdated information. It was brought back to life by Elaine Gottschall. Following the success of the SCD with her daughter, Elaine Gottschall over the years helped numerous people, suffering from Crohn's disease, ulcerative colitis, celiac disease, diverticulitis and various types of chronic diarrhea. But also young sufferers with behavioral abnormalities, such as autism, hyperactivity and night terrors.

Campbell-McBride adopted this plan. But both she and Gottschall have missed the crucial point of changing diet, which is that *everyone's ideal diet is different*. You can't expect generalized plans to work for everyone. It's important to work out the exact well-tolerated diet for every individual. In my vast clinical experience I have had patients made very ill by lettuce, potato, onions, tomato, cabbage, carrots and a whole host of other supposedly healthy foods. It is wrong to make assumptions or generalize. Each person's ideal diet has to be explored and established by proper eating challenge tests [see earlier in section 5.2]

Identifying unique individual food allergens, done properly, can work miracles and over the years I have seen tens of thousands of amazing turnarounds, including severe psychiatric disturbances solved: schizophrenia due entirely to wheat allergy, smoking or cheese (three different patients, that is), major depressive disorder (MDD) from potato, epilepsy due to foods from the carrot family, murderous violence due to potato and beef, hyperkinetic syndrome from sugar, corn, anxiety and fibromyalgia from many common *organic whole foods* and even sexually dangerous and inappropriate behavior from ingesting specific foods.

It starts with a "Stone Age" elimination diet, for a couple of weeks, which is a test diet. But once the patient's individual food sensitivities are known, the maintenance diet is far less stressful and may only boil down to one or two foods. Sticking to major restrictions like the GAPS diet or even just gluten and casein free, if it isn't necessary, doesn't make any sense. It's important to know exactly *which foods* cause a psychiatric patient's problems, and avoid those.

Eating a hunter-gatherer diet has numerous benefits, one of which being these are our natural foods. We know that tribal and Stone Age peoples have a pretty good bowel flora. It's our modern refined and vitiated foods that lead to dysbiosis.

If you are vegetarian, you may like to try excluding all animal products for a time. I'm not recommending veganism as a way of life, though it works for some; but short term modifications and eliminations can often point the way to which foods suit an individual and which don't.[282]

Epidemiological studies have reported that more traditional dietary patterns are associated with good mental health and lowered risk of depression.

My Own View: We are not vegetarians by nature or design; but man in the wild didn't eat so much meat! It's a myth of the Stone Age man out to feed the tribe. Women actually gathered over 60% of the calories cavemen ate (while the men sat around). Try to eat about 75 percent plant-based food: fruits, nuts, vegetables and seeds.[283] [284]

Short-term intervention studies show that traditional dietary patterns can positively influence mental outlook, cognition and chronic fatigue. The Mediterranean diet can be a good call, if you find a full paleo-exclusion diet too challenging. It's associated in the main with robust mental and physical health.[285]

Fermented foods too are good. These have been a human dietary staple for thousands of years, from sour milk to saukraut and everything in between: khefir, yogurt, buttermilk, kapusta, kvass, borscht, etc. These are famously found in Russia and the Balkans, where Élie Metchnikoff (1845 - 1916) did his famous work on yoghurt.

Yoghurt is probably the weakest of the group, despite the current yogurt mania. Don't get carried away by the health claims of manufacturers and suppliers, not even the big ones. In 2010, Dannon had to pay a $21 million settlement to the FTC, for overstating the benefits of its Activia brand.

Fermented foods are not just a European tradition and soured milk not the only source. Early writings show that Chinese workers ate acid-fermented vegetables while building the Great Wall of China. The Japanese have routinely served a small serving of pickled vegetable with their meals. Centuries ago, the Koreans developed kimchi by acid-fermenting cabbage and other vegetables.

The Ancient Greeks wrote about the health benefits of fermented cabbage. The Romans used sauerkraut to treat and prevent intestinal infections. Captain Cook used sauerkraut and lime juice to prevent scurvy on his three-year journey around the world. Many African cultures still routinely use lactic acid-fermentation as a way of preserving gruels made from corn and sorghum. Even the people of India use the juice of sauerkraut.

Prebiotics: probably of far more use than taking probiotics is to eat plenty of pre-biotics. That means foods that provide a nurturing background for natural bowel flora to flourish. As I keep saying, swallowing your probiotics isn't the way to go. Changing what you eat helps your bowel flora improve itself. Key to that is to eat fibrous, healthy foods that provide a matrix in which natural microbes can grow.

Pre-biotics include: Jerusalem artichokes (the star), beans, leeks, asparagus, garlic, onions, brown rice, sweet potatoes, bananas, oatmeal, bran and the fermented vegetables described above.

Although the last word is far from written, it is clear that dietary patterns and specific combinations of nutrients such as omega-3 fatty acids, zinc, magnesium and plant phytochemicals are of relevance to depression and other mental disorders.

In any event eat only whole, unprocessed foods and strictly avoid manufactured foods. If it's in a tin, packet or jar, it's been messed with. You will never restore mental health on such junk.

5.8 Leaky Gut Disorder

You've probably heard of "Leaky Gut Syndrome". Back in the 1980s, we used to think we had it wrapped up: we knew the story, understood the mechanics and had a good treatment modality going.

Unfortunately, we were almost totally wrong, as you will see!

It's not like we thought. Even I didn't realize what was coming down the turnpike! What is surprising is that in the intervening years, orthodox medicine has taken us rapidly forward on the theme of leaky gut, with the discovery of "tight junctions"

First let's quickly re-run the "traditional" story...

The Supposed Mechanism

The idea was that our guts are inflamed by food allergies, dysbiosis, Candida, parasites, heavy metal poisoning etc. So they "leak', meaning they let through molecules they shouldn't. Instead of waiting till proteins, for example, were properly digested down to peptides or even smaller (amino acids), the much larger protein molecules appeared in the blood, not properly digested.

As a result, we got an allergic reaction to the "wheat", or "eggs" in the blood, which shouldn't be there.

It helps to understand a little of the normal digestive process. Here's a quick summary:

Digestion is a pretty impressive process, designed to break down all kinds of foodstuffs and turn these into useful fuel for the cells. It does this by means of chemical reagents we call enzymes. These are remarkable substances, which enable complex chemical processes to take place quickly at body temperature.

In the mouth, ptyalin (salivary amylase) is added to our food, a starch digester, which begins to break down carbohydrates, even as we chew.

In the stomach hydrochloric acid is secreted, together with pepsin, which starts to break down proteins, and rennin, for the digestion of milk. One other important stomach secretion to mention is intrinsic factor, without which we cannot properly absorb vitamin B12. Lack of stomach acid (called achlorhydria) often goes along with a B12 deficiency, which leads to a condition called pernicious anemia (because it really was fatal, until the cause was discovered).

As soon as the sloppy, half-digested food mass exits the stomach, it reaches the duodenum, then two more very important organs come into play: the pancreas and gallbladder. The pancreas adds some industrial-strength enzymes, for the digestion of fats, proteins and carbohydrates. At the same time secretion of bicarbonate turns the liquefied food back to an alkaline mix, or chyle, as it is known. Bile salts, secreted by the liver, are stored in the gall bladder and ejected into the gut whenever fat shows up.

Bile acids are vital because they enable fats to emulsify. The term emulsion means fats in suspension as tiny droplets in a watery liquid (milk is an emulsion). The duodenum (which literally means "twelve fingers," named for its length) has been likened to a second stomach. It is a good analogy. Many animals, as you know, have more than one stomach. Most of the digestive process takes place here, leaving mainly simple sugars, amino acids, simplified peptides and fatty acids.

From there on down the rest of the gut, absorption is the name of the game. The wall of the small intestine is lined with tiny hair-like growths called villi, which increase the absorption area. These can be damaged, causing difficulty in absorption. If the loss of functional capacity is severe enough, as in celiac disease, the patient may simply waste away and die. Nowadays we know the cause is gluten allergy and, by avoiding gluten, the individuals' gut returns to normal and once again absorbs quite satisfactorily.

Beyond the small intestine, food waste enters the large bowel (colon). There water is re-absorbed, to help counter dehydration, resulting in the familiar solid waste or *feces*, to give it its Latin name.

That's it in a few words but it is a mighty fascinating process. Moreover, it can easily go wrong.

Not enough enzymes, for example, can hamper the digestion of foods. In the lower gut, anything which causes damage or inflammation may stop the gut lining working properly and poor absorption results.

That we call malabsorption. I'll come to that in a moment.

Leaky gut, on the other hand, is absorbing partly-digested substances that are really not ready to enter the blood and lymph streams. Thus wheat, corn, milk, egg, banana, etc. are carried around the body and set up what are called "immune complexes" or, in every day terms, food allergy particles, which are highly inflammatory, especially to the brain.

I'm simplifying this but are you beginning to get the picture?

OK, Let's start with malabsorption.

Malabsorption

An inflamed gut cannot do its job properly. The billions of tiny hairs or villi disappear and then the surface area available for absorption diminishes greatly.

All kinds of offenders can cause this inflammatory process, from food allergies, to infestation with parasites; heavy metals to dysbiosis; lactose intolerance to alcohol abuse. It's important to identify the correct cause and eradicate it properly. Otherwise, treatments do no good.

It is important to note that impaired digestion of foodstuffs can also lead to malabsorption. Undigested food molecules are too large to absorb efficiently. Thus lack of proper digestive enzymes is a major cause of malabsorption. Then leaky gut could help, letting through these larger molecules; but it's not really the solution we want...

It is particularly important to detect malabsorption, otherwise medications and supplements are almost worthless, because they are simply not being absorbed! It is a standard joke among those who rent latrines for sporting events and other public gatherings that, when it comes to cleaning the units, large numbers of pills and capsules are left behind, showing they were never even digested, much less absorbed.

Fortunately, we can correct that, as you will see.

The New Leaky Gut Model

The modern-day shock, demonstrated to us by our orthodox colleagues, is that so-called leaky gut is not so much a function of inflammation and damage, as we once thought. It's more a question of tiny trapdoors, controlled by the enteric nervous system, that open and shut to allow different-sized molecules to pass through into the blood! We call these portals "tight junctions" because they should be closed tightly, not loose and open.

The most startling aspect of this discovery is that change takes place very fast; in minutes even. It's not a matter of months or years of relentless damage and malfunction! It's more like a trapdoor function.

Tight junctions are created by protein complexes that work like a glue. Their control is complex and uses chemical signalers, working via the so-called "Gut Brain" or second brain. When closed, tight junctions prevent molecules above a certain size from passing through. But in minutes, a nerve signal can open them wide, letting everything through! The point is that nobody ever saw the fact that opening of otherwise "tight junctions" directly caused leaky gut. Now even orthodox medicine is on the case!

What can we do? Keep the gut brain happy!

- Colostrum
- Probiotics
- Pre-biotics
- Reduce inflammatory foods
- Clean up heavy metal poisoning
- Eliminate parasites
- Detox and cleansing homeopathics

Zonulin

And now the zonulin story. We've got yet another new hormone to worry about; it's called zonulin. Zonulin is a signaling molecule that blows tight junctions wide open. It appears to be triggered by gluten and is raised in celiacs. That's all that orthodox doctors are seeing at the moment; they haven't heard of other cyclical food allergies, so tight junctions couldn't be affected by anything other than gluten, right?

Well, the mechanism is clear; the fact that they haven't yet seen it will apply to all causes of bowel irritation, not just gluten, doesn't alter the mechanics of this. Eventually, they will catch up in their slow, dull way...

Thing is, Dr. Alesso Fasano, in a 2006 study showed that celiac patients who had been off gluten for a number of years, still had high zonulin levels (up to 30 times the amount of controls). Moreover, the leakiness factor was up by a factor of 3 in celiacs, again *even if he or she had been off all gluten* for 2 years or more.[286]

What does this tell us? That zonulin isn't the only control mechanism, or that zonulin is controlled by a number of unknown epigenetic factors. Guess what those are? Food allergies (other than gluten), dysbiosis, heavy metal poisoning, parasites, and all the things I've been telling you here which cause cognitive dysfunction.

How Do We Tell Which Is Which?

Is there any way to tell apart these two critical conditions, which are similar but completely opposite in effects? Fortunately, yes.

For malabsorption, we use D-xylose test (a small sugar molecule): the patient drinks the xylose, and urine or blood are collected. Low urinary xylose suggests poor absorption. It's not getting into the blood, so it doesn't show up in the urine.

For leaky gut, we use the mannitol sugar test (mannitol is a large molecule): The patient drinks the mannitol, and urine or blood are collected. Mannitol appearing in the blood or urine tells us that large molecules are coming through.

Also to be considered are:

- Stool samples looking for undigested fat.
- A breath test to detect lactose intolerance or bacterial overgrowth in the small intestine.

Obviously testing of this type will depend on the skill of the attendant physician in interpreting what's found.

5.9 Pyrroluria Disorder

The late Carl C. Pfeiffer MD PhD was noted for his work on pyrroluria and related nutritional topics concerned with mental illness, especially schizophrenia. His writings are a seminal source of ideas for future researchers. Pfeiffer made famous the 'mauve factor', though in fact it was identified by doctors Hoffer and Mahon in 1961.

Before them, in 1958, Dr. A.N. Payza, a Canadian physician, conducted research by generating a psychosis with LSD in healthy volunteers and alcoholics, and subsequently investigating the urine for indoles and indole-like compounds (pyrrole is an indole).

During this research Payza found bufotenin, a weak hallucinogen, related to serotonin with effects similar to LSD. It was present in the urine of many psychiatric patients who had never taken any LSD.

Abram Hoffer and M Mahon (no-one alive now seems to know who M Mahon was) discovered that when an indole test reagent (known as Erhlich's reagent) was added to the urine of 39 schizophrenic patients, 27 patients' urine samples turned mauve, hence: mauve factor.[287]

The actual substance present in the urine that caused this change is called pyrrole and the condition is more clumsily known as 'pyrroluria' or 'pyrrole disorder' (also known as "kryptopyrrole" (KP) or "hemepyrrole").

It is worth pointing out also that pyrroles were originally found in the urine of several patients undergoing severe LSD psychosis, not unlike schizophrenia. This probably tells us something, but as yet we don't know what.

The fact that pyrroles can interfere with serotonin metabolism and induce strange hallucinations and delusions makes it of great interest in studying schizophrenia, a very difficult and extreme form of mental illness as we have seen (section 2.2). The identification of metabolic factors that may play a role in its causation and can be modified would transform the whole approach to this condition.

But do remember, not all patients with pyrroluria suffer from this extreme disease.

Pyrrole disorder is often seen in children and adolescents who have previously been diagnosed with ADHD, autism, Asperger's syndrome, anxiety, Tourette syndrome, behavioral disorders (including OCD), fears/phobias, sensory processing disorders, and learning disorders. Severe tantrums, bizarre shifts in mood/behavior, and poor response to small stressors are some of the hallmark symptoms of pyrrole disorder in youngsters and adolescents.

Pfeiffer even identified subjects from history who were said to manifest the symptoms of pyrroluria – being withdrawn, melancholic, experiencing blinding headaches, nervous exhaustion (neurasthenia), abnormal sensitivity (one might almost say paranoia) about stressful changes and outside influences, palpitations and digestive disorders, even handwriting abnormalities – naming Charles Darwin, Charles Dickens and Emily Dickinson as possible sufferers, among others.

Nutrient Deficiencies

Pyrroles have no known function in the body. We all constantly excrete pyrroles in our urine. In a typical person this is not a problem, but a person with pyrrole disorder can become deficient in zinc and B6 when excess pyrroles are being excreted. This is because pyrroles have an affinity for zinc and vitamin B6 and attach to them, resulting in increased urinary excretion of these nutrients.

Note that heavy metal exposure, smoking, drugs (medical or recreational) and alcohol can also increase pyrrole levels and hence increase excretion. This explains why the symptoms of pyrrole disorder sufferers tend to get worse for 24 to 72 hours after a big night out drinking or after recreational drug use.

Zinc and B6 are essential for production of neurotransmitters such as serotonin, melatonin (the sleep hormone), GABA (relaxation), and acetylcholine (good for memory). These two nutrients are also involved in production of our steroid hormones such as cortisol (our anti-inflammatory, anti-allergy and stress hormone), among other vital functions.

Deficiencies are thus likely to cause disturbance in mood and thinking.

Large supplements of these two essential nutrients may thus be beneficial to those with schizophrenia and pyrroluria. Suggested quantities are:

- B6 – enough for nightly dream recall but not exceeding 2,000 mg (this level is dangerous, where there is no deficiency of B6, and should only be attempted under skilled medical supervision)

- zinc – 30 mg night and morning; and

- manganese gluconate 10 mg, night and morning.

It is vital to search for pyrrole disorder in all psychiatric cases, but especially schizophrenia. Mainstream medicine does not acknowledge this important condition, because the only way to rectify the problem is by improving the sufferer's nutritional status, digestion, diet and stress levels. There's no profit in that.

Instead they want to suppress symptoms, using drugs, which will only make conditions worse.

So you are on your own!

Conquering Pyroluria, the website of Dr. Greg Newson ND (who can't spell it properly) offers a pyrrole disorder test kit (you can find the link to it in the **Valuable Resources** section at the back of the book). It includes comprehensive instructions and an informative video on how to collect your urine sample and send it off for testing. When the test results are sent to you, you will receive a detailed pyrrole disorder treatment plan, including suggested lifestyle, dietary and nutritional recommendations, which can be very helpful to the lay person.

On an historical note, a strong case has been made for the madness of King George III, that he was suffering from porphyria, a condition which recurred in several royal houses throughout Europe. Pyrroles are not porphyrins; but porphyrins are made from four pyrrole molecules tacked together. There could be something in this. You may have read about King George's blue urine. But don't be misled. That is likely to be due to his treatment, a compound related to gentian which is, of course, radiant blue!

Histamine Disorders (Carl Pfeiffer Again)

In addition to his ground-breaking work in pyrroluria, Carl Pfeiffer also stressed the possible role of histamine in mental disorders. Histamine is a key allergic reagent, produced by the body during allergic reactions. Its presence is recognized by skin wheals, flushing of the skin, headache and, ultimately, shock, due to widespread permeability of the capillaries (fluid "leaking" into the tissues, shrinking blood volume).

Pfeiffer hypothesized two types of individual, according to blood levels of free histamine. Fifty percent of tested schizophrenics, he said, had low serum histamine (histapenia). Twenty percent had high levels (histadelia).

Histapenics, he said, usually have high copper levels as well. Since this may occasionally be primary, it is essential to remove any environmental source of copper pollution, such as in the plumbing. Zinc is then administered, because it counters copper effects.

Pfeiffer gave symptoms for the histapenic patient, which included difficulty achieving orgasm, increased body hair, the absence of allergies and headaches and some of the symptoms suggesting schizophrenia itself, such as the feeling of being mind–controlled by other people, seeing or hearing things abnormally and undue suspicions: in other words, anxiety, hallucinations and paranoia.

Histapenic patients, he said, respond well to nutritional supplements, as given below :

- Niacin, 100 mg twice a day
- Niacinamide 250-500 mg twice a day
- Folic acid 1 mg daily
- B12 by injection
- L-tryptophan, 1,000 mg at bedtime
- Zinc 15 mg and manganese 5 mg daily
- A high protein diet

The histadelic patient, on the other hand, will feel effects referable to the presence of excess histamine. It mimics allergies. Symptoms would include sneezing in bright sunlight, seasonal allergies and headaches, itching, restlessness, excess salivation, nausea, shyness and over-sensitivity as a teenager, given to tears and emotional reactions, backaches, stomach cramps, ease in achieving orgasm, tensions, fears and phobias, with suicidal depressions.

Pfeiffer cited Marilyn Monroe and Judy Garland as likely histadelics.[288]

Histadelics should be treated with:

- a low-protein, complex carbohydrate diet (whole grains)

- calcium supplements (500 mg twice a day)

- methionine 500 mgm night and morning and

- possibly the judicious use of anti-convulsant drugs, if depressed, but that is outside the scope of this text.

Other Psycho-Nutrient Factors

The benefits of B6 and zinc supplementation have already been noted in certain schizophrenics. *It is important to point out that one sub-group in this illness is made worse by the addition of these two nutrients and a physician would have to be alert to this possibility and discontinue treatment immediately.*

Other trace element deficiencies have also been considered. In 1927 Dr Reiter in Denmark treated 30 schizophrenic patients with intravenous manganese chloride injections and reported improvements in 23 of them. In 1929, Dr English of Brookville, Ontario, tried manganese again with 181 patients and about 50 percent of them improved. Then Dr Hoskins of the Worcester Foundation tried it, using intramuscular injections of a different, non-absorbable form of manganese, manganese oxide suspension, and found no effect. Manganese was promptly forgotten.

An IV push of manganese chloride should therefore be tried in suitable cases.

Manganese 0.1 mg/mL (Manganese Chloride Injection, USP) contains 0.1 mg manganese/mL and is administered intravenously only after dilution. No recommended dietary allowances (RDA) for manganese have been established.

When there is no recommended dietary allowance (RDA) for a nutrient, the Adequate Intake (AI) is used as a guide. The AI is the estimated amount of the nutrient that is used by a group of healthy people and assumed to be adequate. The daily Adequate Intake (AI) levels for manganese are: infants birth to 6 months, 3 mcg; 7 to 12 months, 600 mcg; children 1 to 3 years, 1.2 mg; 4 to 8 years 1.5 mg; boys 9 to 13 years, 1.9 mg; boys 14 to 18 years, 2.2 mg; girls 9 to 18 years, 1.6 mg; men age 19 and older, 2.3 mg; women 19 and older, 1.8 mg; pregnant women age 14 to 50, 2 mg; breastfeeding women, 2.6 mg.

Tolerable Upper Intake Levels (UL), the highest level of intake at which unwanted side effects are not expected, for manganese have been established. The daily ULs for manganese are: children 1 to 3 years, 2 mg; 4 to 8 years, 3 mg; 9 to 13 years, 6 mg; 14 to 18 years (including pregnant and breastfeeding women), 9 mg; for adults 19 years and older (including pregnant and breast-feeding women), 11 mg.

This could only be administered by a qualified medical professional, of course. Good luck with that when you say it's an attempted schizophrenia remedy!

Periodic monitoring of manganese plasma levels is suggested as a guideline for subsequent administration.

If such help is not available, at the very least, take 10 mgm. manganese gluconate, night and morning (adult oral dose).

The psychiatric profession is currently investigating abnormal metabolic pathways involving a number of neurologically active 'transmitters' such as dopamine and serotonin. There is much complex pharmacology here, enough to maintain center stage for many decades to come at the expense of more holistic approaches.

Only in one area is 'nutrient therapy' the fashion and that is in treating mania. It has been found that lithium calms manic patients. It will not stop hallucination and mania once developed, but it makes these symptoms less likely to develop. This may mean that only a reduced amount of a more 'orthodox' psychotropic drug is necessary or, in some cases, no drug at all. Because of the marked Parkinsonism–like side effects of some of these drugs, this is a welcome aspect.

It isn't possible to accord lithium the status of a nutritional trace element, but it is close. Animal studies have shown its efficacy and 'essential' status and psychiatrists are in danger of joining nutritionists and clinical ecologists in so-called orthomolecular medicine.

Lithium carbonate is manufactured as Liskonium, Camcolit, Priadel and Phasal.

Conventional thinking says lithium therapy should only be administered where regular checks on blood levels are available. Pfeiffer claimed it is safe in dosages as high as 300 mg lithium carbonate twice daily, without any such monitoring.

You can buy smaller-dose lithium on the Internet and it is now clear that it's not just for serious brain disorders—we ALL need it!

Startling new research reveals that low doses of lithium—available without a prescription—should be taken by most everyone who wants to grow new "gray matter"; restore and rejuvenate brain cells; boost memory; and stay mentally sharp for years to come.

Indeed the *New York Times* recently published an article titled, "Should We All Take a Bit of Lithium?" In it, they report that "relatively tiny doses of lithium can have beneficial effects"...including promoting brain health and improving mood.

5.10 Hypoglycemia

The word hypoglycaemia simply means 'low blood sugar'. Glucose circulating in the bloodstream is a vital metabolic nutrient: all organs combust it with oxygen to release energy for life processes. The brain is especially susceptible to a lack of it, and the consequences if glucose levels fall too low can be almost as serious as those resulting from a lack of oxygen.

The symptoms of hypoglycaemia mimic many conditions including multiple allergy and psychiatric problems. In fact hypoglycaemia often exists side-by-side with other conditions and can be inextricably linked to them. For example, one of the effects of an allergic reaction may be to induce a sudden drop in blood glucose supply.

I have already referred to smoking bringing about profound hypoglycemia (more on that below).

The pancreas gland, a key organ in food allergy syndromes, is implicated. Hypoglycaemia is often described in terms of insulin abnormality and indeed it may very well be a pre-diabetic (a precursor of diabetes). But the real culprit organs are probably the adrenal glands. They too secrete glucose-regulating hormones (glucocorticoids) and are part of the front line of our response to shock. Thus hypoglycaemia is sometimes known as adrenal stress syndrome.

Symptoms Attributable To Hypoglycaemia

Almost any symptom can result from hypoglycaemia, particularly if it causes neurological impairment. Some of the more common symptoms are listed in the table below.

As with all such lists, the reader is warned that many symptoms can have other causes and many do. But taken overall these may give you some clues as to the presence of hypoglycaemia:

- Sudden hunger pangs
- Urgent desire for something sweet
- Feeling tired late morning
- Feeling exhausted late afternoon
- Waking in the night to raid the refrigerator
- Panic attacks
- Rapid heartbeat and palpitations
- Shaking and inner trembling
- Double vision
- Incoherant speech, tendency to slur words or gabble

- Outbursts of temper
- Extreme depression
- Drowsiness
- Negativism
- Difficulty concentrating
- Personality changes
- Lack of co-ordination
- Emotional instability
- Mental confusion
- Light-headedness
- Insomnia
- Poor academic performance
- Premenstrual tension
- Headache or migraine
- Frequent nightmares
- Suicidal thoughts
- Addictions
- Alcoholism
- Antisocial behavior
- Joint pains
- Anxiety
- Manic or restless behavior
- Irritability
- Leg cramps
- Symptoms relieved by food, especially something sweet

As well as diverse symptoms, there are several disorders that may be caused or made worse by hypoglycemia. These include schizophrenia, epilepsy, depression, migraine and asthma. Obviously, it is important to investigate this possibility in any form of mental distress or disorder.

A characteristic feature of this condition is the way symptoms are relieved by sugar and sweet foods. The relief may only be temporary but the need drives the patient mercilessly. Many feel guilty for succumbing to their cravings but they needn't: it is not simply a matter of will power. *The desire for sugar is sometimes so overwhelming it cannot be resisted.* The brain will not tolerate lack of glucose, any more than it will tolerate lack of oxygen. The need is powerful and deep.

I have on occasion heard a patient claim 'I could kill for a bar of chocolate'. These words alone are sufficient to tell me that hypoglycemia is at work.

The Mechanism

Ironically, the consumption of too much carbohydrate food causes hypoglycemia. The exact progress of events is as follows:

1. Consumption of excess sugary food.

   Typical hypoglycemia sufferers eat a poor breakfast, such as cereal with sugar, sweetened coffee and toast with jam or marmalade (or even worse, no breakfast at all, which moves the patient straight to step 3).

2. This raises the blood sugar level rapidly.

   The body responds by releasing insulin and other glucose-regulating hormones from the adrenal glands

3. Blood sugar is lowered, but usually too fast.

   There is an overcompensation and the level falls too low. This is hypoglycemia.

4. There is craving for more sweet food, soon after the previous meal.

   By mid-morning sufferers need a snack, usually cake, biscuits or sweetened drinks and this triggers renewed hypoglycemia in a matter of 10 to 60 minutes (remember the '11 o'clock gap' promoted by a well-known chocolate manufacturer?)

5. The new intake sets off the cycle all over again. Blood sugar levels roller-coaster up and down many times a day.

6. Eventually the body's ability to cope with these continuous rushes of sugar becomes exhausted. It cannot cope with or regulate the ever-circling demand and so the regulation mechanism breaks down completely.

Even doctors sometimes get it wrong and advise the patient to eat sugar, or will prescribe dextrose tablets as the solution. These methods are incorrect and only exacerbate the condition although appearing to bring temporary relief. I repeat: sugar is the *cause* of hypoglycemia.

Diagnosis

Any doctor should be able to diagnose this condition purely on the basis of the patent's history: it is glaringly obvious if you know what to look for.

Laboratory confirmation, where warranted, can come from a six-hour glucose tolerance test.

The normal curve rises steadily to a peak and then subsides back to normal within 6 hours.

The characteristic of a diabetic curve is that it goes high and stays high, falling only very sluggishly, because the body has lost the ability to deal with carbohydrates.

Note that the blood glucose started with a sharp rise to over 50 percent of the starting value within one hour. Then it fell steadily, but at no stage did it fall below the fasting level, which is taken as the baseline.

The characteristic of a diabetic curve is that it goes high and stays high, falling only very sluggishly, because the body has lost the ability to deal with carbohydrate.

Finally, here is a curve showing a tendency to hypoglycemia: note that the graph rose as it should

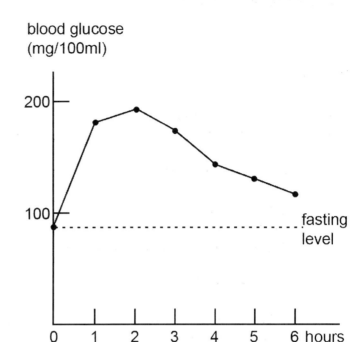

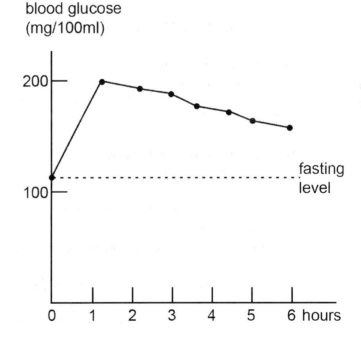

during the first hour and appeared to be normal until the third hour when it suddenly fell very steeply. Within an hour it had dropped by over 70 units. Moreover, from then onwards it remained below the fasting level for a considerable time before returning to 'baseline'. The rapid fall in the third or fourth hour is often accompanied by pronounced subjective symptoms.

This is why it is important to carry out the test over a six-hour period. The usual shorter glucose tolerance test would miss the tendency entirely!

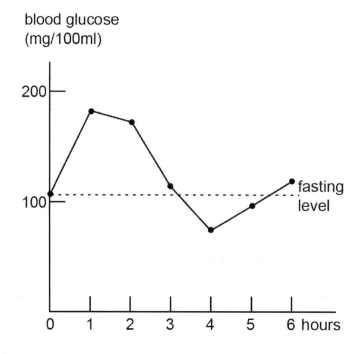

Diagnosing Hypoglycaemia from GTT Results

There are several possible responses to a six-hour glucose tolerance test that would suggest hypoglycemia, either actual or latent:

1. The blood sugar fails to rise more than 50 percent above the fasting level (this is rarely encountered).

2. The glucose curve falls to 20 percent below the fasting level.

3. The blood sugar falls 50 mg per 100 ml. or more during any one hour of the test (usually following a rapid rise of 50 mg percent in the first half hour).

4. The absolute blood sugar level falls in the range of 50 mg percent or lower (anything below 65 mg percent is suspicious).

5. Clinical symptoms such as dizziness, headache, confusion, palpitations, depression and so on appear during the course of a glucose tolerance test-regardless of what the blood sugar readings may be.

Bear these criteria in mind if you ever have a GTT. Your doctor is not likely to be familiar with them, and it may help you to interpret your own results.

Important note: my old mentor, the late Theron Randolph MD, doyen of all the clinical ecology movement back in the 1980s, was always insistent that this test was not so much a test of sugar tolerance but of corn allergy (most commercially-available glucose is made from corn starch).

Treatment

Treatment depends on three key changes you should make in your eating habits. Results may be slow in coming; you need to be patient and work at it for a few weeks, the rewards will come.

1. Eat Less Carbohydrate

You must stop eating and drinking all refined carbohydrate forthwith. This means sugar, white flour and corn sweeteners (as used in cordials, squashes, sodas, colas, doughnuts and so on). These are stress foods in just the same way that allergens are, and with all the same liabilities. Honey and untreated raw sugar are much gentler on the system, but for the time being avoid these also.

Limit your carbohydrate intake to 60 to 80 g per day, depending on your size; a child should be able to manage with 50g. The simplest way of working out your intake is to buy one of those excellent little books on the market with the title Carbohydrate Counter or similar. You will soon learn to regulate your diet without looking up every item. Many foods have a zero carbohydrate content and can be eaten freely without affecting the daily score: for example, any meats, cheese, most vegetables, fish and so on.

2. Eat a Substantial, Cooked Breakfast

There is no doubt that breakfast is crucial if you want to avoid hypoglycemia. The average British morning intake—cornflakes, toast and marmalade, plus tea or coffee (often also sweetened)—is a recipe for disaster. It will rocket your blood sugar and trigger the compensatory plunge by mid-morning, which results in symptoms.

A good breakfast will release glucose slowly from the stomach and so sustain blood levels for a number of hours, without any spikes or dips. By a good breakfast I mean a meal such as chops, liver, kidneys, egg or fish, perhaps accompanied by tomatoes and mushrooms, with fruit to follow. Gradually steer your breakfast habits away from the usual carbohydrate excess.

Remember this maxim: *if you feel hungry before about 1.00 pm, your breakfast is faulty or inadequate.*

The fatty part of the meal should not be omitted. There is a very good reason for this: fat slows down digestion and causes a slow release of digested products from the intestine.

Naturally, you will only breakfast on foods that are safe in allergy terms (section 5.2), but that will still leave you plenty of scope for a good, sound meal.

A lot of patients complain they are unable to face a large meal in the morning. Persist anyway. The usual cause of a poor appetite at breakfast-time is a big meal the evening before. Cut it down; you don't need it then if all you do is sit around watching TV.

3. Eat Little and Often

Don't go more than about three hours without food, preferably not more than two hours. Eat something. That doesn't mean chocolates or sweets but, for example, a piece of fruit, some nuts, some ham or other meat, a carrot or whatever you like to nibble.

Learn to take in fewer, smaller meals - hardly meals at all. The Americans have coined the term 'grazing' for this type of eating. I like this expression, since it helps to fix in the patient's mind what is wanted. There is now a website dedicated to grazing: www.graze.com

Supplements

Certain dietary additions will help to combat the effects of hypoglycemia. Chromium, sometimes known as the glucose tolerance factor, is vital: take 400 mcg. Niacin is also helpful but doses over 100 mg often cause unpleasant flushing. You can learn more about overcoming this problem in the section on nutritional supplements for mental health (section 5.14).

Incidentally, zinc competes for receptors with chromium, so make sure you don't cause a relative deficiency by supplementing one without the other.

Too Little Carbohydrate

It is not wise to continue on a restricted carbohydrate diet for too long. Eventually this too will cause problems. The body only has limited resources for making carbohydrate from protein. If you chronically starve yourself of carbohydrate you may find yourself getting hypoglycemic for the opposite reason. The same symptoms of tiredness, weakness, shaking, etc., will begin to return.

If you go way too far, you will enter a condition called ketosis. While fanatic dieters try to create this state on purpose, to speed the weight loss process, it is not safe long term.

The correct thing to do, after you have defeated the addiction to refined starches and white sugar, is gradually to allow the carbohydrate levels to rise. However, it is important, as before, to stay off refined sugar and flours. Eat only whole grain starches. These are digested slowly in the stomach and do not precipitate the rush of glucose to the blood, which would trigger the hypoglycemia response.

Suggested levels are 120 to 150 g of carbohydrate daily. You can allow more if you are engaged in heavy physical work.

Smoking and Hypoglycemia

I have already referred to the work of William H Phillpott and Dwight D Kalita, relating extreme disordered blood sugar control to the act of smoking (section 2.2). This has been confirmed and extended by more modern research.

A recent study published in the June 2007 edition of *Diabetes Care* looked at people with Type 1 diabetes and found a link between smoking and severe hypoglycemia (dangerously low blood glucose levels). ... The researchers theorized that smoking may possibly cause too much insulin to build up in the blood, leading to low blood glucose levels.

After adjusting for factors such as age, sex, HbA1c, alcohol consumption, waist-to-hip ratio, intensive insulin treatment, and history of severe hypoglycemia, the researchers found that people who currently smoked had almost three times the risk of experiencing severe hypoglycemia than those who had never smoked. For the purposes of the study, severe hypoglycemia was defined as loss of consciousness or being hospitalized overnight because of hypoglycemia.

The researchers theorized that smoking may possibly cause too much insulin to build up in the blood, leading to low blood glucose levels. In addition, smoking can increase the body's secretion of certain hormones that work against the action of insulin, leading smokers to need to inject more insulin, thereby increasing their risk of hypoglycemia.[289]

Exactly as Philpott and Kalita wrote, the effect can be to drive UP blood glucose too. Blood glucose levels were determined before smoking and 15, 30 and 60 minutes after the smoking of two cigarettes, compared to non-smoker controls. Both groups showed an increase of blood glucose following smoking, more marked, however, in the group of diabetics.

In 16 cases the experience was repeated once more, and an even higher increase of the blood glucose values was recorded as a result of the new nicotine charge. Conversely, there was no change in the blood glucose level after smoking nicotine-free cigarettes nor after smoking tobacco cigarettes but without inhaling the smoke.

The increase of blood glucose after smoking is assumed to be due to the mobilization of catecholamines and the stimulation of growth hormone and cortisol production. Growth hormone is known to increase blood sugar levels. Cortisol also mobilized sugar reserves, releasing glucose from glycogen storage deposits.

The authors concluded that this reaction seems to be more marked in diabetics than in metabolically normal subjects.[290]

5.11 Hormonal Imbalances

The idea that hormone variability causes profound disturbances of mood, cognition and behavior is hardly a medical secret. Yet ignorance and folly abound, even within the profession.

One of the laughable aspects of modern so-called "science" is when some science-trained dodo makes a pronouncement—which is nothing more than an opinion—and then this is passed off as actual science.

Case in point: the place of oxytocin in interpersonal reactions. Who doesn't know this is the "love hormone" or the "cuddle chemical"? Yet seriously ignorant Professor Mike Ludwig at Edinburgh University, UK, says it's all "hype".[291]

Professor or not, Ludwig seems not to have read about the actual functions of oxytocin. He's fussing about the fact that no-one has replicated the 2005 study which showed that sniffing oxytocin spray increased generosity, cooperation and trust has never been replicated (only because no-one has tried, dolt, not that all attempts have failed!)

The fact is that the role of oxytocin can reduce anxiety, create calm, trust and inward peace. Moreover, low oxytocin levels have been definitely identified in autism, ADHD, depression, anxiety, addictions (including gambling) and schizophrenia.

Moreover, Ludwig complains that it has not been shown that oxytocin can cross the blood-brain barrier. Well, it has actually, in a 2013 paper from Germany. But not to a standard that a nit-picky prejudiced and pretty ignorant professor would demand, especially one that rates his own opinions over the facts-so-far.[292]

Hormones and Mood

So, having got the rant over, I might as well turn my attention to the role of hormones in mood and thinking.

PMS is a great example. Most men have had the experience of being ready to break up with a woman, till he/she realized that it was a certain time of the month!

I have joked for decades that "Many men suffer from PMS!"

Prickly comedienne Roseanne Barr similarly joked: "Women complain about PMS, but I think of it as the only time of the month when I can be myself."

I don't think anyone is in any doubt of the effect. In 1892 Lizzie Borden was famously acquitted of murdering her father and stepmother with an axe, on the grounds she was psychotic with PMS.

Lizzie Borden took an axe, and gave her mother forty whacks.

When she saw what she had done, she gave her father forty-one.

(children's rhyme)

But which hormones are to blame? It's not easy to figure out, since women's hormone levels change constantly and every woman is unique.

Estradiol, undoubtedly, and progesterone seem to be the two main offenders. Bad moods may relate more to a sudden drop in estrogen levels—or maybe to excessively high levels just before the menses.

High progesterone levels have been linked to increased activity in the amygdala; which is part of the limbic system within the brain, responsible for emotions, survival instincts, and memory. It is involved in the processing of emotions such as fear, anger, and pleasure.

Working Up A Hormonal Profile

A full explanation of a woman's physiology, particularly in relation to the menses and pregnancies, is beyond the scope of this work. I am simply going to expand on the theme of checking for faulty hormone levels and building up a working profile of what is happening inside a woman's body.

None of the remarks I make here exclude females post-menopause, nor strictly exclude youngsters before the menarche (onset of puberty). But obviously, grown women in the child-bearing years are most at risk from the floods of hormones that come and go in her tissues.

Most notorious is estrogen and its many offshoots (estriol, estradiol, etc.) There is no question that when estrogen is present in excess, unpleasant symptoms arise, such as water retention, mood changes (particularly depression or irritability), decreased sex drive, breast swelling and tenderness, headaches and irregular or otherwise abnormal menstrual periods. We call this estrogen dominance.

It's problem enough. But matters are made much worse in this day and age, due to estrogen-like substances present in the environment, so-called xenoestrogens: Bisphenol A, phthalates (in plastics) and parabens (in personal care products).

The environmental presence of these chemical "hormone disruptors" as they are sometimes called is so bad that they are even beginning to affect men, reducing their virility, sperm count and secondary sex characteristics.

So when a woman is tested for her hormone levels, it makes more sense if she spends a month drinking only filtered water, or bottled water from glass bottles, and eating foods guaranteed free of these substances, before taking the test. Even then the lifespan presence of these chemicals in her body has to be factored in.

Even some foods are hormone disruptors: phytoestrogens in soya, dioxins in meat, and BHA/BHT (deliberate food additives), for example.

Testing For Hormones

Blood draw and urine collection testing has been the only standard for years. It works in a hospital environment but is little suited to holistic management of cases.

Two simple alternative tests, in skilled hands, are easy to do, non-invasive and accurate (effective) ways of estimating hormone levels in men and women. That is by measuring saliva levels (spitting into a small ampoule) or what is called a dried urine sample (peeing onto a sheet of paper, which is dried and then posted directly to the lab).

Thousands of studies using salivary hormone analysis have already been published, with more being added on a regular basis. This method can be used to identify existing hormone excesses or deficiencies. For example, finding out that a woman lacks sufficient progesterone to balance high estradiol levels or that high cortisol levels are interfering with the action of progesterone and testosterone.

The DUTCH test (dried urine for testing comprehensive hormones) is newer and less established but may well become the more common of the two methods. Monitoring shows that a dried urine sample is every bit as accurate as liquid urine but far easier to handle (shipping). You can find the links to it in the **Valuable Resources** section at the back of the book.

Both saliva and dried urine testing correlate very well with each other's measurements. But the DUTCH test can also provide more comprehensive information, by measuring metabolites of hormones, and thereby indicating what is going wrong. For example protective methylation may be at fault, allowing the accumulation of un-metabolized estrogens. Or free cortisol may appear low, but production of cortisol is actually high and being cleared too quickly.

In the USA, which is micro-controlled by mindless laws, you will need a licensed medical officer to order the test.

Once a hormone imbalance has been accurately identified, nutritional or bio-identical hormone therapy may be indicated. Again the actual techniques are beyond this text. But many practitioners today practice holistic intervention, using so-called bio-identical hormone replacement therapy, avoiding the patented synthetic hormones sold by Big Pharma. Many of these manufactured "hormones" do not exist in nature and therefore do NOT work (progestin, for example, sounds like progesterone—but it isn't).

Progestins stimulate the progesterone receptors but then block them, so no further progesterone activity takes place and estrogen is allowed unopposed dominance. John R. Lee MD calls progestins the great imposters.

Engine Speed! The Thyroid Gland

The big dividing line in healing philosophy between staid conventional colleagues and doctors like myself, is that we believe the patient more than we believe laboratory tests. If there is a conflict, we assume the patient is a more accurate monitor of disease than blood tests. I mean, how crazy is it to state to a patient (happens often) that, "We have done all the tests and there is nothing wrong," when the patient says she feels awful?

Take the treatment and investigation of thyroid disease as an example. Doctors who don't think for themselves, but rely solely on the blood tests, will ignore striking symptoms such as fatigue, depression, sensitivity to cold, weight-gain, dry skin, hair loss in a middle-aged or older person, if the thyroid markers are "normal". Good holistic doctors will follow the symptoms and treat the clinical deficiency condition, which clearly exists.

The fact is that up to 20% of the population is probably suffering from some degree of hypothyroidism (low thyroid function), though in some territories it could be much higher. The opposite—hyperthyroidism, or overactivity of the gland—is actually relatively rare. The older you get, the more prone you are to low thyroid function; it's part of natural ageing. *But it is still pathological and it should be treated!*

Part of the problem is that the tests are pretty crude and disease has to become pretty serious before it shows up as altered blood levels. Also the usually quoted range is so wide it is relatively meaningless and you could be 50% down on "average" and still said to be within normal limits.

The real point is that a person can be functionally hypothyroid without any other abnormal markers than symptoms and signs of disease. It's a test of a doctor's skill to recognize and treat the disease they see, whether or not the laboratory is helpful in confirming the diagnosis.

It is vital that all doctors start to think more often of thyroid problems. Because it's not just a "quality of life" issue: your risk of heart disease is significantly increased and the confusion and lethargy which comes on may even be mistaken for senility or depression and the patient put on a completely inappropriate program.

It's not just adults: thyroid problems are common in children with autism, and psychiatrist Dr. Suruchi Chandra believes that thyroid hormone disrupting chemicals such as BPA and flame retardants are affecting the thyroid, and that even small changes in thyroid hormone levels may be causing irreversible changes to the brain.

Immunity

What very few doctors seem to know is that the thyroid gland is wrapped up in the process of immunity. Several studies have shown that a patient with thyroid problems is more likely to develop cancer (cancer is best considered a disease of the immune system). This doesn't mean only thyroid cancer; any cancer could be involved!

I first came across the connection between thyroid and immunity in my work as an allergy guru. Time and again patients would present the symptoms of thyroid disease, along with their allergy problems. This was especially true of women and there is a very good reason. Women have a high incidence of a clinical condition called Hashimoto's disease, in which the body makes antibodies against the thyroid gland and hormones (auto-immune thyroiditis). It's one of those allergy-against-yourself diseases.

It must be mentioned in passing that there is another kind of thyroiditis. This is not caused by anti-bodies but a virus, typically mumps or Coxsackie. Usually it resolves clinically but may be the source of chronic hypothyroidism.

Pioneer, the late, Dr Broda O. Barnes reckoned that hypothyroidism underpinned a huge range of diseases in the West, from heart disease, to allergies; cancer to apparent parasitism; loss of sexual function to visual acuity. Notice, by the way, how those are like a catalogue of aging problems!

But it's not just about pseudo-aging: for women, all kinds of menstrual difficulties—notably heavy flow—can be attributed to hypothyroidism, as can emotional and behavior problems in children. Indeed, there is a clear link between hypothyroidism and autism spectrum disorder.

In terms of psychiatric patients, the symptoms that can masquerade as mental illness but are actually caused by thyroid dysfunction are many and varied, including (but not limited to): anxiety, excessive fear, mood swings like bi-polar, rage, irritability, paranoid schizophrenia, confusion, dementia, obsessive/compulsive disorders (OCD), and mental aberrations. These reactions are made worse when the adrenals too are underperforming adrenals (see HPA axis disorder below: 5.9).

What most doctors don't seem to get is that T3 (the most important and active of the thyroid hormone family) is actually a neurotransmitter that regulates the action of serotonin, norepinephrine, and GABA (gamma aminobutyric acid). GABA is an inhibitory neurotransmitter that is important for quelling anxiety. Thus, if you don't have enough T3, or if its action is blocked, an entire cascade of neurotransmitter abnormalities may ensue and can lead to mood and energy changes, including anxiety states and depression.

And another thing: brain cells have more T3 receptors than any other tissues. Why do you suppose that is? Well it means for sure that a proper uptake of thyroid hormone is essential for the brain cells to work properly.

One article I read on the PubMed article database actually coined the term "Myxedema Madness" (myxedema is another name for hypothyroid function). According to the authors:

The clinical presentations of thyroid hormone deficiency are diverse, complicated, and often overlooked... Psychiatric presentations include cognitive dysfunction, affective disorders, and psychosis. The realization that hypothyroidism might be the cause of an assortment of symptoms is critical in the identification and treatment of the hypothyroid patient. Once hypothyroidism is identified, symptoms usually respond to appropriate thyroid hormone supplementation.

The article presented a case of clinical hypothyroidism that came to clinical attention due to psychotic symptoms consisting of auditory and visual hallucinations. That patient could have easily been diagnosed as schizophrenia, submerged in potent but unhelpful drugs, and lost forever to family and friends.

In summary, the authors Thomas W. Heinrich MD and Garth Grahm MD stated:

There is little doubt that thyroid hormone plays a major role in the regulation of mood, cognition, and behavior. As a result, persons with thyroid dysfunction frequently experience a wide variety of neuropsychiatric sequelae [*what follows on*, KSM]. The range of physical and psychiatric presentations and their potential subtle manifestations make hypothyroidism a diagnosis that is easy to miss. Behavioral changes may occur in the absence of the classical physical signs and symptoms of the disorder. As a result, it is imperative to remember that many patients presenting with psychiatric disorders may have alterations in endocrine function. The endocrine dysfunction may be the cause of the presenting complaint, a factor complicating the management of an underlying illness, or a consequence of treatment.[293]

Accelerating Problem

What's worrying is the theory that thyroid disorders are getting worse with every generation. One of the important reasons for such widespread hypothyroid problems in Western civilization is the fact that it is in large part due to the toxic overload that we all bear.

Nothing suffers quite so much as the thyroid gland from loading with pesticides, pollutants and toxic heavy metals (see section 5.11: heavy metals). With each generation, the toxic overload accumulates steadily, much like chemicals accumulate moving up the food chain (remember, we are at the top of many food chains).

But the thyroid dysfunction multiplies too; each parent generation starting their kids off with an already compromised organ, who pass it on to their kids, even more disadvantaged still—and so it goes on.

If this is true, we would be facing thyroid misery of almost epidemic proportions. And you know what? That's exactly what we holistic doctors are seeing. But the medical profession is not getting it—because they rely entirely on stupid and unworkable tests; nothing shows, so there is "no problem".

The Broda Barnes Temperature Test

Blood tests for thyroid hormones, as I implied, are totally unreliable; a patient may have normal thyroid hormone levels but, if the body is not responding to those hormones, a deficiency equivalent is the result.

Here is a simple DIY test for thyroid function—the so-called Broda Barnes test—named after the doctor who first wrote about it. It means taking your basal temperature on a daily basis and observing if it is too low.

Basal temperature means while at absolute rest. In ordinary terms that means first thing on waking, after the body has been lying still overnight. Temperature drops to its lowest at this point. To measure your own basal temperature, use a clinical thermometer, keep it under your tongue, before getting out of bed or any activity whatsoever, for at least three minutes without opening your mouth. Record the results.

Generally, if it is running at 36.5 C (97.5 F) or less, that is presumptive evidence of low thyroid function. Allowance may need to be made for women who are ovulating, since the temperature naturally rises about 0.5 of a degree at this time. I will help the patient interpret what is found.

Other Tests

Bio-energetic testing, such as electro-acupuncture, may be yet another route by which poor thyroid function is called to the attention of the physician.

This also often shows us that other hormonal disturbance is present too, even if subtle and represented only at the energetic level. Furthermore we often learn that these hormone disruptions are the results of long standing energetic "shadows", some of which go back to childhood illnesses and vaccinations.

All very controversial.

But fortunately the new magic of electronic bio-energetic testing (see my book *Medicine Beyond*) also often shows us effective herbal, homeopathic and other holistic remedies which will work in the presence of low thyroid function.

Also, something I learned back in my mega-allergy doctor days: women appear to be allergic to their own hormones sometimes... meaning that if we intra-dermally allergy tested thyroid, estrogen or progesterone, there would sometimes be a significant skin flare, indicating an antibody response. That would be just another kind of auto-immune response. Obviously, the implications of this are pretty big, if that's happening. Mega-allergy doctor? I don't want to detract from your skills and experience but that sounds a bit over the top to me. We can discuss if you want more detail

That's over and above the known autoimmune response of Hashimoto's disease (antibodies to the actual thyroid gland).

Treatment

In my practice I used a several-fold approach. The simplest, if the signs are early enough and the patient is otherwise vigorous, is homeopathic thyroid stimulant. I use a product called *Thyroidea compositum* from Germany. It is one of the most powerful and useful non-drug substances I have in my repertoire. Such is its impact on immunity I find myself prescribing it often for my cancer patients seeking alternative remedies.

If a trial of this substance and related compounds appears ineffective, then supplementation with the hormone can be considered. Conventional colleagues would not normally approach things this way, feeling that if the blood levels are adequate then supplementation is pointless.

The stupidity of this attitude is that they then have nothing to offer the patient, beyond palliative treatment. Often this means prescribing anti-depressants for the lethargy and giving him or her a good ticking off about being overweight!

This is the worst possible kind of psychiatric intervention, because it's misdirection.

A better approach is to use what we call a "therapeutic trial". The patient then becomes his or her own test bed. If taking the hormone results in a rapid return to normal, with renewed zest, fading of mental disturbance and loss of weight encumbrance, is that not adequate intellectual evidence that the thyroid was indeed, in some way, under-performing?

Please bear in mind that the thyroid makes five hormones: T4, T3, T2, T1 and calcitonin. T4, also called thyroxine, is simply a storage hormone meant to convert to T3, the active hormone. But the use of T4 only, as in most medical practice, makes you dependent on the conversion process from T4 to T3, the really active form of thyroid hormone. If that conversion process is impaired, you become hypothyroid, no matter how much T4 you are prescribed!

Yet T4 is the standard medication version. T4 only means you are basically missing out on the other four thyroid hormones, especially the important T3. Duh! Orthodox replacement therapy, using T4-only, has many names: Synthroid, Levoxyl, Levothyroxine, Unithroid, Eltroxin, Levaxin, Norton, Eutrosig, Oroxine, Tirosint, for example.

Synthetic vs. Natural Replacement

Even worse, the usual thyroid hormone replacement (levothyroxine or Synthroid) is synthetically produced. The natural product is better, even though mainstream doctors try to denigrate it. This means supplementing dried thyroid extract from animal sources (pig instead of beef, because of BSE). If Hashimoto's disease is the problem, synthetic products may arguably be better, because the body doesn't react to them in the same way as foreign animal protein.

But best I found was desiccated thyroid extract by Armour. Desiccated (dried) thyroid is a thyroid hormone replacement drug, prepared from the thyroid gland from pigs—also known as "porcine" or *suis* thyroid (*suis*: Latin, pig). Other brand names of natural products include Nature-throid, and Westhroid.

Desiccated natural thyroid preparation has been on the market and safely used for more than 100 years. When synthetic thyroxine was introduced, there was a great deal of baloney and marketing hype about how modern it was, compared to "old-fashioned" desiccated thyroid—and many doctors switched patients over to the synthetic medication. When the patient went into a steep decline as a result, he or she was told "It's your age."

You should know that Synthroid has been sponsor of medical meetings, golf outings, symposia, research grants, and speakers' fees, and is the chief provider of lunches at medical offices, patient literature, pens, pads, mugs, and other freebies, giveaways, and marketing items for decades.

We now have several generations of doctors who have been trained to believe that synthetic levothyroxine—and specifically Synthroid—is the only thyroid replacement medication available or worth using. They simply don't know anything else. They hear ridiculous rumors on a regular basis—spread by drug reps for competitive levothyroxine drugs—that desiccated thyroid is going off the market.

None of this is true. Desiccated porcine thyroid extract remains one of the most powerful and natural psychiatric meds of all time. Don't miss out on it, if you need it.

Tests

Here's where is gets ugly. Today, the medical profession has such an obsession with blood tests and lab work—and such a total belief in their accuracy and supremacy—that it has become considered quackery to override or ignore them. A doctor who administers thyroid supplements to a patient, when the blood tests are "normal", faces censure and loss of the right to practice medicine.

To treat a patient properly with clinical severe hypothyroidism may be as much as a physician's license is worth. To diagnose by the signs of the disease (the only reliable diagnostic method) is a lost art and patients face having their symptoms put down to aging and inadequacy. Some patients are even taken off thyroid replacement therapy because they "don't need it any more"; the blood tests have normalized, they are told.

So the poor patient's worthwhile life is ended, crucified on the cross of stupid and ignorant dogma. He or she declines in energy, looks, vitality, joy and sexuality. Weight gain is relentless; cholesterol soars; a heart attack becomes almost inevitable.

The trouble is that patients who are hypothyroid every so often have normal levels of thyroid hormones, such as T4, T3 and the infamous TSH. The latter is taken as the absolute benchmark of thyroid performance. If it is normal, you don't have hypothyroidism, they say.

Yet this situation (which is very common indeed) has parallels with diabetes type II, in which there is plenty of insulin—actually an excess—yet the body is not responding to it. What difference does it make if the body's thyroid hormone levels are "normal", if the cells in the tissues do not and cannot respond to it?

High levels could even be an indicator that the body is secreting excess hormone, to try and drive the cells, which are not actually responding. In other words, proof something is wrong!

So, bear all this in mind when you ask to see your thyroid test results AND FIGHT YOUR CORNER!

Dosing

Bear in mind the natural desiccated thyroid extract is giving your body all five thyroid hormones: T4, T3, T2, T1 and calcitonin. That takes some getting used to. It may be wise to start with a modest dose, such as 1 grain (or even 0.5 grain). A grain is 65 mgm, give or take.

But you will need to raise the dose quite soon, otherwise hypothyroid symptoms can return, due to the internal feedback loop in your body, which can happen if you stay on a low dose too long. Go to 2 grains in 2 – 3 weeks, providing there are no negative consequences. Then 3 grains for a further 4 weeks, to give the T4 time to build (which can take 4-6 weeks). Tweak it from there, monitoring the response. It's unlikely indeed that anyone would need more than 5 grains.

You can just swallow the grains or take them sublingually. When taking desiccated thyroid extract, it is important to avoid iron, estrogen and calcium supplements at the same time, since all bind the thyroid hormones to some degree (take them separately).

There may be other issues which can reveal themselves as the dose increases, such as sluggish adrenals or low iron levels. These must be competently corrected first, otherwise serious side-effects may ensue or, at the very least, the treatment might fail.

Insufficient iron levels alter and reduce the conversion of T4 to T3, besides binding T3. Additionally, low iron levels can increase circulating concentrations of TSH (thyroid stimulating hormone). Problems with either will cause T3 to pool high in your blood and not your cells. So repeat labs are a good idea after about 5- 6 weeks. The final dosage levels vary, of course, but 3 – 5 grains is not unusual.

Suppliers

If you search the Internet, you'll see Armour by Forest Labs, the oldest on the market, then Naturethroid and Westhroid which came into the picture in the late 1930s–by RLC Labs.

A new generic by Acella, NP Thyroid, hit the picture by late 2010 and is popular. There is Thyroid-S or "Thiroyd" from Thailand with excellent results, and Erfa's Thyroid from Canada. Australia uses compounded desiccated thyroid powder and there are many compounding (traditional) pharmacies around the world, which can help you.

You are looking for the removal of your hypothyroid symptoms, an afternoon temp of 98.6, a morning before-rising temp of 97.8 – 98.2 (held under arm ten minutes), good heart rate and blood pressure, good energy, clearing of brain fog, etc. When optimal, you will notice your free T3 is at the top of the range, and free T4 is midrange. Note: if your free T3 is at the top of the range and you still feel horrible, time to test your iron (with blood) and cortisol levels (via saliva, NOT blood).

Warning: This is not really a go-it-alone area for self-help. You need your blood levels monitored. Thyroid hormone is potentially harmful, even dangerous, and you would be wise to seek out a qualified medical practitioner of the open-minded sort, who can help and steer you.

However, if you are desperate and help is not forthcoming, visit the website run by Janie Bowthorpe (link in the **Valuable Resources** section in the back of the book). She knows more than me! (She should, she suffered thyroid Hell herself and has made a career out of learning the full thyroid story). I cannot recommend Janie's site highly enough.

Low-T

Whenever I hear of men in their late 60s or beyond being depressed, low energy, irritable, fatigued and low self-esteem, I think immediately of testosterone levels. Low-T, as it is called, can trigger a whole host of negative psychological moods and perceptions.

There's good and bad in that. If nobody thinks of the right diagnosis, the man is headed for a miserable old age. The wife too, incidentally, if she sticks with him. That's bad. Yet the instigation of weekly testosterone shots can lift the man's mood almost instantly. It can seem miraculous. That's good!

Serum testosterone is a standard test, conducted by most labs, and is reported as nanograms per deciliter (ng/dL). I'm talking free testosterone here, not the bound form or so-called "total testosterone". Optimum would be around 1,000 ng/dL, which is typical for a young man. 300 – 1100 ng/dL is an acceptable range.

Below 300, testosterone supplementation is required and the humane thing to do. No honest examination of an older man's true psychological state could be entertained, without first normalizing testosterone levels. And that extends to senility and dementia.

Please be aware also of a sad condition called involutional melancholia. It can strike men as young as their 40s and 50s. The man suddenly loses all meaning in his life, everything becomes hopeless and depressing, money may have become an anxiety, nothing will lift him from the gloom. It's a true psychosis, because he begins to believe that things are so hopeless generally that there is no point in his wife and offspring going on living either.

This is the individual who will shoot his entire family and then turn the gun on himself. Stories like this occur often and are usually under-reported. No-one pays much attention to this sort of tragedy. Very sad.

I prescribe testosterone enanthate injections. This is also a kind of therapeutic trial meaning, if the problem is low-T, the individual will respond within days!

Typical doses would be in the range of 200-250 mg per week.

Note also you can raise testosterone levels by supplementing with DHEA and with the herb *Tribulus terrestris*. These supplements are sometimes sufficient to totally normalize testosterone levels.

Note: if you raise testosterone levels without taking steps to counter the conversion to SHBG (sex-hormone binding globulin), which has estrogen-like properties, the man will feminize (loss of drive, man boobs etc.) This xeno-estrogen effect is countered by saw palmetto and zinc: you MUST take at least 300 mg of saw palmetto and 50 mg of zinc daily.

Bear in mind, a 59-year old man has, on average, more estrogen then a 59-year old woman. We don't want any more! If SHBG goes high, this tricks the pituitary and interferes with the secretion of LH (luteinising hormone), which then scores low. LH is meant to stimulate the testes to secrete testosterone. But if LH is high and testosterone low, the regulation pathway is clearly not working.

Chrysin (passion flower), available as capsules or cream also has a definite beneficial effect in this context. Avena sativa (oats) is also said by some to increase free testosterone.

Myths About Testosterone

It's supposed to make men aggressive and violent. But that's not entirely true. A study published in 2016 found that high-testosterone men responded according to social norms. They were more likely to punish someone who had treated them unfairly. But were equally likely to be generous in sport, if their opponent was also generous.[294] What matters is that when testosterone is missing in an aging man, this causes low energy, depression, a lack of sex drive, and erectile dysfunction. You replace testosterone in appropriate doses and all of that normalizes. The reason for that is that many key organs, including the brain, have testosterone receptors. They need to be activated regularly by testosterone for normal organ function.

Women need a small amount of testosterone as well to feel normal and to maintain their libido.

Alcohol, unfortunately, diminishes testosterone on the blood; perhaps another scientific angle on Shakespeare's famous quote, that alcohol "promotes the desire but takes away the performance"! (Macbeth, the porter, speaking in act 2 scene 3)

Adrenal Exhaustion

A rather corny journal I am reading (or I should say the underperforming writer and a lazy editor) says that adrenal fatigue is merely a "nugget of internet wisdom" that "is easy to diagnose online but neither doctors nor scientists recognize such a condition".

This dismissive generalization makes liars out of careful doctors like me who recognize the condition as real and important enough to treat. Doctors who don't know adrenal insufficiency are dangerously ignorant.

These are the published symptoms of adrenal insufficiency, taken from the government National Institute of Diabetes and Digestive and Kidney Disease (NIDDK) website:

- chronic, or long lasting, fatigue
- muscle weakness
- loss of appetite
- weight loss

- abdominal pain
- nausea
- vomiting
- diarrhea
- low blood pressure that drops further when a person stands up, causing dizziness or fainting
- irritability and depression
- craving salty foods
- hypoglycemia, or low blood sugar
- headache
- sweating
- irregular or absent menstrual periods
- in women, loss of interest in sex[295]

A number of these, as you see, are emotional in nature.

Can Stress Hormones Be Protective?

An intriguing possibility is being debated: higher levels of estrogen in women and testosterone in men may have protective effects against PTSD (post-traumatic stress disorder). For example, women who had been raped but took an emergency contraceptive hormone (progesterone based) afterwards seemed to have less likelihood of developing PTSD than those who took no abortive estrogen.

And studies of men with high testosterone and cortisol levels before battle were found to be less likely to develop battlefield PTSD.

These findings suggest the administration of hormones immediately after a stressful event could lower the incidence of PTSD developing.

And, you will have noticed, further point up the real nature of adrenal insufficiency and how dangerous it is.

All Act Together

It is important in reading this review to understand that all hormones are interactive. It would be very rare to get significant changes in one and not have it affect the others.

All endocrine glands (the ones without ducts that secrete hormones directly into the blood) are controlled by the pituitary gland, which in turn is subject to rule from the hypothalamus, which is dominated by our thoughts and emotions. The hypothalamic pituitary pathway has profound influences on our hormonal and emotional state.

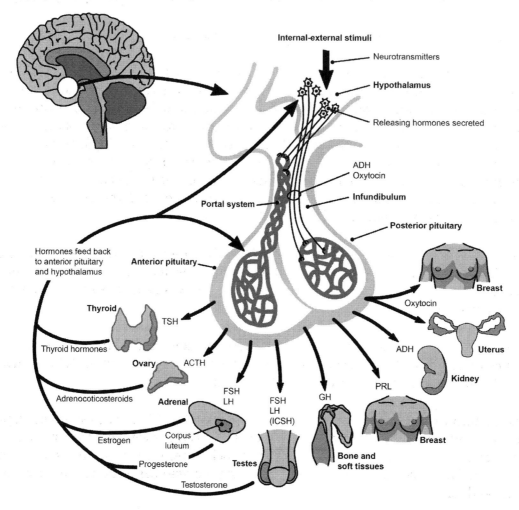

Key: GH growth hormone, FSH follicle stimulating hormone, LH luteinizing hormone, PRL prolactin, TSH thyroid stimulating hormone, ADH antidiuretic hormone.

HPA Axis (from Wiki)

The HPA axis is a major hormonal regulation system involved in the neurobiology of mood disorders and functional illnesses, including anxiety disorder, bipolar disorder, insomnia, posttraumatic stress disorder (PTSD), borderline personality disorder, ADHD, major depressive disorder (MDD), burnout, chronic fatigue syndrome, fibromyalgia, irritable bowel syndrome, and alcoholism.[296]

That's a pretty comprehensive list of psychiatric conditions.

HPA stands for hypothalamus-pituitary-adrenal axis. It denotes the fact that our moods and emotions, via the hypothalamus, are directly connected with the hormone master-control gland, the pituitary. In fact the two are just millimeters apart, sitting at the base of the brain. This "secret" lock-step between the brain and the pituitary is the reason our moods so closely influence our hormones and, indeed, our whole body physiology.

Indeed, this is a major aspect of the body-mind connection.

The third link in this chain, the adrenal glands (two of them, one sat atop each kidney, hence the name) is one of our primary energizers, releasing cortisol, adrenalin (epinephrine to the Americans), noradrenalin (norepinephrine), so-called mineralocorticoids, of which aldosterone is the most important (helps regulate salt and water balance), and finally a raft of androgens (male sex-related hormones), mainly dehydroepiandrosterone (DHEA) and testosterone. All have weak effects, but play a role in early development of the male sex organs in childhood, and in women during puberty. These are involved in creating and maintaining the differences character differences between men and women (Mars and Venus stuff).

Pretty important, all in all. And, sure enough, if the adrenal glands fail (Addison's disease) the individual will surely die, if not rescued by artificial hormone supplements. President J F Kennedy had Addison's disease (a big secret) but he was kept alive by daily doses of adrenal hormones.

Cortisol has a bad rap, being known as the "stress hormone" and high levels in chronic stress can kill. But without adequate cortisol, we cannot adapt to stress. PTSD is made worse, for example, if cortisol levels are not adequate.

Several neurotransmitters are important in regulating the HPA axis, especially dopamine, serotonin and norepinephrine (noradrenaline). There is evidence that an increase in oxytocin, resulting for instance from positive social interactions, acts to suppress the HPA axis and thereby counteracts stress, promoting positive health effects such as wound healing and relaxation.

Studies on people show that the HPA axis is activated in different ways during chronic stress depending on the type of stressor, the person's response to the stressor and other factors. Stressors that are uncontrollable, threaten physical integrity, or involve trauma tend to have a high, flat diurnal profile of cortisol release (with lower-than-normal levels of cortisol in the morning and higher-than-normal levels in the evening) resulting in a high overall level of daily cortisol release.

On the other hand, controllable stressors tend to produce higher-than-normal morning cortisol. Stress hormone release tends to decline gradually after a stressor occurs. In post-traumatic stress disorder there appears to be lower-than-normal cortisol release, and it is thought that a blunted hormonal response to stress may even predispose a person to develop PTSD. [Miller GE, Chen E, Zhou ES (January 2007). "If it goes up, must it come down? Chronic stress and the hypothalamic–pituitary–adrenocortical axis in humans".[297] Investigating The HPA Axis

The reader will readily see that measuring sex hormones may not cut it at all. A thorough investigation of HPA axis function is required in any patient showing signs of chronic stress, which means, in effect, any seriously impaired psychiatric patient. To omit this vital step is criminal neglect.

HPA axis dysfunction as it's called is very real and has diagnostic criteria. It may be a better term than "adrenal exhaustion", which points the finger too harshly at the adrenals only, forgetting the rest of the control mechanism.

Instead of measuring only the output of the adrenal glands, it makes more sense to investigate also the pituitary hormones, which are supposed to stimulate their release.

The relationship of hypothalamic-pituitary-adrenal (HPA) axis activity and resilience (resistance to stress) can be measured using the generally-accepted Resilience Scale for Adults. Resilience, of course, is seen as a positive response to stressors. According to the bio-psycho-social model, resilience is influenced by self-esteem, coping strategies and personality traits. In schizophrenic patients, resilience seems to affect real-life functioning (a vertical), while in mood disorders, resilience influences the longitudinal course of the disorder, reducing the frequency of relapses and improving drugs response.

The overall ability to handle stress clearly depends on the individual's HPA axis responsiveness, which in turn has been found to predict the likelihood of developing neuropsychiatric disorders such as addiction. However, under chronic stress this feedback becomes dysregulated, leading to the variety of psychological syndromes, such as anxiety, various forms of depressive disorders and addiction, including alcohol dependence as a coping mechanism. So this is very important stuff to psychiatrists.

Interestingly, I found a major paper in the journal *Frontiers of Psychiatry*. It discussed the function of cortisol receptors (glucocorticoid receptors, or GRs) and the ability of a substance mifepristone, also known as RU486, to block them. This resulted in a significant reduction in substance addiction, notably amphetamine, cocaine, morphine and alcohol. The authors concluded that mifepristone offered a promising way to temporarily reset the stress response system that has become maladapted following chronic and long-term alcohol consumption and a variety of neurological and psychological disorders. I quote the study here merely to reinforce the very significant effect that the HPA axis has upon stress-related pathology.[298]

Adaptogens

There has emerged in recent years the concept of "adaptogens", meaning substances that can enhance health in general and create adaptability, or resilience. This unique group of herbal ingredients work by improving HPA axis and adrenal function, thereby, as we have seen, managing your body's hormonal response to stress and the ability to cope with anxiety and fight fatigue.

The term 'adaptogen' was originally established by N. V. Lazarev (1947) to refer to a substance which was claimed to increase "non-specific" resistance to adverse influences to organism (biological integrity) and stress. The term "stress" is used here in the classic sense as defined by Hans Selye (1936, 1950) as a state of threatened homeostasis.

Adaptogens should be differentiated from so-called "tonics" and stimulants. The defining factor is that performance improves after both stimulants, tonics and adaptogens have been ingested, but only remains high after the adaptogens (meaning some significant physiological change has taken place).

The concept is new to Western medicine. In fact the European Medicines Agency stated in 2008 that the concept requires additional clinical and preclinical research, and is therefore not accepted into current medical terminology. But remedies of this type have been around for millennia and in common use in Chinese herbal medicine and Ayurveda.[299]

Generally, these work better than sugar, caffeine or alcohol, so are well worth taking a look! It could be argued these are a better first line of treatment for many psychiatric disorders than current pharmaceuticals.

There isn't space here to expound the topic in full. But a list of possible adaptogenic substances would certainly include:

- Asian Ginseng
- Holy Basil
- Milk Thistle
- Ashwagandha
- Rhodiola Rosea
- Ginseng Eleuthero
- Rosemary
- Aloe Vera
- Gotu Kola
- Astragalus
- Moringa Oleifera
- Schisandra
- Bacopa
- Licorice Root

The one to be careful of is ashwaganda. It can make some people very sick. That's an idiosyncratic response, meaning it doesn't apply to most people. But it does mean you must be cautious. Try a little first. In fact that may be good advice for any of these herbs.

My favorite is holy basil or Tulsi tea, which I drink every day!

Oxytocin The "Love Hormone"

Oxytocin is a powerful hormone, meaning it is secreted by an endocrine gland; in this case the pituitary gland. But it also acts as a neurotransmitter (like serotonin and dopamine). It seems to be consistently associated with bonding, nurturing, love and peace. Bring it on!

Oxytocin regulates social interaction and sexual reproduction, playing a role in behaviors from maternal-infant bonding and milk release to empathy, generosity, and orgasm. When we hug or kiss a loved one, oxytocin levels increase; hence, oxytocin is often called "the love hormone" or "cuddle hormone". In fact, the hormone plays a huge role in all pair bonding. The hormone is greatly stimulated during sex, birth, and breastfeeding. Oxytocin is the hormone that underlies trust. It is also an antidote to depressive feelings.

It's been shown that certain psychological states are associated with (I do not say caused by...) a deficiency of oxytocin. These include:

- Autism spectrum disorder
- ADHD
- Depression
- Anxiety
- Addiction
- Gambling
- Schizophrenia

Aren't those conditions which would just turnaround with lots of love? I think so!

For all its positivity, however, oxytocin has a dark side. Or, better stated, it plays a more complex role in human behavior than is commonly thought.

It does help groups to bond. But there is a tendency for such groups to unite against outsiders (different tribes), giving rise to envy, prejudice, and possibly aggression.

Moreover, excess oxytocin is associated with psychopaths. Does that make sense? Yes, these people love only themselves; they are lonely and detached.

Oxytocin may also play a role in anger management. Research has indicated that certain variants (polymorphisms) of the oxytocin receptor (OXTR) gene are associated with an increased tendency to react angrily to situations. In particular, differences in OXTR gene expression appear to affect the regulation of the relationship between alcohol and aggressive behavior.

Oxytocin in women

Oxytocin is a particularly important hormone for women. The hormone causes uterine contractions during labor and helps shrink the uterus after delivery. When an infant suckles at his or her mother's breast, the stimulation causes a release of oxytocin, which, in turn, orders the body to "let down" milk for the baby to drink.

Oxytocin also promotes mother-child bonding. Studies show that virgin female rats don't like pups (baby rats). But once they give birth, the attitude is transformed, so those female rats find the pups irresistible. And similar findings are seen in human women; the ones who go all gooey at the sight of a baby are usually not virgins.[300]

A 2007 study published in the journal *Psychological Science* found that the higher a mom's oxytocin levels in the first trimester of pregnancy, the more likely she was to engage in bonding behaviors such as singing to or bathing her baby.

It seems the baby's oxytocin levels rise too.[301]

Maybe it's time we paid especial attention to oxytocin in psychological disorders and distress sates of all kinds. After all, most disharmony starts as the feeling of loneliness, not belonging or rejection. In other words, *a lack of love.*

Oxytocin in men

In men, as in women, oxytocin facilitates bonding. Dads who got a boost of oxytocin via a nasal spray played more closely with their 5-month-old babies than dads who didn't get the hormone zap, a 2012 study found. (There is a second hormone, called vasopressin, which plays a stronger role in men.)

Another study found that men in relationships given a burst of oxytocin spray stood farther away from an attractive woman than men who weren't given any oxytocin. Single men didn't see any effect from the hormone, suggesting oxytocin may work as a fidelity booster for guys who are already bonded with another woman. That's very odd![302]

In another study, published in PNAS in 2010, men were given a dose of oxytocin and asked to write about their mothers. Those with secure relationships described their moms as more caring after the hormone dose. Those with troubled relationships actually saw their mothers as less caring. The hormone may help with the formation of social memories, according to the study researchers, so a whiff strengthens previous associations, whether good or bad.[303]

Oxytocin Administration

Oxytocin nasal sprays are marketed widely on the internet. It has to be said that the science is not all that good and the claims are mainly just hype. It's hard even to be sure they contain any oxytocin!

There are no long-term studies on the side effects of the legitimate oxytocin sprays used in hormone research; most studies give people one dose of the hormone only.

A better idea is a development by one of holistic medicine's founding fathers, C. Normal Shealy MD, PhD. It's one I've tried and shared personally and it DOES work. We can persuade the body to release its own oxytocin and therefore bypass all issues of purity, cost and safety!

Norman developed a wonderful stimulant essential oil mix he calls "Air Bliss'. It does smell heavenly!

Applied as Norman prescribes, it is said to stimulate the release of oxytocin in generous pharmacological levels. I think it should be in everyone's medicine cabinet and considered an essential tool for any kind of psychiatric disorder, from schizophrenia and anxiety, to depression and autism, which all must, by their very nature, include an element of isolation and disconnection.

The secret is to apply the Air Bliss to a series of related acupuncture points, which Norman calls the "Ring of Air", as follows:

Spleen 1 A, bilaterally

Liver 3, bilaterally

Stomach 36, bilaterally

Governing Vessel 1, 16 and 20

Gall Bladder 20, bilaterally

Lung 1, bilaterally

You can find these points and order yourself an ampoule of wonderful "Air Bliss" oil at Norman's website (see below).

Incidentally, using a GHz stimulator, the Shealy PainPro, for 3 minute stimulation of each pair of points, he discovered a significant increase in Neurotensin, a natural neuroleptic (substance that melts away mental troubles) and anti-nocioceptic (a substance that melts away physical pain)—in one person the rise was 600%!

Neurotensin has been implicated in the modulation of dopamine signaling, and produces a spectrum of pharmacological effects resembling those of antipsychotic drugs, leading to the suggestion that neurotensin may be an endogenous neuroleptic; that is: a class of medication primarily used to manage psychosis (including delusions, hallucinations, paranoia or disordered thought), principally in schizophrenia and bipolar disorder. But neuroleptics are increasingly being used in the management of non-psychotic disorders. Very helpful stuff, in other words, and far safer and more effective the antipsychotic drugs, with their hideous side-effects).

"Some years later I had a sudden intuitive hit that the Ring of Air would also raise oxytocin and I have now proven that this is true," says Norman. *"And, even more re-markably, I have discovered an essential oil blend, Air BLISS, which works when placed on the points! It is significantly helpful in relieving depression and anxiety and early reports show improvement in autism and Asperger's syndrome."*

Visit the website (located in the **Valuable Resources** section at the back of the book). I use it myself whenever I feel stressed and hassled, so it has very widespread potential.

The Last Word On Oxytocin?

Let's end this look at the "love hormone" with one of the most beautiful assemblage of words on the subject of love I have ever encountered. The quote is by New York preacher Emmet Fox, from his book *Sermon On The Mount*. I enjoy reading and quoting it often:

There is no difficulty that enough love will not conquer;
No disease that enough love will not heal;
No door that enough love will not open;
No gulf that enough love will not bridge;
No wall that enough love will not throw down;
No sin that enough love will not redeem....
It makes no difference how deeply seated may be the trouble;
How hopeless the outlook;
How muddled the tangle;
How great the mistake....
A sufficient realization of love will dissolve it all

It is, in every sense, the ultimate psychiatric prescription, which renders all else of secondary consequence.

Pregnenolone

This has been called the happiness hormone, because of its effect in raising overall mood. Interestingly, pregnenolone levels in the healthy brain are some 10 times greater than DHEA levels (see next).

Nicknamed "the mother hormone," pregnenolone is a vital building block in the making of other hormones, such as dehydroepiandrosterone (DHEA), testosterone, progesterone, estrogen, and cortisol.

Pregnenolone has been found to be 100 times more effective for memory enhancement than any other steroids or steroid-precursors in animal laboratory tests. Based upon this, pregnenolone appears to be the most potent memory enhancer of all.

Scientists have been studying the impact of hormones on learning and memory for many years. Various studies have found that pregnenolone significantly enhances motivation, the ability to acquire knowledge, and long-term memory. A research group of industrial psychologists conducted studies in the 1940's to test pregnenolone on students and workers for the ability to enhance job performance. They found that the students/workers had a markedly improved ability to learn and remember difficult tasks.

In medical studies it has been demonstrated to enhance performance on the job and dramatically increase mental alertness while helping to relieve both stress and fatigue simultaneously.

What seems to be happening is that pregnenolone stimulates the NMDA (N-methyl-D-aspartate) channels (or receptors), without the excitotoxin effect that characterizes too much glutamate.

We know that, while glutamate is critical for normal learning, too much excitation by glutamate over time can damage neurons and is thought to be one of the underlying factors in neurodegenerative disorders such as Alzheimer's disease.[304]

When all is working properly, pregnenolone seems to play a pivotal role both in laying down memories in the first place, and then preventing their loss by directly protecting the nerve networks that store them! This exciting new and controversial science is a crucial element in a text on holistic psychiatry.

But as I said, it doesn't just make people sharper, it makes them happier too. It was, in a very real sense, a wonder hormone. So guess what happened?

Research on pregnenolone halted in the 1950's when Merck brought out its synthetic cortisone, which they billed as an immediate cure-all. Soon after cortisone and cortisol came into use, the synthetic steroid hormone dexamethasone was introduced, followed by prednisone. Remember, these steroids are hundreds of times more powerful than pregnenolone (or DHEA for that matter). Big Pharma wanted pregnenolone buried, because it cannot be patented and therefore had no financial advantage.

Patients suffering from depression have been found to have pregnenolone levels less than half those found in non-depressed persons. These decreased levels of pregnenolone have been found in both unipolar and bipolar depression (the manic-depressive disorder).

Overall, pregnenolone seems to have a pleasant stimulatory effect on the brain, without overstimulation.

Suggested dose: 50 mg daily. Discontinue this powerful substance if you have any kind of a negative response, such as rapid heartbeat, anxiety or insomnia. You may be more comfortable using it only on an "as needed" basis, for example, when you are stressed, fatigued, depressed.

DHEA

This is not a book about hormones, though hormones are powerful modulators of mental function, as I have been at pains to demonstrate. Perhaps one other hormone is worthy of space in this book of fecund and startling ideas! DHEA.

It is probably the most abundant steroidal hormone substance in the body. Levels are especially high in the brain. DHEA is the biochemical precursor to a number of other hormones, notably estrogen, progesterone and testosterone, which may explain in part why it benefits depressed patients.

In a randomized, placebo-controlled, double-blind study that lasted for six years, researchers tested 90 mg DHEA daily for 3 weeks and 450 mg/d for 3 weeks as a monotherapy for both mild and severe depression. They found that DHEA therapy resulted in a significant improvement in symptoms, compared with placebo.[305]

DHEA has been shown to effectively lower evening cortisol levels and improve mood, by a double-blind placebo-controlled trial. So it is an important influence on the HPA axis.[306]

Dose: 10-50 mg per day to start (men), 10-30 mg per day to start (women); and if possible to assess effect via repeat blood test. Note that DHEA often causes greasy facial skin in women and dosage may need to be reduced accordingly.

Hormone Labs

All that I have written in this section would be useless without some means of measuring levels of different hormones. How can we do that?

There are three basic measurements: blood, urine and saliva testing.

Most critical hormones are easily measured by a simple saliva test from laboratories such as Diagnos-techs. It is important to measure all hormones and when supplementing, even with so-called bio-identical hormones, to bear in mind that they all inter- react with each other. The aim is to restore hormone levels to those of a healthy young adult.

There's a helpful lab link in the **Valuable Resources** section in the back of the book.

5.12 Hyperventilation

The subject of hyperventilation is of considerable importance to knowledgeable holistic doctors. In the 1980s, it was talked about a lot. Today it is less widely known and appreciated, which means it has become a "missing" or forgotten diagnosis.

Along with many sections in this remarkable book, I urge that conscientious practitioners study and learn more about it. In doing so, you will uncover more and more cases of it and, as a result, be able to help many people who would otherwise baffle those who practice the healing arts!

The point of introducing it to this text is that hyperventilation may also be a source of obscure and unusual psychiatric complaints.

What Is Hyperventilation?

The word means overbreathing: that is, breathing in excess of physiological re-quirements.

In the normal course of events air is drawn into the lungs. Oxygen is removed into the blood and, at the same time, carbon dioxide is given off as a waste product in the exhaled breath. We call this process respiration or, more correctly, external respiration.

The uptake of oxygen need not concern us here. The oxygen is tightly bound to hemoglobin (the red blood pigment) and remains at a fairly constant level provided the lungs are working normally. Carbon dioxide, on the other hand, dissolves directly into the plasma. A simple chemical reaction takes place, which may be represented by the equation:

$$CO_2 \quad + \quad H_2O \quad = \quad H_2CO_3$$

$$\text{Carbon dioxide} \quad + \quad \text{water} \quad = \quad \text{carbonic acid}$$

Carbonic acid dissociates into H^+ ions and HCO_3^- (bicarbonate) ions and this affects the acidity of the blood (the blood's pH, for those with scientific knowledge).

Both the kidneys and the lungs control bicarbonate levels, the kidneys by selective excretion and the lungs by blowing off extra carbon dioxide. There are chemicals called *buffers* present in the blood that are able, to a certain extent, to 'mop up' excess acidic and alkaline ions, but there is a limit to how much they can regulate the body's acid-alkali equilibrium.

You will now readily see that over-breathing will lower the carbon dioxide levels excessively, which will deplete blood bicarbonate and will in turn upset the body's acid-base equilibrium enough to cause symptoms in susceptible patients.

Those who perpetuate the acid-alkali foods and water myth need to get a grasp of the crucial physiology. The body does not like pH values outside a very narrow range and the kidneys will restore the imbalance created by any substance that causes a major departure from normal values, whether acid foods or "alkaline water", etc.

Of course, we are talking about un-conscious involuntary overbreathing now, not something indulged in temporarily to order to play the bagpipes or some similar act. It is a bad habit that has become elevated to the status of a disease process.

Symptoms

The brain is susceptible even to tiny drops in carbon dioxide levels. It is not surprising, therefore, that a number of subjective symptoms can be produced, including major psychological disorders, as well as objective responses. The table below lists the common symptoms that must lead to the consideration of hyperventilation as a diagnosis.

For each category score 1 point for each symptom even if only one symptom within the category applies to you. Do not increase your score if you suffer from more than one of the symptoms in a category.

Mental States

- Sensation of floating (feeling 'spaced out', 'unreal' or 'distant')
- Difficulty with memory
- Difficulty concentrating
- Mental confusion ('racing thoughts')
- Tension
- Anxiety
- Panic attacks
- Fear of crowds, shops, queues, stuffy places, artificial lights, lifts, trains, underground trains, etc. Feel physically ill, tight-chested, prone to collapse when faced by the above situation

- Temporary delusion
- Seeing things that are not there (hallucination)
- Quick temper
- Quick/easy tears
- Coma, stupor or convulsions-if hyperventilation is severe

Sleep

- Vivid/frightening dreams
- Waking in morning feeling 'drugged'/headachy/fatigued/lethargic/with aching muscles
- Waking in the night choking/breathless/panicky
- Waking repeatedly soon after going to sleep
- Sleep apnea

Eyes

- Blurred or double vision
- Distortion of perspective ('the room tilts away')
- Sensitivity to bright lights

Ears

- Vertigo (dizziness)
- Tinnitus (ringing/buzzing in ears) which varies from hour to hour
- Sounds seem distant or unusually loud
- Sensitivity to loud noises

Nervous System

- Lack of co-ordination/bumping into things/clumsiness 'Tension headache/thick head/hangover-like state for large part of many days
- Headache during 'attacks'/caused by exercise
- Migraine attacks
- Numbness/'deadness'/tingling in extremities, limbs, lips, face, tongue
- Feeling 'electric' – but not the electric shock one can get by making contact with an object
- Unpleasant sensations in skin/just below surface of the skin

- Cold/burning/aching/ 'creeping' feeling, commonly in the thighs/buttocks/ feet but maybe other parts of body

Autonomic Nervous System

- Emotional sweating/sweaty palms/armpits
- Easily blushing or going very pale
- Cold hands/feet (when rest of body is warm)
- Raynaud's disease

Respiratory System

- Unreasonable breathlessness/air hunger/feeling of restricted chest
- 'I do exercises to improve my breathing'
- 'I do not breathe enough/breathe deeply enough'
- 'Sometimes I stop breathing/have to remember to breath'
- Frequent sighs/yawns
- Cigarette smoke provokes other symptoms listed on this chart
- Singing voice becomes off key/tuneless/husky
- Speaking/singing loudly provokes symptoms listed on this chart
- Speaking voice goes husky/feels strained
- Throat dry/'rough'/sore
- Asthma attacks now/in the past

Heart

- Rapid, slow or irregular heartbeat
- Blood-pressure changes easily
- Dull pain/ache in center of chest
- Angina/ coronary pain, but medical investigations prove negative
- Profound/ frequent fainting spells

Muscles

- Weakness/fatigue
- Exercise has to stop due to sudden unreasonable exhaustion
- Sudden loss of strength

- Hard exercise improves symptoms
- Muscles feel stiff or 'in spasm'
- Muscles ache (feeling 'beaten up' or as if 'been in a fight')
- Tense jaw muscles (may cause headache)
- Muscle tremors
- Muscle twitching
- Tightness around eyes/mouth

Throat

- Globus (sensation of pressure or lump in throat or at root of neck)
- Sensation of restricted throat
- Difficulty swallowing

Gastrointestinal System

- Excessive belching, swallowing air
- Discomfort/tension/sinking feeling/distress just below tip of breast-bone
- Distended stomach
- During attacks of other symptoms: urgent/uncontrolled bowel movement

Urinary Tract

- Frequent need to pass urine
- Discomfort at neck of bladder
- Severe urge to pass urine/incontinence, when accompanied by any of the other symptoms in this table

Reproductive System

- Orgasm during cult activities ('unusual' sexual practices)
- Premature ejaculation
- Sex provoking prolonged exhaustion
- Sex improving all symptoms for a few hours

Interpretation

Less than 15: Unlikely to be overbreathing;
15-20: Symptoms may be caused by hyperventilation.

Tests

There are no laboratory tests to detect hyperventilation, though patients subject to it may have chronically low serum phosphorus and this is well worth checking. The only real way to diagnose it for certain is for the patient deliberately to overbreathe by way of a test.

This should be done with the patient lying down and preferably accompanied by someone who understands his or her condition. The overbreathing needs to be kept up for several minutes; the patient should be quite tired as a result. If the familiar group of symptoms appear, the diagnosis is obvious.

Treatment

Drug treatment is quite inappropriate.

The real answer lies in retraining the patient to breathe correctly. Help from an expert physiotherapist is invaluable but beware: many physiotherapists make the problem worse by teaching the patient how to breathe deeply and efficiently, which is fine for someone with asthma but the exact opposite of that is wanted here.

During severe panic attacks the old trick of breathing into a paper bag is as valid as ever. Or, if the patient can be reasoned with, get him or her to breathe out, count for six long seconds then breathe in slowly, out again, hold for six more seconds, and so on. It should be possible to slow the respiration down to about ten breaths per minute or less.

The Buteyko Method

This reminds me of the Buteyko method, named for Russian Dr Konstantin Buteyko, which is excellent for correcting hyperventilation. It was originally developed as a treatment for asthma and other obstructive airways disease.

The patient *and doctor* get this wrong and believe the way to compensate for a tight chest or wheezing attack is to force deep breathing. It doesn't work. In fact the depletion in carbon dioxide levels and the resulting plasma acidity lowers the stimulus to breathe and makes things worse.

Buteyko found that the correct thing to do is *the exact opposite*: to reduce breath intake, to take smaller and more frequent inhalations and exhalations.

It takes practice to restore a normal breathing pattern but proponents point to the many benefits of the Buteyko method, which far exceed merely helping asthma cases.

Chronic hyperventilation is less visible but a major indicator of chronic stress. It has a long-term effect on general health, because less oxygen is delivered to your tissues (Bohr effect). This can cause pain, inflammation, or other malfunctions throughout the body. For example, less oxygen reaching your brain can cause you to make mistakes, or to have headaches, confusion, panic, or difficulty remembering things. When the body is threatened by the lack of oxygen, stress levels rise, further increasing the heart rate, sweating and other normal responses to stress. This creates a vicious circle.

Test Your Control Pause

Buteyko practitioners estimate the degree of chronic hyperventilation by what is called the control pause (CP).

Here's how to do the test:

Sit down and adopt a reasonably straight posture;

Take a small breath in and let a small breath out (the breath should not be noticeable);

Hold your nose on the exhalation. Your lungs should be mostly empty but not completely devoid of air. Holding your nose is necessary to prevent air entering into the airways;

Count how many seconds you can comfortably hold your breath before you need to take a breath in. *Please note that this is not a test of how long you can hold your breath using willpower, but simply until you feel the first physical urges to breathe.*

Release your nose and breathe in through it;

Continue to breathe normally through your nose. Your first intake of breath after the Control Pause should be no greater than your breath prior to taking measurement. If you need to take a much bigger breath after measuring the Control Pause, that fact alone is a sign that you have held your breath for too long.

The level of carbon dioxide in the body determines the length of time the breath can be held; a higher level of carbon dioxide corresponds to a longer breath hold. Increasing levels of carbon dioxide in the blood helps to reduce the symptoms of over-breathing and lower breathing volume to a normal level.

The closer your CP is to 40 seconds, the better the match between breathing volume and metabolic requirements, and the greater the oxygenation of the body. In hyperventilation cases, the CP is low (less than 20 seconds). It is common for people in the Western world to have a Control Pause of between 5 and 15 seconds, indicating a prevalence of habitual over-breathing.

By practising the Buteyko Method using books, DVDs, or with the tutelage of a Buteyko practitioner, you should be able to increase your CP until you have reduced or completely eradicated the symptoms associated with chronic hyperventilation.

5.13 Heavy Metal Poisoning

At first the idea of toxic metals, like mercury, cadmium and lead causing cognitive impairment (never mind psychosis) might seem strange. But a moment's reflection will show you that you already know part of the story. Even if you have never read Lewis Carroll's classic children's tale *Alice in Wonderland*, you will certainly have come across the Mad Hatter character. It's a case of mercury poisoning and was well-known in Carroll's day.

The phrase "mad as a hatter" was in use 30 years prior to the publication of Carroll's novel, and is associated with industrial felt hat workers in 19th-century England. Hatters cured animal fur to make felt with a salt called mercuric nitrate. Over the years of occupational exposure, they commonly developed mercury poisoning, which included such symptoms as tremors, irritability, and mental instability.

During his relatively long lifetime, Sir Isaac Newton (1642-1727), perhaps the greatest scientist that ever lived, suffered two serious bouts of uncharacteristically erratic behavior (to put it politely). Some historians now believe he suffered from a mild form of mercury poisoning. They point out that Newton was conducting experiments with mercury at the time of both occurrences.

Today we have Minamata disease, named for the Japanese port where fish contaminated with mercury from a nearby industrial plant were brought ashore and sold. The local population had many cases of poisoning with methyl mercury, the deadliest form. Victims suffered from very high fever, convulsions, psychosis, tremors, loss of consciousness, coma, and finally death.[307]

Local bird life as well as domesticated animals also perished. In all, 900 people died and 2,265 Minamata residents have been certified as having directly suffered from mercury poisoning in the years since 1956.

A similar pollution crisis occurred in Sweden when farmers used methyl mercury as a crop dusting and fed treated seeds to animals. Swedish food produce became heavily contaminated. The government responded quickly and, to this day, Sweden leads the world in concern about the issues surrounding mercury.

The tuna fishing industry was especially hard hit with several of these scares in the 1960s. Even today, with strict guidelines as to allowed mercury levels in food, confidence hasn't fully returned. The limit set by the American Food and Drug Administration is 0.5 parts per million: the truth is, we just don't know what safe levels are.

Elemental mercury occurs naturally and is present in the earth's crust. Exposure to mercury affects the skin, kidney, eye, and nervous system, and the respiratory system if inhaled. Telltale signs of mercury poisoning are emotional instability, cognitive and memory loss, shyness, speech problems, and the characteristic tremors.[308]

Mercury is one of the most toxic substances known to humanity, particularly when combined with other atoms and molecules, such as the chloride or methyl forms. These have far greater biological penetration. Brain tissue is especially at risk.

The United States Public Health Service banned use of mercury in the felt industry in 1941, not so much for health risks but because mercury fulminate was needed for World War II detonators.[309]

So, with these facts under our belt, we can investigate the possible role of heavy metal poisoning in our holistic journey towards mental wholeness.

Let's finish up the mercury story...

Matter Hatter disease is known officially as erethism. The most obvious cause is occupational exposure (eg. dentists), now strictly controlled. But other sources include contaminated seafood (not just from Minamata Bay), dental amalgam, vaccines containing thiomersol salt (which the Americans insists on calling thimerosal), in some thermometers, barometers, switches, thermostats, and electrical switches.

Moreover, according to the US National Research Council, combustion processes, especially coal-fired power plants, are major sources of mercury contamination in the environment. The U.S. Environmental Protection Agency (EPA) is considering regulating mercury emissions from those plants.

In the first half of the 20th century, we saw infants with "pink disease" (infantile acrodynia). It was caused by exposure to teething powders, which contained elemental mercury, would you believe! Sure, 20/20 hindsight and all that. But that's no excuse: mercury has been known since the dawn of history as extremely poisonous. Gram for gram, it's one of the most toxic substances we pull out of the earth.

The problem with mercury is that if humans are exposed to any of the forms of mercury, depending on the amount (dose), route (ingestion, skin contact, inhalation), duration (time) of exposure, it can be toxic.

People with erethism experience behavioral changes such as irritability, low self-confidence, depression, apathy and shyness. There may be delerium, personality changes and memory loss can occur as a result They find it difficult to interact socially with others (social phobia). All this puts the patient at risk of being diagnosed as a psychiatric case and the true cause never found, because it is not searched for.

Although most of the effects of erethism are neurological, some physical problems arise as well, including a decrease in physical strength, "headaches, general pain, and tremors after exposure to metallic mercury, as well as irregular heartbeat. It has been documented that "the tremor in the hands can be so severe that the victim is unable to hold a glass of water without spilling its contents."

You can read more about this fascinating story by accessing the link in the Valuable Resources section in the back of the book.

Threefold Problem

There are really three issues where mercury is concerned. The first is the tendency of mercury to concentrate electrical fields. This is an ordinary biophysical effect and explains why people with too many dental fillings cannot work in areas where large field currents are developed.

The second is hypersensitivity. This is really more or less an allergic reaction to mercury and various estimates place this as applying to between 1 and 15 percent of the population. Anyone in prolonged contact with mercury tends to develop such a sensitivity; thus dental students show a sharp increase in the percentage of positive patch tests for mercury sensitivity as they progress through their studies.

In passing, it should be noted that similar sensitivities can occur with other metals, notably nickel, chromium, cobalt and gold, though these are rare.

The third and most important effect has been talked about already: that is toxicity. We inhale mercury vapor from our dental amalgam and swallow its compounds. This release of mercury is increased by chewing hot or salty foods.

Unfortunately, mercury from the teeth has an especially great affinity for brain tissue but it also lodges in other body organs. It can have a disastrous effect on the nervous and immune systems.

What To Do?

Right, let's talk about diagnosis and solutions. What is written in this next section can provide a good framework in which to investigate any other source of toxic metal poisoning (lead, aluminium, etc.)

Rule one: anyone with mental, neurological or psychological problems who is even under suspicion of exposure to mercury (occupational, dietary or dental amalgams, etc.) should be investigated as a matter of course.

A hair mineral analysis may be a helpful place to start. Hair can be a good indicator of exposure because it grows slowly and incorporates toxic metals into its structure over a long period of time, and therefore may be a better measure of actual tissue levels. It has its weaknesses but certainly, if levels are raised in the hair, providing the cause is not an external contaminant such as hair dye, that implies toxic overload. Unfortunately, negative or low levels found in hair does not rule out mercury poisoning.

Instead, I would prefer a meaningful mercury challenge test. The theory in the past was that, if we challenge the body with a chelation agent such as DMPS (see below), if mercury appears in subsequent urine samples, we have "proved" that the body has a raised burden of mercury.

I prefer to accept the critique of Christopher W. Shade PhD of Quicksilver Scientific, that there are several flaws with this traditional interpretation. The truth is, the measurement of mercury in the body and extrapolation to body burden and toxic conditions is a very complicated field, requiring acute clinical discernment, including integration of patient history, current exposures, symptomology, and effect of co-morbidities. The extreme simplification of the challenge test is no longer serving the evolution of the field of clinical metals toxicology, and it is now time for the adoption of better tools.

Moreover, recently, challenge tests have come under fire from federal authorities as a diagnostic tool.

Shade points to 3 main flaws, which cannot be ignored by anyone aspiring to be fully scientific:

1. The supposition that the mercury pool identified by the challenge is the whole body burden. Even worse: the supposition that it uniquely reflects the neurological burden.

2. There is no widely-accepted reference range to compare the challenged test results to. This is probably the biggest problem from a regulatory standpoint since there is such obvious potential for over-treatment

3. The lack of standardization of the challenge procedure, including agreed upon conditions.

Christopher W. Shade has an excellent document you can download for more information. You'll find the link in the **Valuable Resources** section in the back of the book.

A number of practitioners refuse to accept Shade's criticisms of the conventional challenge test and go on doing what they have always done.

But Quicksilver Scientific now offers a "Mercury Tri-Test". The tri- comes from the three body compartments tested: blood, hair and urine. It effects to measure two separate forms of mercury: methyl mercury and inorganic mercury. The point is that QS claims their instruments are sensitive enough to measure the presence of mercury in each of these compartments, without needing to do a challenge test.

Removing Mercury

Dental amalgams are a special problem. Safe removal is very difficult. If you undertake this treatment, be sure your dentists knows, understands *and follows* the protocols developed by the International Academy of Oral Medicine and Toxicology (the "good guys" in holistic dentistry).

The dentist must use a rubber dam around the tooth and provide efficient air extraction to prevent the patient swallowing mercury vapor. It is also a good idea for the patient to take charcoal tablets before and after amalgam extraction, to adsorb any stray mercury.

Even better is to run an IV and have high-dose vitamin C in the line, to help with detox.

For sicker patients, it may be a good idea to go on a hypoallergenic diet and take vitamin and mineral supplements through this period, starting a few days before the first visit to the dentist.

It needs to be understood that the alternative replacement materials cannot be expected to be as durable as the mercury amalgam. Patients are advised to go to a dentist who has had a lot of practice with these alternative types of filling.

The Role Of Drugs In Treating Mercury Toxicity

My advice is to ignore claims for seaweed, cilantro, pectin and algae (eg. chlorella). These are too slow and far too hit-and-miss for the seriousness of a psychiatric disorder. Time is of the essence, if the patient is at risk of a brutal drug assault or hospitalization. When mercury is an issue, we need it GONE, as fast as possible.

Two drugs are useful to use to chelate mercury. Research in several countries has shown them to be generally safe and effective, though they must be administered and controlled by competent MDs (I hold a board certificate in chelation from the American Academy for The Advancement of Medicine). The first, meso-dimercapto-succinic acid (DMSA), is taken orally and has been shown effective in removing mercury from all organs, except the kidneys.

The second drug, 2,3, dimercapto 1, propanesulphonic acid (DMPS), is potentially more toxic and has to be administered by intra-muscular injection. DMPS is better at removing elemental mercury, which is the kind chiefly encountered when the toxicity comes from dental amalgam. However, it should not be used where brain toxicity is suspected since it cannot itself be removed but is instead bound into brain tissues, with its mercury load.

DMSA, on the other hand, does not bind to neurological tissue and is the drug of choice in such cases.

Treatment with either drug is made more successful with proper preparation: the patient should go on an oligo-antigenic diet, avoid chemicals and other toxins and follow a supplement detoxification program, as outlined elsewhere in this book.

EDTA chelation is the new established treatment for chelation of certain metals, but not mercury. EDTA stands for ethylene diamine tetraacetic acid and is safe enough to be recognized as a food additive.

Given intravenously, it can pull out heavy metals and get them excreted, via the kidneys. The excitement in recent years has been the so-called TACT trial (Trial to Assess Chelation Therapy), which showed a resounding success, much to the dismay of its critics, who wanted the trial halted (never mind the truth!)

The potential hazard of all forms of chelation is that it may cause redistribution of mercury into organs, including the brain.

There is no space to tackle such an ambitious subject on this book. But you can find plenty of references online, starting with some I've provided in the **Valuable Resources** section at the back.

Lead

OK, moving on. This is another neurological biggie. I think most people know that lead is capable of lowering IQ and impairing cognitive performance, especially in children, who are most at risk.

"Plumbism", the disease, is from *plumbum*, Latin for lead, (which also gave us the word plumber, since these men formerly dealt mainly in lead piping and water channels) has numerous characteristics that medical students have to memorize. I remember lead poisoning as "the dangles with dry colic"! The dangles refers to peripheral nerve paralysis, which causes wrist drop. The dry colic means abdominal pain without diarrhea. It was also known as "potters colic" since lead pottery glazes were used a great deal, before the hazard became clear.

You probably know the theory that the vast Roman empire finally fell apart, because the citizens and leaders were mentally incapacitated by accumulations of lead, caused by their lead baths, plumbing, etc.

Today, routes of exposure to lead include contaminated air, water, soil, food, and consumer products. Lead paints have always been a source too but in the USA and other countries, lead paints are now banned.

Leaded gasoline was also a former hazard. Although the law now excludes such petroleum products, it's naïve not to recognize that roadside dust everywhere continues to contain significant quantities of lead. Just walking the streets could be a lead hazard!

Today, lead levels in bone are probably the number one accurate predictor of death. So be warned.

The Damage

Peripheral nervous system effects (the paralysis) are more prominent in adults. In children, central nervous system effects (brain impairment) are more prominent in children. Lead causes the axons of nerve cells to degenerate and lose their myelin coats (which is what happens in multiple sclerosis).

Lead exposure damages cells in the hippocampus, a part of the brain involved in memory.

Lead can interfere with the release of neurotransmitters, so the reader will readily see the potential for psychiatric symptoms. It also interferes with the release of glutamate, a neurotransmitter important in many functions including learning, by blocking NMDA receptors.

The targeting of NMDA receptors is thought to be one of the main causes for lead's toxicity to neurons. In addition, lead has been found in animal studies to cause programmed cell death (apoptosis) in brain cells.

Dioscorides, a Greek physician who lived in the 1st century AD, wrote that lead makes the mind "give way".

One study I found on PubMed showed young adults with higher blood lead were more likely to suffer a major depression and panic disorder. Exposure to lead at levels generally considered safe could result in adverse mental health outcomes.[310]

Effects of lead on the central nervous system are not typically reversible. While peripheral effects in adults often go away when lead exposure ceases, evidence suggests that most of the effects of lead on a child's central nervous system are irreversible. Children with lead poisoning may thus have adverse health, cognitive, and behavioral effects that follow them into adulthood.

This is bad news, all the way!

Eliminate Lead

Recommended steps by individuals to reduce the blood lead levels of children include increasing their frequency of hand washing and their intake of calcium and iron, discouraging them from putting their hands to their mouths, vacuuming frequently, and eliminating the presence of lead-containing objects such as blinds and jewelry in the house.

In houses with lead pipes or plumbing solder, these can be replaced. Less permanent but cheaper methods include running water in the morning to flush out the most contaminated water, or adjusting the water's chemistry to prevent corrosion of pipes.

Household lead testing kits are commercially available. Swabs wiped over surfaces turn red in the presence of lead.[311]

Other treatments include restoration of iron, calcium, and zinc deficiencies, which are associated with increased lead absorption.

Removal Of Lead Burdens

Chelation is the best and only really effective method of extracting lead from the body. Again, it's not worth bothering with trivial chelators, such as seaweed and pectin. Calcium EDTA intravenously is the treatment of choice. Other agents include dimercaprol (BAL or British Anti-Lewisite), which are injected, and succimer and d-penicillamine, which are administered orally.

Yet again, chelation of toxic heavy metals is only recommended under the care of a boarded or otherwise certified MD specialists in the procedure. This is not for enthusiastic meddlers. I have seen patients put into a wheelchair by erroneous practices. One even came in on a stretcher. Beware!

While chelation treatment of patients with frank symptoms of lead poisoning is plauded by orthodox doctors, treatment of raised blood levels is more controversial. Some doctors have been disciplined for attempting it.

Arsenic

According to Mike Adams' Natural News site, history's largest mass poisoning of a human population has occurred in Bangladesh. Because of it, 35 million people have been exposed to lethal levels of arsenic. Mortality rates are estimated at 13 per 1000, which means that this poisoning has ended as many at 455,000 lives.

It happened simply enough. In the late 1960s and 1970s, UNICEF and the World Bank, concerned that surface water in the area was causing too many cases of fatal diarrhea, funded the drilling of new wells. These deeper wells provided an abundance of fresh water to the booming population of Bangladesh and West Bengal.

Unfortunately, the new wells were heavily contaminated with arsenic.

Groundwater contamination with arsenic is a major public health concern in some countries.

Although the literature is sparse on this topic, studies in China and Bangladesh have shown unequivocally that mental health problems (e.g. depression, PTSD, anxiety) are more common among the people affected by arsenic contamination.

In addition, experiences with animals have pointed out that perinatal arsenic exposure was associated with depressive-like behaviors in the affected mouse offspring.[312]

You should know that in the US there is a heavy load of arsenic poisoning carried to humans via chickens (and to some extent pigs). Roxarsone is the most common arsenic-based additive used in chicken feed, used to promote growth, kill parasites and improve the color of chicken meat. It is normally benign, but under certain conditions that can occur within live chickens or on farm land, the compound converts into more toxic inorganic arsenic.

Even if you don't eat chicken, don't think you are safe: chicken manure is used as fertilizer on vegetable farms and this contains arsenic which then contaminates the vegetables. Arsenic is everywhere.

Aluminium (non-US spelling, note)

Why the Americans call it aluminum is beyond me. They don't say sodum (sodium) or potassum (potassium) so why aluminum? To the rest of the world, it's aluminium and so it remains in this book!

Aluminium is the most widely distributed metal on the planet and it's used in the production of many every-day products. Cook pans and cooking trays are often made from aluminium, soda cans are aluminium, and aluminium foil is found in most kitchens. Aluminium is also in antacids, aspirin, vaccines, and even flour.

In fact it is virtually impossible to avoid significant exposure.

There was strong evidence to implicate aluminium in Alzheimer's disease (AD). Then the fashion turned against this idea. Cookpot manufacturers were quick to exploit the weakness in science and claim that aluminium is safe in their wares. Don't listen!

We already know that the aluminium content of brain tissue in late-onset or sporadic Alzheimer's disease is significantly higher than is found in age-matched controls. So, in-

383

dividuals who develop Alzheimer's disease in their late sixties and older also accumulate more aluminium in their brain tissue than individuals of the same age without the disease. Just remember the old dictum: association does not mean causation.

But latterly, a new study published in the *Journal Of Trace Elements In Medicine and Biology*, in March 2017, has made us come back to the theme. Researchers found "extremely high" levels of aluminium in donated AD brains; in fact "some of the highest values recorded for individual samples of human brain tissue."

The authors concluded as follows: "Aluminium is neurotoxic and the concentrations of aluminium found in these familial AD brains are unlikely to be benign and indeed are highly likely to have contributed to both the onset and the aggressive nature of any ongoing AD in these individuals. These data lend support to the recent conclusion that brain aluminium will contribute towards all forms of AD under certain conditions."[313]

This book wishes to point out that, logically, other mental disturbances could also be precipitated by aluminium exposure. It has to be borne in mind.

Research studies are not conclusive, but suggest that aluminium inhibits cholinergic functioning and may inhibit synaptic uptake of dopamine, norepinephrine and 5-hydroxytryptamine (serotonin). So cognitive skills and mood are bound to be compromised.

Notice that dialysis patients eventually manifest dementia and this is known to be due to the accumulation of aluminium. It is prevented by using only de-ionised water.

Listen Up

You need to grasp the tremendous importance of heavy metals toxic overload. And the direct inflammatory effect on the brain (called encephalitis). I'm shortly going to run out of further space here. So let me finish with an important tabulation of the neurotoxic effects of heavy metals and their psychiatric implications...

According to psychiatrist James S. Brown, Jr., MD, MPH, the neurotoxic (nerve poisoning) heavy metals of greatest notoriety and importance to clinical practice are aluminum, arsenic, lead, manganese, mercury, thallium, and tin. Exposure to all of these metals can cause agitation, poor concentration, personality change, and memory loss.[314]

Additional symptoms include:

- Mood swings: Aluminum, lead, manganese, and mercury
- Depression: Aluminum, lead, mercury, thallium, and tin
- Anxiety: Aluminum, arsenic, lead, manganese, mercury, and thallium
- Irritability: Aluminum, arsenic, mercury, thallium, and tin
- Laughing/Crying: manganese

- Mania: lead, mercury, and tin

- Violence: Aluminum, lead, mercury, thallium, and tin

- Shyness/Social Withdrawal: Mercury

- Bizarre behavior- Aluminum, and arsenic

- Suicidal- Aluminum, arsenic, lead, and mercury

- Homicidal- Aluminum and mercury

- Confusion- Aluminum, lead, thallium, and tin

- Hallucinations- Aluminum, arsenic, lead, manganese, thallium, and tin

- Insomnia- Aluminum, lead, manganese, thallium, and tin

- Developmental delay-Lead, thallium, and tin

Note that Dr. Brown does not include **cadmium**.

The New York University Department of Medicine lists no mental health symptoms associated with cadmium exposure or toxicity. However, because many authors consider cadmium to be associated with heavier metals such as zinc and mercury, it is believed to cause similar symptoms as those associated with heavy metal toxicity, such as:

- Anxiety and irritability

- Difficulty concentrating, or "brain fog"

- Depression

- Fatigue

- Insomnia

- Memory loss or forgetfulness

The chief source of cadmium poisoning is smoking; it's a contaminant of tobacco.

5.14 Stealth Pathogens Including True Lyme Disease

In the 1970s we started speaking about "smoldering viruses"; also sometimes referred to as "slow viruses". This meant sub-clinical virus opportunists that got under the radar of the immune system and couldn't be dislodged.

Instead, they hung on and lingered, often for the entire lifetime of infected individuals, setting up chronic, damaging inflammation throughout the body. Diseases of aging and autoimmunity (see below), such as atherosclerosis, Alzheimer's, multiple sclerosis, rheumatoid arthritis and many other deadly ailments have been linked to chronic stealth infections.

Once again, it was the clinical ecologists and alternative community who first spotted what was going on. We were open to think laterally and outside the box.

We started to talk about "post-viral fatigue syndrome", since the debility would not go away after the acute infectious episode. Fibromyalgia (ME in Europe) is typical of the pattern of symptoms for post-viral syndrome. Attention to allergies and intolerance often aided recovery a great deal. This pointed to a disordered immune response. But in my 1988 book The Allergy Handbook, I began asking "Is it not that we get the viruses because the immune system is poor or incompetent, rather than we get the immune dysfunction because of the virus?"

I started thinking along the lines that environmental toxins debilitate the immune system, which then leads to the stealth virus. I have not yet been proved wrong. We just don't know.

Since those early years, so-called stealth-adapted viruses have been recovered from multiple tissues, including blood, cerebrospinal fluid, urine, throat swabs, breast milk, brain biopsies and tumor samples from patients with various neurological, psychiatric, auto-immune, allergic and cancerous diseases.

Take the Epstein-Barr virus, a large lymphotrophic DNA virus that establishes life-long residency in the infected host and is associated with a number of human tumors. I had a serious attack of it ("glandular fever" aka. infectious mononucleosis) when I was 17 years old and went down heavily, with a damaged liver and jaundice. But usually it's not so dramatic. EBV can slip in under the radar and sneakily manipulate the host's DNA and the methylation processes, to escape detection and destruction. The result may be chronic fatigue, depression, and autoimmune disease, including hashimoto's thyroiditis.

EBV also causes an estimated 200,000 cancers across the world every year, including lymphomas, liver cancer, nasopharyngeal cancers, and some stomach cancers. So this is a serious issue. And it is not confined to viruses.

Examples of neurological illnesses which could have this sort of basis include autism, attention deficit and behavioral disorders in children; depression, schizophrenia, amyotrophic lateral sclerosis (Lou Gehrig), multiple sclerosis, chronic fatigue and fibromyalgia in adults; and neurodegenerative illnesses in the elderly, such as Shy-Drager and multiple system atrophy.

By following individual patients over several years, it has been found that there may be lateral transfer, leading to related but diverse illnesses within a family. Even pets may be affected.

The strange bone disorder called Paget's disease is now recognized as a "slow" version of the canine distemper virus. The actual disease emerges decades after the initial infection.

Other examples of the guilty viruses are Coxsackie, cytomegalovirus, enterovirus and herpes viruses, notably human herpes virus 6 (HHV-6).

Other organisms that can become stealth pathogens include molds (section 5.4), myco-plasma, and bacteria, such as *Chalamydia pneumoniae*, Bartonella species and *Borrelia bugdorferii* (true Lyme disease).

It is now known that stealth pathogens can infect almost any organ, but that the brain is especially prone to manifest the effects of even limited localized cellular damage. Toxo-plasmosis, for example (section coming up) is known to erode brain cells, resulting in loss of brain tissue. That will give rise to a whole host of hard-to-diagnose psychiatric complaints.

Numerous studies document that infections, such as pediatric autoimmune neuropsy-chiatric disorders associated with streptococcal infections, syphilis, hepatitis C, and zoo-notic (transmitted from animals) diseases, can cause mental illness. Does this line make sense?[315]

The same syndrome may be caused by different infections in different individuals, and the same infection can cause different syndromes in different individuals. For example, obsessive-compulsive disorder has been caused by infection with Streptococcus, B burg-dorferi, Japanese B encephalitis virus, herpes simplex virus, Borna disease virus, Ep-stein-Barr virus, and Mycoplasma, as well as by the pandemic influenza of 1918.

Robert C Bransfield MD in a 2007 article in *Psychiatric Times*, reports having observed cases caused by Hong Kong influenza and coxsackie virus infection. Of course, many stealth infections have also been shown to cause other psychiatric and somatic symp-toms. Some infections result in residual injury even after the infection itself no longer persists, while other infections may persist in a chronic relapsing and remitting state.[316]

Unfortunately, there are no reliable tests to date and stealth pathogens are notorious for imitating other organisms, so their true nature goes often unidentified.

This makes them especially difficult to even study, never mind eliminate.

Lyme Disease is The New Syphilis

Before the advent of antibiotics, syphilis was one of the most common infections in the Western World, afflicting up to 10% of the adult populations.

In 1927 Julius Wagner-Jauregg was given the first and only Nobel Prize awarded to a psychiatrist. This was for work done in 1917 in which Wagner-Jauregg had exposed three neurosyphilitic patients to malaria drawn from the blood of a wounded soldier. The re-sulting high fever killed the syphilis bacterium, leading to their recovery! Given that there were few cures for anything in 1917, Wagner-Jauregg's achievement was a milestone in psychiatric and medical science. There was now a reliable, albeit risky, cure for neu-rosyphilis.

When I went to med school there was a saying: "To know syphilis is to know medicine," meaning that the bacterial spirochete responsible for syphilis—a twirling spiral-shaped organism or "spirochete" called *Treponema pallidum*—was a great imposter and could mimic almost any medical condition in the textbooks, including major psychiatric disorders.

Indeed, if I had attempted this book fifty years ago, syphilis would have had its own chapter as a leading psychiatric and neurological disorder.

Today, that same description of "the great imposter" or mimic would have to go to Lyme disease and other tick-borne comorbidities. The only real difference is that syphilis is a sexually-transmitted disease (STD); Lyme is a tick-borne infection.

Just like syphilis, Lyme disease is caused by a spirochete with a multitude of possible manifestations (*Borrelia bugdorferi*) and, just like syphilis, has 3 identical stages: early with dermatological symptoms, disseminated, and a late stage. The late stages of syphilis were very impressive to the young medical student: general paresis of the insane (GPI), an outrageous grandiose madness; and tabes dorsalis, a progressive paralytic condition, with agonizing pains down the spine and limbs.

Both were sometimes lumped together as neurosyphilis, which may not emerge till up to 20 years after the initial infection, making diagnosis sometimes difficult. For that reason, all medical students were taught that for atypical behavioral and psychiatric symptoms, neurosyphilis should always be considered. I wonder if students are taught that today?

Syphilis is still with us and continues to be a major global health issue. Worldwide, 36.4 million people were estimated to be infected with *Treponema pallidum*, and 10.6 million new cases of syphilis were reported in 2008 alone.[317]

I'd Rather Get Lyme

Lyme is not perhaps so cruel in its later stages but there is no doubt whatever it can cause a great deal of confusion and uncertainty, leading to mis-diagnosis and incorrect treatments.

The trouble is that, unlike *Treponema pallidum*, the causative agent of Lyme disease, *Borrelia burgdorferi*, can be much more difficult to eliminate, diagnostic testing is less reliable, and interactive copathogens are major contributors in the pathophysiology.

B. burgdorferi is a highly adaptable organism, with 6 times as many genes as T. pallidum and 3 times as many plasmids (loose bits of DNA) as any other bacteria, which allow it to evolve rapid genetic adaptations.

It is an arch stealth pathogen that can evade the immune system and pathophysiological defense mechanisms. Knowingly or not, most psychiatrists have at some point been perplexed by patients with late-stage psychiatric manifestations of Lyme borreliosis.[318]

The classic patient is an individual who did not have psychosomatic symptoms in the past and was not hypochondriacal, now complains of an increasing number of somatic, cognitive, neurological, and psychiatric symptoms. Although Lyme disease may be suspected, the laboratory tests available to most clinicians often lack sensitivity and thus are read as negative for Lyme disease. Fibromyalgia, chronic fatigue syndrome, or multiple sclerosis (MS) may be erroneously diagnosed.

The major symptoms encountered include fatigue, multiple cognitive impairments, depression, anxiety, irritability, headaches, and a multitude of neurobiological and somatic symptoms.

In keeping with the rest of this book, it is good to remind readers that most common human diseases, including neuro-psychiatric disorders, are caused by the interaction of environmental insults (overload) and genes (susceptibility), that frequently results in a pathological interaction including inflammation, oxidative stress, mitochondrial dysfunction, and excitotoxicity, which in turn can lead to brain dysfunction.[319]

Diagnosis and Treatment

Obviously successful treatment starts with a correct diagnosis. Getting the right label may be difficult and patients face much hostility and are suspected of malingering, psychosomatic weakness, hypochondria and hysteria (whatever that is!)

But if you or your family member can wade diligently through the obstacles thrown in your path, you should get a result. *B. bugdorferi* and other stealth pathogens, whether classical in presentation, or appearing as a strange and bizarre psychiatric condition, can be vanquished. Antibiotics commonly used for oral treatment include doxycycline, amoxicillin, or cefuroxime axetil. Patients with certain neurological or cardiac forms of illness may require intravenous treatment with drugs such as ceftriaxone or penicillin.[320] Antimicrobials alone are rarely sufficient. It is vital to co-treat all aspects of immunity, overload (section 4.2) and psychological burdens. Any sort of unburdening will benefit the fight against stealth pathogens, be they viral, bacterial or other classes of pathogen (eg. Mycoplasmas).

The CDC says that, though 80-90% of the cases reported are considered resolved with the treatment of antibiotics, 10-20% of patients go on to develop the chronic form, which is a persistent and sometimes devastating illness that can harm any organ of the body, including the brain and the nervous system.

Killing The Resistant Form

The reason for the resistant cases is that the Borrelia spirochete can morph into other hard-to-kill forms, such as spheroplasts (or L-form), round bodies, and biofilms, when conditions are hostile. When conditions are favorable, however, it can shift back to its spirochete form.

However, you need to know one surprise substance that will destroy these harder-to-kill forms and that's stevia. Yes, the natural sweetener *Stevia Rebaudiana* has the potential to terminate late state or chronic Lyme disease!

Research conducted at the Department of Biology and Environmental Science at the University of New Haven in West Haven, Connecticut, concluded that "Stevia whole leaf extract, as an individual agent, was effective against all known morphological forms of B. burgdorferi."

Stevia leaf extract is rich in many phytonutrients that are known antimicrobial agents. For this study, the antimicrobial effect of stevia extracts was examined in comparison to doxycycline, cefoperazone, daptomycin, as well as a combinations of these antibiotics, as they were revealed to be effective against the persistent forms of Lyme disease. Results showed that the stevia leaf extract was effective against all forms of the bacteria in lab tests.

The stevia extract was found to work against even the most antibiotic-resistant of the bacteria, known as the biofilm. The individual antibiotics, on the other hand, actually increased the biofilm rather than eliminating it.

TO FINISH: Some clinicians still believe that there is no late-stage encephalopathy in Lyme disease and maintain the original, highly restrictive definition of the disease from 1975. This is naïve at best and abusive in most contexts. The fact is that many reports have discussed the expanded complexity of the clinical presentations and pathophysiology, and the role of tick-borne and non-tick-borne interactive co-infections.[321]

"Lyme neuropsychiatry" is here to stay.

Think Toxo

Toxoplasmosis is a disease that results from infection with the *Toxoplasma gondii*, a single-celled parasitic organism that can infect most animals and birds. Toxo, as it's called for short, is one of the world's most common parasites. Between 30 and 50 percent of the world's population is believed to be infected with the *Toxoplasma gondii* parasite, but very few people have symptoms because the immune system usually keeps the parasite from causing illness. The obligatory host is the domestic cat.

Infection usually occurs by eating undercooked contaminated meat, exposure from infected cat feces, or mother-to-child transmission during pregnancy.

Most newly infected individuals experience mild flu-like symptoms before it goes into a chronic and dormant phase. But the disease can be fatal in people with weakened immune systems and in fetuses, which can be infected through the mother. This is why women are advised to avoid contact with cat litter boxes while pregnant.

But it is emerging that symptoms can be very subtle and easily mistaken for a psychiatric disorder. Some studies have shown that schizophrenia, depression and anxiety are more common in people with toxoplasmosis, while others have suggested that the disease can influence a person's levels of aggression, extroversion and risk-taking, researchers from the Karolinska Institute in Sweden pointed out.[322]

The weird thing about toxo is that it makes mice behave suicidally weird; they literally seem to seek out death in the jaws of a cat; a "fatal feline attraction" as it's been called. This of course suits the parasite admirably, since cats are the definitive host.

Scientific studies in mice have shown that the wily parasite forces the body, especially the immune system, to secrete the neurotransmitter GABA. Among its roles, GABA inhibits feelings of fear and anxiety. That explains why the mice get reckless.

Unfortunately, disturbances of the GABA system occur in people with depression, schizophrenia, bipolar diseases, anxiety syndrome, obsessive-compulsive disorder, attention-deficit hyperactivity disorder, mood disorders and other mental health conditions.[323]

So think toxo: it could be a prime suspect in any of these disorders.

But there's more. These parasites are dazzlingly clever and sophisticated. Toxo has two genes that allow it to crank up production of the neurotransmitter dopamine in the host brain. Dopamine is a critical signaling molecule involved in fear, pleasure, and attention. Furthermore, dopamine is known to be jacked up in people with schizophrenia—another one of those strange observations about the disease, like its tendency to erode gray matter, that have long puzzled medical researchers. Antipsychotic medicine designed to quell schizophrenic delusions is claimed to block the action of dopamine, which is doubtful. But it might really be thwarting the parasite!

Scientists have shown that adding antipsychotic medicine to a petri dish where T. gondii is happily dividing will stunt the organism's growth. Subsequent tests in which researchers fed the antipsychotic drug to rats newly infected with toxo, showed they didn't develop fatal feline attraction!

Suddenly, attributing human psychological and behavioral changes to toxoplasmosis seemed much more plausible.

Epstein-Barr virus, mumps, rubella, and other infectious agents, have also been linked to schizophrenia—and there are probably more as yet unidentified triggers, including many that have nothing to do with pathogens. But for now, according to psychiatrist E. Fuller Torrey, Toxo remains the strongest environmental factor implicated in the disorder. "If I had to guess," says Torrey, "I'd say 75 percent of cases of schizophrenia are associated with infectious agents, and Toxo would be involved in a significant subset of those."[324]

Toxoplasmosis, arguably, is the sneakiest stealth pathogen of all. We are only just beginning to wake up to it's appalling potential for mind and brain disorders. We have been naïve in believing it to be an animal problem, just because it's primary life-cycle is played out in animals. Toxo has to be kept in mind to have any chance of being diagnosed. A simply antibody test will usually confirm the diagnosis.

Conventional, unimaginative, treatment is with the use of Pyrimethamine (Daraprim). This medication, typically used for malaria, is a folic acid antagonist. It may prevent your body from absorbing the B vitamin folate (folic acid, vitamin B-9), especially when you take high doses over a long period. For that reason, your doctor may recommend taking additional folic acid.

The Toxoplasma gondii parasite needs vitamin B complex to live. Pyrimethamine stops B vitamin uptake and it is usually administered with sulfadiazine, which also prevents the parasites from using it. Of course it stops you getting any too, so the side-effects can be severe, and potentially worsen any psychiatric symptoms!

With this combination of drugs over 80% of people show improvement within two to three weeks. But be warned: it will return if the immune system is not enhanced. So a better idea is a full holistic restoration of general health and immune competence. This will include unburdening, change of diet, nutritional supplements, oxygen enhancement and possibly psychotherapy or hypnotherapy.

Specific treatments can include wormwood (artemisinin), black walnut husks, berberine (a natural plant alkaloid toxic to most parasites, available from powdered Oregon grape), nutmeg (this may turn out to be a number one toxo fighter), thyme oil and Bunium persicum (a relative of the cumin plant).

Homeopathy has much to offer, though you will see it rubbished widely on the Internet (even some holistic practitioners join in the mockery and ignorance).

A 2015 double-blind, controlled, randomized study using animal subjects showed that a homeopathic remedy made from the cysts of the T. gondii parasites effectively reduced the number of cysts inside of the animal's bodies due to toxoplasmosis, which is promising for humans.

Incidentally, the higher dilutions (called potencies) worked better; a fact which drives orthodox scientists wild![325]

5.15 Meteorological Stress

It is beyond doubt that weather conditions act as a stressor to some people, though it may be anything but easy to see why. Most doctors pay scant attention to patients who say they are worse during certain types of weather. Their 'training' and textbooks tell them boldly this cannot be so; therefore the patient is assumed to be a humbug or hypochondriac. This is a great pity.

Weather effects can include a wide range of psychological and somatic changes such as migraine, headache, mood swings, tension, increased accident-proneness and even heart attacks. Tests have shown that sodium is lost from the tissues and glucocorticoid hormones are released from the adrenals to cope with this kind of stress, like any other. There are several well-known examples of atmospheric conditions making people ill. Hot, dry winds seem to be the chief offenders, possibly due to static build up. Positively-charged ions, most inimical to well-being, are generated in the upper atmosphere by the sun's radiation. They tend to reside there but can be brought down by certain freak pressure combinations, causing downwinds with devastating effects.

Some of these winds affect mood and temperament and have even been said to drive people crazy. Examples include the *sharav* of Israel, the *sirocco* of southern Europe and the North African *khamsin*.

Northern Europe and North America do not suffer such climatic extremes. Nevertheless, minor disturbances occur from positive ions coming down to fill low-pressure areas. This probably accounts for the widespread tendency for people to find overcast days 'heavy' and 'oppressive'.

It is common knowledge among homoeopaths – who take careful case histories – that some people are adversely affected by the lead-up to thunder storms. Once again, static build-up is the key. Electrical fields before a storm can reach up to 50,000 V/m. volts per metre.

Sometimes the cause isn't quite as obvious as it looks. Some patients experience unpleasant symptoms prior to the onset of cloudy and rainy weather. This may give an important clue to mold sensitivity (section 5.4). Molds spore in advance of the damp conditions and patients may begin to react at this time. Those who claim they can tell when it will rain because their nose twitches may be speaking from experience based in scientific fact, not folk nonsense.

SPACE WEATHER The Forecast!

It's hotting up and likely to get worse is the forecast! Well, that's said as a joke. But it is true that scientific interest in the Sun as a health hazard is hotting up.

In my 1988 book *The Allergy Handbook* I devoted a whole chapter to the fact that we are living in an intense electro-magnetic environment. In scale, it makes the levels of cell phone radiation we worry about so much seem like a wet firecracker to a hydrogen bomb. There is a plasma layer up there in the sky that is hotted up to many millions of volts. Solar storms intensify this plasma layer. We are, in effect living in the center of an active dynamo: as the Earth turns, its massive iron core rotates in this intense electromagnetic field.

It's a wonder we are not fried in mere seconds. Indeed, we would be, except for certain in-built protections, like the ozone layer and the Van Allen belts, which shield us from the most violent solar storms. But once in a while, even the protective layers fail and when the Sun gets pissy and spits out (a so-called coronal mass ejection or CME), it can literally fry electrical equipment here at the surface.

In 1859 the Earth at night lit up like a Christmas tree, and people ran out on to the sidewalk to watch the sky glow. Some individuals were so confused they got dressed and set off for work, thinking it was morning! The "Carrington Event," as it was known, came after the sun unleashed a large coronal mass ejection, a burst of charged plasma aimed directly at the Earth. When the particles hit our magnetosphere, they triggered an especially fierce geomagnetic storm that lit up the sky and frazzled communication wires around the world. Telegraphs in Philadelphia were spitting out "fantastical and unreadable messages," one paper reported, with some systems unusable for hours.

Does It Affect Humans?

You might think this is an obvious question, but it's been a long time in coming, the recognition that all this energy activity might just have some effect on human life! Scientists scoffed at the notion and lumped such an idea along with astrology as nonsense. Indeed, many still do.

However Russian scientist Alexander Chizhevsky suggested in 1915 that solar storms directly cause conflict, wars and even death among humans on Earth. His work was continued by Professor Raymond Wheeler of the University of Kansas. In the 1930's Wheeler began a lifetime study that analyzed world climate and cultural activities back to the dawn of recorded civilization. He presented his research in his book, *Climate: The Key To Understanding Business Cycles.*

There is no doubt according to Wheeler that weather does affect us.

Scientific Studies

Pretending there is nothing happening is an untenable position today. We now have many studies showing that human health is markedly impacted by celestial events.

The first real study, which startled the world, was published in 1961; in it, researchers had found a clear link between a rise in mental hospital admissions and geo-Solar magnetic activity.[326] This was no fluke and was repeated again in 1994, when R.W. Kay published a study in the *British Journal of Psychiatry*, linking hospital admissions due to depression with days of geomagnetic activity. The researcher found a "36.2% increase in male hospital admissions with a diagnosis of depressed phase, manic-depressive illness in the second week following such storms compared with geomagnetically quiet control periods."[327]

So the effect of the Sun's activity on mental health is beyond question. Only the ignorant dodos would deny it.

Heliobiology

They are now calling it "heliobiology", from *helios*, the Greek for Sun. Obvious effects include mental status (mood), heart attacks, strokes and migraines.

In a 2012 study, electrocardiograms of functionally healthy persons, who were digitally registered at the Laboratory of Heliobiology located in the Medical Centre INAM (Baku, Azerbaijan), were studied in relation to different levels of cosmic ray activity and geomagnetic field disturbances.

In total, 1,673 daily digital data of heart rate values and time series of beat-to-beat heart rate intervals were registered for the time period July 15, 2006–March 31, 2008, which includes the period of December 2006, when intense cosmic ray events and strong geomagnetic disturbances occurred.

Results revealed that heart rate increased in proportion to the rise of geomagnetic activity but that large cosmic ray intensity decreases were also a trigger factor, to which the heart responds. Moreover, heart rate increased on the days before, during and after geomagnetic storms with high intensities and on the days preceding, and following cosmic ray intensity decreases.[328]Heart Affected

At least three studies correlate a strong link between the occurrence of geomagnetic storms and heart attacks (myocardial infarctions). It appears that strong magnetic pulses from geomagnetic storms interfere with the electric impulses that stimulate the heart muscle to contract.

According to these studies, the number of hospitalizations due to heart attacks peak during storm activities. In one study, the number more than doubled, and in another study, the number of fatal heart attacks increased by 70%.

Researchers also noticed a very significant rise in hospital admissions for strokes, correlated with Solar activity (130% rise). So whatever way you look at it, solar activity creates biological stress down here on Earth and changes of mood and behaviors, sometimes very dramatic, are a common observation in stressed patients.[329] [330]

Headaches

Headaches and migraines also rise significantly when there is a Solar "storm" blowing. That fits very well with the known effects down here of a high concentration of positively charged particles, blown in by winds such as the Santa Ana winds (Los Angeles), The Khamsin (Middle East), The Mistral (France) and the Chinook (North American prairies).

People sometimes go completely crazy; headache and feeling lousy is commonplace.

Researchers studied the relationship between the migraine triggers of 40 patients and meteorological elements such as humidity, temperature and geomagnetic activity. They recorded the meteorological data and frequency changes of geomagnetic activity and compared them with the onset and severity of the migraine attacks.

The researchers concluded: "Our results indicate a significant correlation between geomagnetic activity and migraine attack frequency."[331]

Studies of traffic accidents in Germany and in Russia show increases of up to four times the normal level, on the days after a solar flare.[332]

How Could We NOT Be Affected?

Climate change is an emerging challenge to the mental health of all of humanity. Several studies, in recent times, have brought to light the adverse public mental health outcomes of extreme weather events for the suffering communities.

With the rising global temperatures, which is a climate related phenomenon, people with mental illness are at increased risk of heat-related deaths. When heat waves happen, the populations may suffer heat strokes which may lead to delirium and neuropsychiatric syndromes with symptoms such as altered consciousness, agitation, restlessness, unconsciousness, and even death, as happened in the 2003 heat wave, when Europe was hotter than at any time since at least 1540. Peer-reviewed analysis places the death toll at more than 70,000.[333]

Moreover, it has been observed that persons with mental illness have greater vulnerability to a heat stroke, is this is of grave concern to the text you are reading.

Some researches have also suggested that there is a causal relationship between heat and violence and that rising global temperatures may be followed by an increase in incidents of violent aggression, as may be seen in increasing rates of assault, rape, robbery, burglary, and larceny, due to more people getting outside their homes as a result of higher temperatures.

Even domestic violence has been found to increase due to natural disasters resulting from frustration and anger related to these unexpected events.

This is not such a crazy idea; it may be due to the fact that more stress hormones are released into the blood due to excessive exposure to heat.

Suicides are up.

"There's every reason to expect that climate change might increase people's tendencies to be more aggressive towards each other, and that might have impacts on mental health" said one Spanish paper.[334] I could go on for many pages with this theme. You can read a well-informed and scholarly article about the health effects of climate change at the Hindawi website (link in the **Valuable Resources** section in the back of the book).[335]

The important point for this text is that you fully grasp that climate conditions can be a mental health factor and you look into it, for yourself or for any member of the family.

It's quite crazy for psychiatrists to put a patient on an antidepressant or antipsychotic drug, if the real problem is sun spots!

I leave it with you.

5.16 Nutritional Supplements for Mind and Brain

By the time the reader has reached this section, he or she should be in no doubt that nutritional deficiencies are a risk that mental patients cannot afford to chance. Moreover, nutritional deficiencies are very common in the population at large. Numerous studies have shown that psychiatric patients are often below even average in the nutrient content of their blood and tissues.

So, how do we make sense out of the incredibly complex needs and interactions of the body's many organs and pathways?

The short answer it that it isn't possible. The best we can hope for is to take a broad view and hope that by producing a substantial suite of supplements, that the patient's own body is able to make the necessary corrections and repairs.

The point is that nature cannot build or repair tissues without adequate healthy building blocks. If the nutrition is not there, the body simply cannot help to correct itself.

There is no question that to get the best of nutrients, you need to eat a quality healthy wholefood diet (having due regard for food allergies and intolerances, naturally).

But in our modern world, just taking food as the sole source of nutrients is not enough. The world we live in demands more.

Nutrition Science Mainly A Fraud

The present science of nutrition is a fraud and needs ousting in place of something with more wisdom and workability.

Recommended Daily Allowance (RDAs) are described as the average daily level of intake sufficient to meet the nutrient requirements of nearly all (97%-98%) healthy people. But these levels were set over 50 years ago, by ignorant scientists who knew next to nothing about the importance of nutrition in building health. They knew that you needed about 1 to 1.5 mg a day of vitamin B1 to avoid getting *beri beri*. So that's it! They set 1.5 mg as the required daily level. BUT THAT HAS NOTHING TO DO WITH OPTIMUM HEALTH. Avoiding *beri beri* is a far cry from being in tip top condition.

Do you suppose that being able to walk only 3 paces a day is the same level of health as a fit athlete who runs several miles a day? Of course not. But these dodos supposed that what was enough to stop you dying was the same as keeping you in optimum health.

There are some fatal problems with this stupid estimation of requirements.

1. It ignores the fact that we are all biologically different (remember the bell curve from earlier: some need a little, some need a great deal and then there is "average"). No two people have the same requirements in respect of nutrients.

2. What is swallowed may bear little or no relation to what is absorbed. All through this text you will hear that malabsorption, leaky gut, dysbiosis and intestinal inflammation blocks the efficient performance of the digestive system.

3. Requirements change from time to time, even in the same individual. A viral infection, for example, will bump up the requirements for vitamin C by up to a hundred-fold; drinking more alcohol than usual will deplete vitamin B levels, requiring extra intake to compensate.

4. We eat food supplied by a crooked agribusiness. They are interested only in profits and do nothing to preserve the nutritional worth of their products. Indeed, they will *always* sacrifice quality in favor of profits.

5. Finally and most importantly we live in a very different world to the days when these silly RDA standards were first published. We are under such a massive toxic overload that our body defense systems are strained to the limit in trying to cope. Our bodies need extra help! Take glutathione: every toxic molecule removed from the body requires the liver to produce a replacement molecule. If we don't take HUGE quantities of N-acetyl cysteine and alpha-lipoic acid (pre-

cursors of glutathione) we have no chance of defending ourselves against this chemical overload which, by conservative estimate, is a million times more than it was fifty years ago.

A classic example of the failure of this RDA estimation system is the needs of a certain subset of schizophrenia patients. As you have read, some of them have been shown to need as much as 2,000 mg of niacin daily, to avoid the symptoms of schizophrenia. But most doctors laugh in their ignorance, scorning the idea that anyone needs more than 16 mg a day for men and 14 mg a day for women.

What's more, they claim this amount is easily obtainable in a varied diet and should prevent deficiency in most people. Try telling that to someone who's brain is wildly inflamed and throwing out strange voices, frightening hallucinations and disordered perceptions. Yet they go on arguing, even when an acutely disturbed patient has calmed to normal, just by adding large doses of niacin, B6 and zinc.

That's not medicine. That's not science. It's pig ignorance.

Minerals Too

Today we realize that optimum health not only relies on optimum doses of vitamins and chemical compounds, such as alpha-lipoic acid (alpha-thioctic acid), but also on the presence of minerals called co-factors. These co-factors make metabolic processes work better.

Because they are inorganic substances, minerals can't be synthesized by the human body. They have to be obtained from the foods we eat and unfortunately, our modern, unhealthy diets are high in low-quality, processed foods. This poor diet, combined with mineral-depleted topsoil and crops, has made it difficult for most people to get adequate amounts of these essential nutrients.

Only small (trace) quantities are needed, so we generally call these essential nutrients "trace elements". These should be distinguished from minerals, which the body needs in substantial quantities – for example calcium, magnesium and potassium.

It's a long list—a book in itself. So here we can only review what there is to look for and what sort of corrective actions can be taken.

Most people know the value of zinc in assisting the immune system to fight infections. Slightly fewer know that chromium helps in the regulation of blood glucose (so-called glucose factor). Well-read students of nutrition know that 200 mcg daily of selenium helps fight the toxic effects of mercury and, coincidentally, virtually blocks the development of cancer.

Here are a few more connections:

Copper: helps to activate the antioxidant enzyme superoxide dismutase and also plays an important role in the healthy formation of red blood cells, proper enzymatic reactions, and maintaining healthy connective tissue, hair, and eyes (connective tissue will help prevent dissecting aneurisms of the aorta, as Joel Wallach tells us).

Manganese: essential for mitochondrial health and sound bone formation. Its possible role in pyrrole disorder has already been discussed (section 5.7). Care is needed not to overdose with manganese.

Molybdenum: is essential to humans and is needed for at least three important enzymes.

See also the list of mineral deficiencies and imbalances in section 2.8 (crime)

Hair Mineral Analysis

One of the most valuable tools to a nutritionist—providing it is interpreted wisely and not too literally—is hair mineral analysis using photospectrometry. It can be helpful for detecting a burden of heavy metal overload, such as lead and mercury though, as I said in section 5.11, a mercury tri-test may be better.

But we can also use hair analysis to infer levels of needed nutrients too. It isn't always accurate to simply take a blood test and suppose that gives an accurate guide (magnesium, for example, is better reflected in the amount within blood cells, instead of plasma levels). A better approach would be to combine investigations into blood levels, urinary excretion and hair samples. Hair grows slowly so, in many situations, it gives a better picture of what the body's content load really is.

Examining hair biopsy specimens is not new. In the 20th century, archaeologists began to study mineral compositions present in the hair of mummies thousands of years old. Moreover, forensic scientists have long known that substances such as arsenic can be concentrated in the hair.

Combined with a sweat test, hair analysis can become very useful. The main drawback with sweat testing is that patients must present themselves in person at the laboratory, unlike the case for hair analysis, where the sample can be sent through the mail. Since there are very few centers equipped to carry out this procedure, for the majority of patients this means considerable travel. It is possible that sweat testing will become more widely available in the future, but until it does, its use is confined to those living near a laboratory or for whom distance is not a deterrent.

Controversy

Advocates of hair mineral analysis have perhaps been a little over-zealous in extolling its accuracy and too willing to ignore the paradoxes and inconsistencies in results. Matters came to a head (no pun intended) when, some decades ago, a cynical journalist sent off samples of the same hair under two separate names and was sent two entirely different results.

The difficulty with interpreting hair analysis results lies in being sure exactly what we are measuring. One source of conflict is that hair biopsy results don't always correlate very well with blood serum levels of a given element. Proponents of hair analysis are not deterred and argue, rightly, that we have no justification for assuming that blood levels are an accurate guide to the total amounts of any substance in the body, let alone of trace elements.

Since the body tends to carefully regulate the levels of substances in the blood, these levels could be high while in fact the body is depleted of the substances and I am of that view. An example would be calcium, for which the body would rob the bones and cause them to become soft and weakened, rather than allow blood levels to fall. So why should the same not be true of copper or selenium?

In any case, workers in this field are quick to point out that the picture given by the blood, which changes almost from hour to hour, could hardly be expected to reflect results in the hair, which represent changes over many months.

Advantages And Disadvantages

One of the great advantages of hair as a biopsy material is that it is easy to collect, the method being non-invasive and therefore painless. Hair also keeps indefinitely under normal conditions without deterioration and its mineral content can be measured relatively easily. Only about one gram is needed, which most people can spare without any visible sign of loss.

Another important point is that the substances being measured may be anything up to two hundred times more concentrated in hair than in the bloodstream. This makes relative measurements (see 'The Ratios', below) much more accurate and minor variations less significant statistically.

Some obvious problems present themselves when using hair in this way. One is contamination. The hair of someone who lives in the city, for example, may contain lead; has this lead come from the body or been deposited by traffic fumes? Of course, the samples are washed carefully to minimize extraneous elements, but vigorous washing may leach out quantities of the minerals that are truly present, rendering any measurements inaccurate.

Cosmetic hair treatments are also a problem. Selenium is believed to be a very important trace mineral and measuring it accurately is of vital concern. Yet it is the chief 'gimmick' ingredient of a number of shampoos. Similarly, hair-darkening compounds such as Grecian 2000 may add spurious lead levels due to their utilization of lead acetate. Bleaching and cold waving will also alter considerably the true picture of chemicals present in the hair.

Identifying Exposure

Yet with all these caveats, hair analysis can yield clinically usable results.

It can identify possible over-exposure to potentially toxic metals such as lead, mercury and aluminium. I have discussed the mental health impact of these metals elsewhere in the book. It has been shown that we have several hundred times the amount of lead and over a thousand times the amount of mercury in our bodies than primitive people had.

Some workers, such as former colleague Professor Bryce-Smith, and Christopher Shade at Quicksilver Diagnostics, are convinced that we are already, most of us, exposed to fully toxic amounts of lead. This is especially true of children, many of whom have smaller body weights and yet the same ambient exposure (higher body concentrations). Routine screening consistently brings back results of lead levels higher than required to affect mentation, and in many cases much higher than could be regarded as safe.

Mercury estimations may be the least accurate, even though the most needed with many patients. Alternatives are very expensive.

Again, I add my caution that hair analysis results be interpreted carefully and without excessive belief in the accuracy of the results.

The Ratios

Although the actual values of necessary trace elements, or the burden of toxic metals, found by hair analysis may be of debatable accuracy, the ratios—that is, the relative proportion of one element to another—are much more reliable. Even though there may be differences in technique from one laboratory to another, this would not affect a ratio.

Knowledge is still in its infancy, but it does appear that some ratios may offer guidance to the performance of certain aspects of physiology. For example, the measured ratio of calcium to phosphorus can provide an important pointer to the possibility of bone deterioration. Sodium and potassium ratios can indicate malfunctioning of the adrenal gland, so-called 'adrenal stress syndrome' found in allergic conditions and hypoglycaemia (section 5.9).

Most important of all seems to be the zinc/copper ratio. High copper/low zinc is common in a number of diverse conditions, including schizophrenia, criminal and violent behavior. Conversely, if zinc supplementation is too vigorous or prolonged there may be a relative lack of copper, leading to deficient blood production, possible impaired liver performance and arteriosclerosis.

What To Do

OK, we need a plan. What can be done about complex nutritional requirements which, as I have already said, vary widely among individuals?

The best answer may be to take multiple-composition formulas. A good liquid mix is particularly valuable. Whereas I prefer (and take myself, daily) a formula called "Passion-4Life", there are several others on the market.

The value of liquid formulas is that they are rapidly and efficiently absorbed. On their website Passion4Life has a video of an fMRI scan, showing brain activity lighting up within just a few minutes of ingesting their preparation (you can find the link in the **Valuable Resources** section in the back).

OK, a marketing ploy. But a brain scan is a brain scan! And of course it would apply to other liquid vitamin and mineral formulas.

The things to look for in choosing a liquid formula are the absolute amounts. Many manufacturers hide behind the RDAs, which I have already described as utterly inadequate, and tell you they are providing 200% of the RDA, or whatever.

Ignore these claims and just look at the absolute amounts (in milligrams or micrograms). How much is present in formula A, compared to formula B?

Also, count up the ingredients supplied. Passion4Life boasts 135 nutrients, from 18 amino acids to resveratrol. There's even aloe vera, wild blueberry extract and prune thrown in, for good measure (I'm never impressed by so-called ORAC values). There's not enough magnesium (20 mg); I'd throw out some berries and up that to 300 mg. But no formula is perfect and there is one thing I can say in support of Passion4Life: they've got the most ingredients, with the highest overall quantities on the market. Yet it sells for less than all the competition (around $40 for a month's supply, at the time of writing).

To get all that good stuff down you would entail swallowing about 60 pills and capsules daily, plus eating 4 cups of spinach, 31 bananas, 25 salmon fillets and 6 cups of mushrooms!

Finally, here's a handy table showing Passion4Life against two major competitors:

	Eniva Vibe Liquid Vitamin	Vemma	Passion 4 Life
Cost one month supply	$63.93	$50.99 + $7.25 Shipping	$39.95
Source	Multi-Level - Marketing Co.	Multi-Level - Marketing Co.	No MLM Direct to Consumer.
Serving Size:	1 Ounce Daily	2 Ounces Daily	1 Ounce Daily
Servings per Bottle:	32	32	30
Calories	24	35	20
Total Carbohydrate	5 g	8 g	5 g
Sugars	3 g	8 g	2 g
Vitamin A	3000 IU	2500 IU	10000 IU
Vitamin C	120 mg	300 mg	1000 mg
Vitamin D	500 IU	1000 IU	1000 IU
Vitamin E	30 IU	60 IU	150 IU
Thiamin (B1)	1.5 mg	1.5 mg	25 mg
Riboflavin (B2)	1.7 mg	1.7 mg	20 mg
Niacin	20 mg	20 mg	20 mg
Vitamin B6	2 mg	5 mg	25 mg
Vitamin B12	6 mcg	15 mcg	250 mcg
Panthothenic Acid	10 mg	10 mg	100 mg
Calcium	100 mg	NO	100 mg
Magnesium	YES	NO	YES
Phosphorus	YES	NO	YES
Zinc	4 mg	NO	24 mg
Selenium	25 mcg	50 mcg	100 mcg
Manganese	1.5 mg	NO	2 mg
Chromium	120 mcg	NO	200 mcg
D-Biotin	300 mcg	300 mcg	300 mcg
Potassium	175 mg	NO	50 mg
Iodine	YES	NO	NO
Copper	0.4 mg	NO	YES
Folic Acid	YES	YES	YES
D-Ribose	NO	NO	200 mg
Organic Sea Vegetation	NO	YES	NO
Plant Source Trace Minerals	YES	YES	YES
Organic Aloe Vera Juice	NO	NO	3000 mg
Liposomal Resveratrol	NO	NO	20 mg
Proprietary Fruit Blend (High ORAC Fruit Blend)	YES	NO	9 mg
Proprietary Long Life Blend (Acai, Goji, Noni, Mangosteen)	NO	NO	25.2 mg
Proprietary Amino Acids Blend	NO	NO	150 mg
Proprietary Power Blend (acai, noni, goji, mangosteen, cat's claw, alpha lipoic acid, vanadium)	NO	NO	YES
HeartPro Proprietary Blend	280 mg	NO	NO
CollaMAX Proprietary Blend	3300 mg	NO	NO
Dietary Fiber	NO	NO	3 g
Proprietary Vegetable Blend	YES	NO	YES

all Information collected from Amazon 12/27/2017

Liquid Mineral Formulas

The same principle can be applied to trace elements supplementation. We need around 90 different mineral nutrients. Just get a liquid mix! I take Joel D. Wallach's Youngevity Plant Derived Minerals™ complex. It tastes disgusting but that's easily disguised with fruit juice! Note: this product is derived from plant sources and should not be confused with Wallach's earlier formulation, made from colloidal metallic minerals (clay, ancient sea beds, rocks and dirt!)

As with the multi-vitamins, it's very easy just to swig an ounce or two a day and that will take care of over 95% of needs. That just leaves the critical ones to tweak.

The Plant Derived Minerals™ is sold via an MLM (link in the **Valuable Resources** section at the back of the book). But you don't have to join. I'm not a member. I just order my requirements directly from the company.

It's less than $50 for a 32 oz. bottle (1 month supply) and you can buy a pack of 4 for only $75, plus shipping. That's outstandingly cheap. And, as I said, I'm not an MLM member, not getting a commission for saying all this. Just trying to make things easy for you.

There are many other multi-mineral formulas out there for you to try, as the fancy takes you.

The Tweaks

So, we are just left with the quirky and oddball requirements.

I have covered schizophrenia high-dose requirements in the body of the text (the Abram Hoffer protocol). Also the needs of pyrrole disorder (Carl C. Pfeiffer) and specials like iodine for thyroid performance and chromium for hypglycemia.

Be sure to get enough omega-3 oils, to fight inflammation (3 gr per day). Plus other anti-inflammatories, like curcumin (not well absorbed), green tea, cat's claw (*Uncaria tomentosa*) and *Boswellia serrata* resin (also known as frankincense).

Adaptogens—substances which help a person fight stress—may have a place. Rhadiola is a good one. Asian ginseng (Panax), maybe. Ashwaganda, which is often pushed by online dealers, may sometimes make a person very ill. I do not recommend it for that reason. You can drink Tulsi tea; I do, every day.

Bacopa is an effective adaptogen and can help you cope with stressful situations and decrease indicators of stress in all regions of the brain. *Bacopa monnieri* is a creeping marsh plant that is traditionally used to tune up the mind (nootropic), for longevity, and to help with anxiety and depression states.[336]

Bacopa promotes communication between neurons by increasing the growth rate of nerve endings. There's some solid research on its effects on memory and can reliably improve memory in both healthy people and those experiencing cognitive decline. Studies show improvements in verbal learning, memory acquisition and improved recall.[337]

Other studies showed an increase in retention of new information, likely from a decrease in forgetting (as opposed to an increase in rate of learning).[338]

For any state of fatigue, inertia and possible depression, Dimethyl glycine (DMG) is a good energizer (see my Mito-Cell Rejuvenator formula). So are *Cordyseps sinensis* and Astragalus.

Don't forget lipoic acid: it's a star.

New evidence suggests that alpha-lipoic acid may help guard against Alzheimer's disease. It may do so by increasing the production of acetylcholine, an essential substance in the creation of memory and something deficient in the brains of Alzheimer's disease victims.[339]

Lipoic acid is able to pass readily into the brain and reach all parts of a nerve cell, which is good. *Experimental studies have shown that animals who received lipoic acid after a stroke effect had a survival rate three times greater than those that did not.*

Some of the protective effects conferred by lipoic acid in promoting healthy nerve function may be related to its ability to regenerate the antioxidant glutathione, which is often significantly depleted by harmful oxidative stress associated with cerebrovascular events such as stroke.[340]

So alpha-lipoic acid is overall brain-friendly, as well as liver-friendly (glutathione). Make sure you supplement it. You'll notice the difference if you do.

Please note, there are two types of alpha-lipoic acid supplement, two types are found in health food stores and online, the R- form and the S- form. All this good stuff applies only to the natural R- form). It is the only form of lipoic acid that is proven to improve memory, reduce brain damage, reverse cognitive dysfunction, and protect the brain from neurodegeneration associated with aging.

When selecting a supplement, be sure to look for 100% R-lipoic acid; otherwise you're probably getting some of the cheaper S- form, which is less bioavailable.

You can also get lipoic acid from the food you eat, it's found in red meats and offal, such as liver, kidney and heart. Dark leafy greens, broccoli, peas, brussels sprouts, spinach, collard greens and brewer's yeast also contain ALA in smaller amounts.[341]

The List Could Go On And On!

This is barely a beginning of nutritional science. You still need to eat well. Something totally overlooked (not even dreamed about) by standard nutritionists and dieticians is the fact that natural foods in their natural state manifest energetic properties that go way beyond their biochemical composition. The whole is more than the part! That's one of the characteristics of organic, living things.

Moreover, what is swallowed does not equate to nutrition. Malabsorption and dysbiosis are rampant, as I explained above. Digestive unwellness is the norm. So there is no guarantee whatever that swallowing supplements equates to fulfilling nutritional requirements.

Then another key principle: no nutrients act alone, they are all interdependent. So studies that say things like "vitamin E doesn't help heart disease" are structured on a lie and therefore, not surprisingly, come up with the wrong result.

We can generalize this to an important principle: *all studies which purport to examine the effects of vitamins and minerals in isolation are likely to be misleading.*

Note, as well as their nutrient content, foodstuffs, notably plants, often contain pharmacologically active substances. The effect of these drug-equivalents can rightly be seen as a sub-function of nutrition (also a complex, vast subject!)

It only remains to say: choose a diet rich in a variety of plant-based foods, eat freshly prepared foods and eat only whole foods.

Eat plenty of vegetables and fruits. That's part of the Mediterranean diet and, remember, in section 2.1 I reported on marvellous new studies that make it clear the Mediterranean diet has powerful benefits to offer those struggling with inner turmoil and labelled as "mentally ill".

Maintain a healthy weight and be physically active.

Drink alcohol only in moderation, if at all.

Prepare and store food safely.

Vitamin L

This is a joke. But it's also serious. The most important vitamin of all, for any human being, sick or well, is LOVE! (vitamin L)

It's an outstanding nutrient that none of us can live without.

Love is the healer of all ills; it's a factor in mental health and longevity: love of self and others; love of life...

Love yourself means live clean and live well, avoid toxic relationships, read only nutritious books and watch only healthy movies and TV shows. Nothing is to be gained from immersing yourself in violence, depravity, crime and gore.

If your main relationship does need a "refresh", to get it out of the toxic zone, you might consider **Supernoetics®** and **"Punk Psychology®"**, described in section 3.12. You can go it alone, or ask for help at info@supernoetics.com

Now, what comes next? Woo...

PART 6

WEIRD STUFF

In this section we'll look at strange mystical and spiritual experiences that are definitely outside the norm (in other words *paranormal*). That's not to say I think of them as pathological. But others might and many a patient has been judged insane for hearing voices, being possessed by demons (supposedly), or having mystical visions. In centuries gone by you might count yourself lucky not to be burned at the stake, especially if you were a woman.

But old prejudices linger and in this world of modern mechanistic science, which claims there is nothing above and beyond material, it argues by definition that people who find themselves experiencing reality in a different way *must be mad*.

We are told we are a brain and nothing but a brain; therefore anyone who finds themselves leaving their body must be deluded. There is no place for this phenomenon in a scientific worldview which says that nothing which is non-material exists. The stupidity of saying so is lost on most would-be scientists: yes, of course things which are non-material do not exist in the normal sense of the word. That doesn't mean they are not there!

I remember a sad case of a lovely patient of mine—a woman in her thirties, Irish, and somewhat prone to romancing—who offered to take me to see fairies nearby. We made all the arrangements and I confess I was quite excited to see if I could see what she saw (or if not, what I would see instead). But as the day dawned I received a phone call from her husband saying, *"She won't be coming. But not to worry. She had been forcefully admitted to a psychiatric hospital and was now on medication. All was well. She is in good hands."*

To say I was incensed would be an understatement. I was incandescent! How DARE they kidnap a person off the street, sequester her against her will, and pump her full of toxic filth, when all she wanted to do was play a while in the etheric?

I had no way of proving there were such things as fairies. But equally, they had *absolutely no proof* that such a phenomenon did not exist. It was psychic fascism and did a lot to harden my heart against psychiatrists.

OK, let's get started on the weird, scary and wonderful!

6.1 Spiritual Emergencies (or The Crisis Of Becoming)

The term spiritual emergency (sometimes called a psychospiritual crisis) was coined by psychiatrist Stanilov Grov and his wife psychotherapist Christina.

For those with a model for spiritual transcendence and peak experiences (Abram Maslow), out-of-body and de-manifestation, these are seen as great surges of Being and awareness; a physical or emotional life-enhancing or awe-inspiring experience. Unfortunately, mainstream psychiatry makes no distinction between spiritual or mystical experiences and mental illness. "Religious or Spiritual Problems" was entered into the infamous DSM-IV as a malady (1994).

This unjustifiable hijacking of experiences of mystical wonder by mainstream medical psychiatry has been challenged by critics from within the field of medical psychiatry itself. R. D. Laing, for example, argued that mental health problems could also be a transcendental experience with healing and spiritual aspects. Arthur J. Deikman further suggested use of the term "mystical psychosis" to characterize first-person accounts of psychotic experiences that are conceptually similar to reports of mystical experiences.[342]

But who is to decide what's true? In the new psychiatry, a person who claimed to have seen an angel needs medicating, to get rid of the delusion. If a man came down from the mountains claiming a bush had spontaneously burst into flame and a voice had spoken from heaven, he would be considered certifiably insane. And what about Buddha? Thirty years sitting under a tree, barely eating: he was obviously severely clinically depressed and would today be a candidate for electro-convulsive therapy!

In his book *Cosmic Consciousness: A Study in the Evolution of the Human Mind*, published in 1901, Richard Bucke writes of "certain men who...are either exalted, by the average self conscious individual, to the rank of gods, or, adopting the other extreme, are adjudged insane." This is the earliest mention I have found of the potential problem inherent in the spiritual growth process: bouts of madness, or at least extreme dysfunction.

Bucke described his own experience, that of contemporaries, most notably Walt Whitman, but also historical figures including Buddha, Jesus, St. Paul, Plotinus, Muhammad, Dante, Francis Bacon, and William Blake.

Better Terminology

Instead of "spiritual emergency", perhaps we can follow the lead of some workers and use the less threatening expression *exceptional human experiences* (EHEs). In many cases, new realms of mystical and spiritual experience enter the person's life suddenly and dramatically, resulting in fear and confusion. This may be mistaken for a panic attack (section 2.4). He or she may feel tremendous anxiety, have difficulty coping with daily life, a job, and relationships, and may even fear for their own sanity, until someone is able to explain to them what is happening.

EHEs can be scary for an individual not experienced in peak states and not expecting it to happen, hence the term spiritual "emergency". But the real crisis is to keep these people out of the hands of psychiatrists, who do not understand, and are likely to treat it as acute psychosis, dosing the person on abominable and unjustified drugs.

If the person suddenly comes close to God, or whatever, why is that even a disease condition, never mind a psychotic state? Well, predictably, the psychiatrists (or the puppets to the Big Pharma trade) have grabbed "religious or spiritual problems" for their infamous *Diagnostic and Statistical Manual*.[343] Mental health professionals are now required to have expert knowledge on religious beliefs, practices and their effects... presumably so they snaffle the ones with unorthodox ideas as "not religious". Seriously, they are trying to make this divide up to a serious scientific proposition.

But as Socrates once said: "Our greatest blessings come to us by way of madness, provided that madness is given us by divine gift".[344]

A spiritual emergency may be triggered by a lack of sleep or matters related to childbirth, miscarriage, or abortion. One of my dear friends had a dematerialization that seemed to be triggered by hypoglycemia. Her body felt light and insubstantial (somewhat transparent). She began to spontaneously levitate later that day. This was witnessed by a medical doctor I know and there is absolutely no justification for scoffing at this experience. It's typical of the level of drama that can occur. This took place in Harrod's store (London), while passing through a turnstile, so there is no special circumstance in which this unworldly experience can or will occur.

Psychotropic drugs can equally trigger a spiritual emergency, especially "bad trips". Extreme sexual indulgence can also result in a spiritual emergency (Tantric sex practitioners would probably call it something else). Being electrocuted or involved in an almost-fatal car crash have been triggers for plenty of EHEs.

Saul's awakening on the road to Damascus is a prime example of something non-pathological, which would have been classified as an acute hallucinatory episode by modern psychiatrists! Mevlevi dervishes deliberately dance until they get a crisis experience! ("whirling dervishes" is a bit pejorative). Muslim *sufis*, the wise ones, also acknowledge these deep spiritual encounters and actively seek them, as do the Zen Buddhists (satori).

Other examples could be Hildegard of Bingen (1098-1179), the brash and brilliant medieval abbess, author, herbalist, composer, prophetess and visionary who ruled her own monastery of Rupertsberg, high on a hill in rural Germany. She had her "visions", in which the Lord spoke directly to her.

We find it sometimes in past-life experiences; encounters with spirit guides; Kundalini rising; near-death experiences and even UFO encounters (see my own book *Medicine Beyond* for at least a plausible scientific explanation for what could be called an "alien abduction").

As I said in the section on schizophrenia (2.2), the diagnosis of "illness" is often based on mere disapproval. The person manifests thoughts, behaviors or utterances that others cannot embrace comfortably and therefore reject as "abnormal".

Lawrence Stevens JD, a lawyer who represents psychiatric "patients", joins me in arguing that labels such as pornography, schizophrenia and mental illness, and many similar terms are indefinable and indicate disapproval of that to which the label is applied and nothing more.

How To Deal With It

Firstly, it's not a problem. We are, as I have said repeatedly, non-material spiritual beings. This has been drummed out of us since childhood, but it hardly hurts to be reminded of our true nature. If managed properly, a spiritual emergency can become a valuable and inspiring life experience. It is, in that sense, a true *emergence*, not an emergency!

In the absence of an enlightened and skilled quality of life coach to help, as for example a Supernoetics® practitioner, a good place to start would be with the International Spiritual Emergence Network. ISEN believes in providing a collaborative platform that connects networks around the world that offer compassionate support to those who understand their experiences to be a spiritual crisis rather than a mental illness, raising awareness of a non-pathological integral framework within the mental health field.

For those of you facing up to any EHE by yourself, I can commend the wisdom of Lynn Woodland (you can find a link to her website in the **Valuable Resources** section in the back of the book):

Stop trying to process your spiritual experience. Stop trying to understand it all at once. Give your mind a rest. Know that in order to assimilate new ideas and especially new paradigms of thought, a period of confusion is necessary. Don't fight it. You don't need to analyze the experience in order to assimilate it. If you try to force understanding prematurely, your interpretations are likely to fall short of the whole truth. Trust that clarity will come to you in time.

Shift your focus of attention from the strangeness/specialness of the spiritual phenomena to the question of how this new energy, awareness or ability can serve you and help you to serve others. What are you feeling drawn to do with this energy? Doing something will help you shift out of self-absorption. Creativity is a great outlet for spiritual energy. Paint a picture, make music, dance, create a beautiful altar space, write a poem or journal about your experience. Do a service for someone. Pray for people. Send a silent blessing to everyone you meet. Do some reflection and journaling on your life purpose. Imagine what you would like your life to be like in five years. These are just a few ideas for directing spiritual energy toward your highest good. Find the outlet that brings you the most satisfaction.

Dark Night Of The Soul

St. John of the Cross (1542-1591), a Christian mystic, coined the phrase and said of this experience, that it; "...puts the sensory spiritual appetites to sleep, deadens them, and deprives them of the ability to find pleasure in anything. It binds the imagination, and impedes it from doing any good discursive work. It makes the memory cease, the intellect become dark and unable to understand anything, and hence it causes the will to become arid and constrained, and all the faculties empty and useless. And over this hangs a dense and burdensome cloud, which afflicts the soul, and keeps it withdrawn from the good."

This is a brilliant insight, given the constraints of the language of the day and crude mediaeval psychology (which was mostly Christian imperatives, rather than real understanding of the mind).

Implicit in this complex metaphor is the accompanying emergence, discovery and self-actualization which follows the profound depths. There seems to be a proportional relationship: the deeper, more searing the pain, the greater the ascension afterwards.

So no matter how tough the transition time, there is a reward for those who can endure.

But how much of a disease of the mind is it, when the individual has sunk into the abyss of despair? Why should hitting hard times, extreme misery, be something that requires medicating? For me, it is certain that trying to block the natural unfolding of this process is to deny the individual something worthy, a reward, growth, something that would make the searing pain worthwhile; an investment if you like!

6.2 Out Of Body Experiences

Sometimes the description of an exceptional human experience makes it clear the person is having some kind of out-of-body experience. Without the normal sensory channels, the person feels very disconnected. Once the body platform has been left behind, any kind of sensory experience can supervene, from telepathic messages, to seeing through walls.

In 1958, Robert Monroe floated out of his body for the first time. It began "without any apparent cause," he wrote. His doctor, predictably, prescribed tranquilizers. A psychologist friend, meanwhile, suggested Monroe try leaving his body again, re-assuring him with the fact that, "some of the fellows who practice yoga and those Eastern religions claim they can do it whenever they want to."

Monroe did try it again—and again and again. He recalls his discoveries in this field in his classic 1971 book *Journeys out of the Body*, which launched the phrase "out-of-body experiences" (OBEs) into public awareness. Monroe died in 1995, but the fascination with out-of-body experiences endures.

Whether you choose to explore this fascinating area of psychology or not, it is important to understand that it is something entirely predictable in the non-material mind model I have been writing about. Since you have the impression you are inside a body only because you elect to preceive things that way, then it takes only a simple shift of viewpoint to alter the feeling to being "outside".

Sometimes the patient loses the ability to move or "work" the body and he or she feels frozen or paralyzed. It is not true paralysis. It is simply a result of trying to control the body from somewhere in the non-material domain. We do this all the time, incidentally—all of us, via the brain—but when you are suddenly "over there" it might seem impossible to make your arms and legs work properly. The brain really does not move your limbs; it is only the relay point. The will-to-move comes from you, in your non-material compartment of mind!

One question people unfamiliar with this phenomenon ask is: can you die from being out of the body (sometimes called astral projection)? People who practice astral projection claim that a "silver cord" connects the astral body to the physical one, which has given rise to the idea that the physical body will die if this silver cord is severed. This is complete nonsense but gets passed from fool to fool and, for some, it becomes "true". Generally speaking, nothing you can do while "outside" will harm your physical body, and because the astral body is immaterial, it can't be physically harmed.

The important thing to bear in mind is that this is not a psychotic episode; don't be frightened; try to relax and enjoy the sensations rather than be scared or phobic. Above all, do not fear that you will not be able to get back. That's an artifical worry and I know of no instance of a person being stranded outside their body. In any event, sleep puts everything to rights. You'll wake up "normal".

Kundalini arousal is a similar experience, often described. The Kundalini, in the Hindu tradition, is a spiritual energy presumed to reside at the base of the spine. When it is awakened, it is said to rise like a serpent up the spine, and opens the psychic centers

Also known as Kundalini awakening, this spiritual emergency most commonly occurs as an unintentional side-effect of yoga, meditation, chi kung or other intensive spiritual, particularly meditative, practices. Some theorists include psychotherapy, giving birth, unrequited love, celibacy, deep sorrow, high fever, and drug intoxication to also be triggers, and some believe kundalini awakening can occur spontaneously without apparent cause.

Many OBEs have been checked for veracity, meaning that someone has checked up on what the person was supposed to have seen when out of body and there have been plenty of corroborations.

The important point is that, today, with what we now know, there is no need for every supposed instance to be proven. This is experience, not physics. So one or several people being mistaken or deluded does NOT disprove the OBE hypothesis (as skeptics like to pretend). Rather, the other way round: *if even just one OBE was confirmed by recording details which subsequently check out, then the possibility of any and all OBEs plus non-material states becomes PROVEN*, if you follow my logic!

Which leads naturally to...

6.3 Peak Experiences

American psychologist and philosopher Abraham H. Maslow (1908-1970) coined this term to describe nonreligious quasi-mystical and mystical experiences. Peak experiences are sudden feelings of intense happiness and well-being, and possibly the awareness of "ultimate truth" and the unity of all things. Accompanying these experiences is a heightened sense of control over the body and emotions, and a wider sense of awareness, as though one was standing upon a sacred mountaintop. The experience fills the individual with wonder and awe. He feels at one with the world; he or she has seen the ultimate truth or the essence of all things. [Corsini, Raymond J. (1998). Encyclopedia of Psychology. United States: John Wiley & Sons] It is a visionary experience that is so intense as to be almost overwhelming. Almost but not quite.

Those who have experienced these mystical moments use remarkably consistent language to describe peak experiences as "rare, exciting, oceanic, deeply moving, exhilarating, elevating experiences that generate an advanced form of perceiving reality, and are even mystic and magical in their effect upon the experimenter." (on the investigator)

There are several unique characteristics of a peak experience, but each element is perceived together in a holistic manner that creates the moment of reaching one's full potential.[345] Peak experiences render therapeutic value as they foster a sense of being lucky or graced; release creative energies; reaffirm the worthiness of life; and change an individual's view of himself or herself. Maslow cautioned against seeking such experiences for their own sake; echoing the advice of the mystics who have pointed out that the sacred exists in the ordinary. Maslow further believed that domestic and public violence, alcoholism, and drug abuse stem from spiritual emptiness, and that even one peak experience might be able to prevent, or at least abate, such ills.

Only in strained circumstances or among the wrong people would such a fortunate event risk being classified as a psychotic or delusional moment. Psychologist James Hillman, a critic of humanistic psychology, observes that peaks and highs say nothing of the worth of the person having them, for they can occur among psychopaths and criminals. Transcendence by means of a high, he says, is a psychopathological state in disguise.[346] Well, isn't that the classic angst-ridden American puritan talking? It's certainly not a valid medical standpoint.

In fact peak experiences are enjoyed as a very positive event and for ever afterwards the lucky person longs to get back to the magic moment.

This next section is an essay about "soul retrieval" I wrote back in the 1990s. It stands as true today as when I wrote it, though it would be better enjoyed and understood, if read in conjunction with the "Complex Of Self" model (section 3.15)

6.4 Mending The Fragmented Self

I turn to the shaman model of healing called soul retrieval, not merely as a curiosity, but in considerable awe and respect for a tradition as old as consciousness and twice as old as other healing arts! It has worked so well for so long among so many peoples, it is in every sense a Super Healing technique. The fact that most of the proponents are supposedly less sophisticated than ourselves does them less than justice and probably turns our blind eye of prejudice away from what may ultimately prove to be the best of all wellness approaches.

Quite simply, there is no real health without true being. We are not a body; therefore to treat only the body is to miss much of the impact and purpose of the healing arts. In the words of Sandra Ingerman, US career-shaman, "For shamans the world over, illness has always been seen as a spiritual predicament".[347] Her lovely book is subtitled *Mending the Fragmented Self*, which says it all. Mechanistic reductionist science has little currency here.

One of the most succinct models for dis-ease in this domain is the "loss of soul" or soul parts. You might prefer the term consciousness particles" to soul parts. The concept is that of parts of the self being torn off and getting lost. This would typically take place at times of extreme suffering. Today we often find soul loss is a result of such traumas as incest, abuse, loss of a loved one, surgery, accident, illness, miscarriage, abortion, bad drug trips and military combat. Even witnessing traumatic events, such as a crime scene or bloody death, can cause loss through shock and horror. Coma, of course, is the most extreme form of soul loss.

The whole of this concept plays to, and is an integral part of, my "cloud consciousness" model and it is very important. In no sense can we regard ourselves as a single discrete consciousness entity, not even a self. We are a cloud of selves! Hold that idea in mind as you read through and practice this.

The Clues

People will often describe feeling as if they are incomplete after the calamity; "something died inside me", "I don't feel myself anymore", "I left my heart behind", "I don't feel all here", "I'm aching and empty inside" and so on. The hippies used to have an expression "feeling untogether", which is a rather poetic way of putting it, though in their case it was often self-inflicted, due to recreational drug abuse.

What seems to happen is the patient loses some of their resources when the part or parts flee. Certain skills, qualities or other desirable character traits are no longer there and so he or she cannot act out these aspects of the self. The same is true in reverse, of course, and the skills and knowledge present at the moment of schism return remarkably when the retrieval procedure is completed. But the break is very real and the homecoming particles sometimes have to be brought up to date regarding what has happened to the patient in the intervening years in order to fully integrate.

Sandra gives a checklist of symptoms which might point to soul loss. I reproduce them here:

- Do you ever have a difficult time staying "present" in your body? Do you sometimes feel as if you're outside your body observing it as you would a movie?

- Do you ever feel numb, apathetic, or deadened?

- Do you suffer from chronic depression?

- Do you have problems with your immune system and have trouble resisting illness?

- Were you chronically ill as a child?

- Do you have gaps in your memory of your life after age five? Do you sense that you may have blacked out significant traumas in your life?

- Do you struggle with addictions to, for example, alcohol, drugs, food, sex, or gambling?

- Do you find yourself looking to external things to fill up an internal void or emptiness?

- Have you had difficulty moving on with your life after a divorce or the death of a loved one?

- Do you suffer from multiple personality syndrome?

If you answer yes to any of these questions, you may be dealing with soul loss. Important parts of your essential core self may not be available to you. If so, the vital energy and gifts of these parts are temporarily inaccessible."[348] History Of Shamanism

The basic technique is remarkably similar and cogent in societies throughout the world which practice soul retrieval. Typically, the shaman was the one who did the travelling to other realities to look for the missing part or parts and invited them home. The technique I now propose to describe is easily done by the subject, with or without accompaniment. I believe it strengthens and educates the person more if they are held less passive and invited to actually experience the procedure for themselves. There is the additional advantage that the person acting as shaman does not need the same depths of transcendental skills. The therapist does not need to visit other worlds or speak to spirits (though it's fine if you can do that successfully).

No ceremonies are needed. We are better off without them. There is always the danger that the methodology becomes identified with the ceremony. This makes it easy for cynics to scoff. If there is drumming, they will argue that drumming cannot make the psyche whole; if there are scents and candles, critics will suppose that there was a trance state. Of course it is the re-integration that makes the person whole, not the accompanying music or rituals.

Additionally, there is no reason to blindly observe ritual and history, beyond its proper context. It seems right to take older practices and modernize them, in accordance with later learning. To do otherwise is to accord too much significance to the act and not enough to the knowledge process. Yet there are people who think to change procedures or improve them is to be "wrong" and that one has become somehow disrespectful.

Gestalt

The psyche, spirit or soul is creative in at least as much as we experience what we want to experience, (often) independently of outer reality. That there are many aspects to the way we react to our surroundings is simple but adequate evidence of a multiple-viewpoint personality. The modern gestalt view that we are a sum of parts and integrated as a greater whole is more or less sufficiently self-evident as to be regarded as axiomatic.

People are naturally whole and integrated. We have all the qualities and resources we need. This needs interpreting with care, however, since we do sometimes find the missing part far into the past (previous incarnation). Such a person was not born whole in this life.

The idea of losing a part of oneself seems quite natural, once the spiritual model is entered. People readily grasp the metaphor of losing a part of "self" leaving it behind in some other place or some other time. Occasionally we find the part has drifted off into other realities (magical zones and fantastic environments).

If you don't like the notion of a soul (many people object to the word because of its identification with a restrictive religious context), you can still get the idea of a personality in many parts. Gurdjieff spoke of many "I"s. To lose one is to lose a part of one's self; to be less than whole. A "part" means an awareness or consciousness fragment or entity - a grouping of personal qualities, attitudes, abilities and emotional feelings that is not complete in itself but can have some of the characteristics of a whole being.

Some people experience many "I"s as an everyday reality. The fact that they tend to be considered mad and treated as such may have more to do with prejudice than exact psychology. However, it is worth observing that such individuals do tend to have difficulty coping with themselves and ordinary reality, so it is not a state one would like to share with them, even if it is true they are seeing deeper into the reality of our nature.

Soul Giving and Soul Theft

The usual cause of this phenomenon, which might logically be called dis-integration, is some powerful emotional trauma. Very little matches up to the psychic violence of continuous abuse or losing a loved one, whether through death or infidelity and separation. Sometimes the things a person says give the game away. We hear expressions like "That man took away my soul", "She stole my heart", "I'll always be with you in some meaningful way", and so on.

The very essence of a loving relationship is that ego boundaries go down and we share "as one". So it is quite natural for bits to end up in the wrong place after a marriage or relationship breaks up. Sometimes a person goes off with a piece of a loved one, stealing it, clinging on to it for their own needs, usually to avoid the sense of desolation which follows. This leaves the part unavailable to the owner and is a major infringement or transgression.

In other cases, the person leaves behind a part of their own soul, a sort of gift (usually unwanted). What manifests here is that the person who is dumped with the gift continues to manifest traits they don't really want; these have come from the departed one. Removing the stuck part and sending it back to its owner is both a kindness (for them) and a release for the patient in question.

It may be obvious from what material you are offered while working that such a phenomenon has taken place. Great compassion and insight is needed in these tricky situations. You often feel like you are dealing with more than one patient! Discuss matters with the client and get her agreement and understanding.

When To Do Soul Retrieval

The most fruitful time to do self re-integration is after you have been cleaning up a stressful event or area of a person's life, using recall therapy (Punk Psychology® for example). The actual technique you are using doesn't much matter, provided it drains off or as we say "flattens" the adverse emotional and spiritual energy (sometimes also called "discharging"). Usually from this sort of regression approach, done properly, you get a resurgence and the individual brightens up considerably. It is as if black energy has been cleaned off and they have been freed up from an area where their attention has been stuck for so long.

However, it is sometimes obvious that, despite the benefits, the individual is still to a degree stuck there. He or she feels "better" or even "great" but they are not congruently clear of it and you can see that doubt or dispersal still lingers.

This happens when a part of the self was shed and the loss has not been spotted. A full recovery would need retrieval of the missing part and re-integrating it.

The detailed and highly effective procedure, taught to me decades ago by the late Alan Wright, is given here:

Step 1. Preliminary

An incident is encountered and reduced by some kind of therapy or de-stressing procedure (abreaction).

A soul retrieval step would be considered if:

the person wasn't balanced, content and whole afterwards

it was "logical" that the soul broke up or parts were lost (NDEs, severe injury, shock, dreadful emotional harm such as abuse cases, threat etc).

Step 2. Investigation

Ask: "During this incident, did a part of you leave?" or "At that time (long period) did a part of you fade or leave?"

If the person says "No" and she has no reality on this concept, you have nothing to do.

If she says "Yes," continue.

If the next action is needed, put on your big-hearted shaman's hat, create a huge amount of loving space which enfolds your subject. Talk gently, wisely and calmly. Proceed as follows:

Step 3. Locating The Missing Part

If the patient/client cannot easily spot the part, say explain, "We will do a journey to locate it".

The part could be in ordinary or non-ordinary space and may be in the past. Bearing in mind you are the shaman, you can participate in the search if you wish. You may even see where the missing part is, before the subject finds it. In shamanic practice the shaman makes the journey alone and retrieves FOR the person. We find that aware individuals do best if they make their own journey.

It's strange but the patient/client always knows where the part is, when asked simply and directly. Nothing mystical is required. "Where does it seem to be?" I asked a distressed woman with an abuse history.

"In the library where I loved to read as a child," she replied. When her pain was unbearable, she could always retreat to the library. No-one minded a child taken to reading a lot; it seemed a totally natural thing to do. For her it was a welcome escape from the abuse at home. The bonus was she had grown up a well-educated woman. But her heart—or part of it—still lingered in her childhood sanctuary.

It's fascinating but the part will often have the age, emotions and attitudes that were appropriate at the time it left. You might be dealing with basically a child psyche. Get into gentle communication and rapport.

We ascertain what other parts of energies are present. Usually these would belong or relate to the other people present in the original traumatic episode. Sometimes there are several fragments and we deal with each one in turn, leaving the patient/client's own part till last.

For the person's own part we might want to ask, "What happened that caused you to separate?" Very importantly, we need to ask, "Would you like to return?"

We also have to ask the patient/client, "Would you like it to return?" "Do you have space for it?" and possibly "Will you honor this part if it comes back?"

We discuss the possible implications of this. Remember this "part" could have the age, emotions and attitudes that were appropriate at the time it left. In other words, be very immature and childlike. Get into gentle communication and rapport.

Say to the part "We are here to help you".

Step 4. Separating The Mixture (Soul Mix)

Almost invariably there are other soul parts, from other beings, mixed up with the subject's own. These would usually be people involved in the original event (see also *soul gifts* and *soul stealing* later).

Tell your subject: "Look at it (the soul part) - are there other parts or energies present?"

Instruct her to unravel "who" is involved. Separate them out, being kindly and gentle. Once unravelled it will be easier to see who is there.

Step 5. Handling The Parts.

NB. Always do the person's own part last, when all the others are gone, otherwise it would be rude.

Explain we want to send each part back home.

"Who do we take up first?" There will be an appropriateness in this, as in all other stages.

Have him or her locate the being with part(s) present, as they are in real time-space (If dead, use other-reality). Have him or her thank the part for its good intentions. Then:

Have the subject mock up "hands" and put the part cupped into one hand and the real-life being in the other. He or she now simply brings the hands together gently. The part will be perceived to have rejoined and leave.

Check for more parts and repeat.

Step 6. The Subject's Own Part.

Ask, "What happened that caused you to separate?"

"Would you like to return?" but don't invite it yet.

Possibly "What resources can you bring that will be beneficial?" but don't imply barter.

Shift of attitude: All this has been done with a loving, calm and gentle manner, with a BIG safe space. Now switch back to therapist mode.

Step 7. Is It Wanted?

Focus on the subject (not the part): "Would you like it to return?"

"Do you have space for it?"

Possibly "Will you honor this part if it comes back?" Discuss the possible implications of this.

Step 8. Ask It Home.

Back to shaman voice and mode:

Run out the part's distress if necessary, otherwise you might bring it along.

Then ask it home. Get the subject to cup the part with "hands" and draw it in, willingly, welcomingly and non-judgmentally. Nine times out of ten it will just come in.

Tell the subject "I would like all your cells to wake up and receive this energy back". Warn her it often fizzes and scintillates. *There will usually be some heavy emotions running at this point.* I have seen patients sob and sob and sob; but eventually the storm calms and the sun begins to come out once more.

Simply wait for a sensible moment to break off and then do a grounding or run some "fresh reality"...

This is a quick and dirty remedy, taken from my Supernoetics® methods, for getting the person back into their body and experiencing normal reality.

Simply guide the person with the following instructions:

"Point out something you like."

"Point to something close at hand."

"Point to something far away."

"Touch that (room object)." (vase, table, picture, wall, etc., etc.)

"Look around here and find something you would like to remain in place."

"Go over to that wall and touch it. Describe its characteristics (temperature, texture, etc.)".

"What is the condition of that (room object)?"

Please note, there are no right or wrong answers. The person's choice is final. Keep it up to a point where the person is grounded and fully present, here and now. It usually doesn't take very long—ten or twenty repetitions maybe. Remember to acknowledge each instruction carried out.

Step 9. Grounding

When the sizzle and storm has passed, take your subject out to open ground and in contact with the earth.

Do the Gaia step. Have the subject make contact with the earth's heart, feel the physical connection, and ask the Earth Goddess to renew her energies and sustain them. Have him or her feel the Gaia energies coming up through the ground.

Step 10. Power Animal

Optional. But if it's never been done before, this is a nice moment for this action...

We go on to produce the power animal learning. It is very simple. Have the person in their new state of awareness run a few swift paces across the earth, leap high into the air and then take up an instinctive gait upon landing. Usually they burst into some kind of stylized movement.

Usually you will get a boisterous shout, "I'm a wolf, I'm a wolf!" (bear, deer, etc.) If there is uncertainty, ask her what animal it feels like.

Tell her to honor and respect this new power animal and use it *often*. It's a use-it-or-lose-it gift. The secret to using your power animal is to take some time (often) to *look out from the animal's own eyes at the world and see what new hidden signals appear.*

Step 11. Finalization

The whole process of re-integration and adjustment can take days, weeks, even months. Many things will change for the individual. Most of it is very holistic and personal but there may be real psychological initiatives too.

It is vital that you instill one or two warnings. The new soul part which came home is often very disoriented. It may have been alone and isolated for decades and be very uncertain of its new environment.

Do not allow your subject to drive or work machinery for a few days. Accidents can happen.

There may also be strange emotional reactions, some of them unpleasant. Ask her to stay calm and talk gently and reassuringly to the new part, as if educating a child (which is basically the case). In fact I suggest the client walk around and point out to the returning fragment of Self, "This is where I live now. This is my husband, Jim. I like ice cream, do you? This is my cat Timmy..." and so on, as appropriate.

Problems with Soul Retrieval

If it gets stuck or won't come home:

Check for other parts that may be stuck to it. Clean them up and then try again.

The part may need more understanding of the present-time situation (explain to it).

Try negotiation: "What would it take for you to come home?"

If still no response, try running its shock incident again.

Ask again: does the subject really want it back? Would he/she honor it and use it? Talk through any rejection, fears or doubts.

In the reverse, make sure the one whose part is left behind wants it returned. If not find out why (you as practitioner are negotiating telepathically, via the subject). Handle what comes across.

Generally, it would be a sense of being rejected or kicked out by someone loved. Talk to the other being like an intelligent fully-formed self and get it to understand it needs all its parts at this time. Whereas the "gift" (if that's what is was) is a wonderful notion, it is time-expired and no longer appropriate.

Finally, you may have to ask it, "Well, what would the God energy want?" or something to jog it back to its senses. Whatever works.

An Example

To get more of a grasp of how this can go, let me outline a soul retrieval session. The patient was a 35-year old female aromatherapist with severe ME (fibromyalgia). There was no couch, no music, no psycho-galvanometer; just the patient sat in an upright chair, relaxed, with her eyes closed. I decided to begin exploring the psychological aspect of her eczema, which continued unresolved. Exploration of life issues revealed the fact that she had been left somewhat bereft since her grandmother had died painfully of cancer a few years previously. Father was evidently quite controlling and domineering and perhaps grandmother had been to a degree able to intervene and protect her, if not physically, then with mental resources at a distance.

We reduced the force of the death and bereavement. There were tears. From what was said it was obvious that the patient was still very connected; her images were of "sailing away in a boat" with grandmother. A soul loss was discussed and this seemed real to the patient, who was very aware of higher consciousness issues (but knew nothing of the soul retrieval model).

On the day in question I re-oriented her to the issue of grandmother and asked directly: At that time did a part of you leave? She affirmed yes. I asked her gently "Reach out and find it... in this space, other space or any universe or dimension, wherever". After quite some time she reported having made contact. I asked her where is the part? She said "up among the stars, playing with grandmother". I told her to say hello and tell it "We are here to try and help". Again, this took some time but eventually she nodded that this had been done. I asked what was happening and she said that grandmother was laughing and playing with the soul part

I said to thank grandma for her good intentions but to ask her respectfully if she would be willing to give back this soul part. The request was denied and grandmother continued to laugh and play. I was careful not to think any judgmental thoughts about grandmother's attitude, in case these were imparted telepathically and closed down the session.

So I instructed the patient to ask grandmother if she would be willing to speak with me directly -- I explained there was no need for magic or mysticism: the patient would be acting as a relay messenger for my words. Yes, grandmother was willing, I was told.

So I asked the patient to explain to her "I am trying to help you (the patient) and that you might need the resources of this other part in order to fully regain your well-being". Grandma apparently understood but was reluctant. I said "Please tell her from me that she might want to move on to another incarnation and work on some more karma". But grandma hesitated and didn't think this was possible. I asked "Is there anything standing in the way of you taking a new incarnation and coming down here again with us?"

The answer was that there was a black sticky cloud hanging around making it difficult. As a shaman, I knew right away what it was and had the patient ask her: "Is this the pain and unhappiness surrounding the final disease?" The answer was yes. The patient now told me Grandma had stopped laughing and fooling around; that she had started to cry and felt confused. Grandma simply didn't know what to do.

Via the patient I explained that I wanted both of the ladies to carry out a task for me, which was to pour glowing bright energies on the blackness and blow it away: "Gold is best but white or blue will do fine". I thought it was a good idea to get the patient helping in this task too, since she loved her grandmother so much and would clearly want to help.

Considerable time passed, in which I watched various facial and energetic phenomena. I encouraged them both with various comments and was kept informed as it was melted away. After a long pause I checked and was told that it had gone but it kept coming back. So I said to explain to grandmother that this black mass was her creation but that it was not her self. She should separate from it and stop putting it there. She had done that bit of karma and wouldn't need it again in the next incarnation, I told her. Yes, she now understood this.

I now turned attention to the missing part and had the patient speak directly to it and ask: "Would you like to come back?" In reply, it said it was unsure. So I left it for a moment and asked the patient: "Would you like the part to come back?" She said yes but I told her not to invite it home yet. I then had her turn back to Gran and ask her: "Would she be willing for the part to come home, that you need it?" Progress; Gran was now fully in agreement!

Back to the patient; I said to her to explain to the part that everything was now OK but that it would now be holding Gran back if it clung on, that she needed to wrap it up here and move on to her next stage of karma. It agreed, reluctantly, to come home.

Setting the stage ready, I had the patient tell Grandma to mock up some beautiful loving hands, ready to hand back the soul part and to mock up some loving hands of her own, ready to receive the part. Ready? Everyone was now poised. "Now take it from her, with love, and say thank you, and then start to pull it towards you".

After some struggle with this move it was obvious there was still some resistance. I asked the question : "Ask the part what would have to happen for it to be happy to come home?" It answered "I want to be able to see grandma when I wish to". A little bit of horse trading was called for here. So I had the patient tell it that Grandma needed to move on, that she had her own purpose to lead, and that if she was truly free she could come down here to earth again and be with those who were dear. I explained that there were many loving couples meet up this way in successive lifetimes and that might be a good answer. I told the part that I had a patient who was the incarnation of her own grandfather.

This seemed to do the trick and the patient at last started to reel it in gently. As the part arrived I saw her face suffuse with a beautiful glow and a smile. I had her welcome it and show it love. This was a very special moment. All that remained was to sign off with Grandma. I told the patient to go out to her again and say that the time was close for the last farewell. "Not this moment but please decide what course you want to follow and I'll leave it to you to break the connection and I will know. And I hope to see you again soon".

Everything seemed OK and, although she was clearly emotional, the patient was smiling with love and sentiment. I ended off and, after giving her the warnings referred to above, took her out for some Gaia energy and a grounding. It seemed like just a matter of moments but the whole thing took about 90 minutes. The following week she reported sparkling fizzy energies, which lasted for several days before calming down.

Her old zestful self seemed to have returned.

6.4 Entities, Possession etc.

Writing about souls and soul parts in this way begs the question: what about entities and possession phenomena? Is there anything to this model?

Well, it happens. It happens a lot. Of course that doesn't make it "normal" but it does mean it is something that needs addressing in the context of personal spiritual wholeness and subjective well-being.

The term 'entity' refers to non-physical beings, presences which come to be attached to human beings and act as psychic parasites, thereby creating various emotional, mental and physical problems ranging from eating disorders and uncontrollable emotions to the most severe diseases.

The topic is both old and new. Old, because in all traditions and folklores of the earth, one finds references to spirits and non-physical beings which can interfere with human beings. Historically we have the sometime presence of *succubi* and *incubi* (non-material entities who like to visit members of the opposite sex in sleep and perform sexual acts). Richard Wagner's opera *Tannhäuser* portrays a love affair between a troubadour and a non-material entity, in this case Venus herself.

In Western medicine, the topic of entities can be regarded as quite new, for it has very rarely been studied seriously. Even though entities appear to play a significant role in a number of mental and health disorders, minor and major, one does not find a systematic way of dealing with them in any of the main forms of therapy presently used. The number of qualified therapists capable of handling entities properly is negligible.

A notable exception is my own subject of Supernoetics® and my model of the "Complex of Self" (section 3.15), in which it can be predicted there will be some interference with "non-self others" in an individual's psychic space. Our method of "spiritual rescue technology" (SRT) developed by David St Lawrence in fact directly addresses this very issue.

Notwithstanding, I was intrigued to come across the traditional Asian model of the "hungry ghost". These are the demon-like creatures described in Buddhist, Taoist, Hindu, Sikh, and Jain texts as the remnants of the dead who are afflicted with insatiable desire, hunger or thirst, supposedly as a result of bad deeds or evil intent carried out in their life times. Hungry ghosts are found in every part of the Far East, from the Philippines to Japan and China, Thailand, Laos, Burma, India and Pakistan, they are universally described as human-like wraiths with mummified skin, narrow withered limbs, grossly bulging stomachs and tiny mouths.

Their craving for satisfaction, be it with food, alcohol or sex, is something that can be imparted to the living. One recurring characteristic is that the possession entity seems to drain the patient's energies.

Even if the feeling was only "as if" something foreign had entered the mind or body, it is still a very vivid reality and the person needs support and some way out of the difficulty.

And there's the first point to make: many people are aware of and talk to separate internal beings they consider "spirit guides" or "personal angels". I have never heard this idea considered a mental dysfunction. Surely it is only a slight shift sideways to suppose it can happen with other beings who come on board and do not necessarily have altruistic motives?

If there is such a thing as a guardian angel, we must allow that there can also be malicious entities? So maybe, apart from the frightening nature of these apparitions and entities, there's no big deal? I think not.

However, let me reassure the reader who has come to this section: entities in the main are foolish and harmless. Yes, you need to get rid of an entity, otherwise it will try and take over your thoughts and actions (that's why it's there).

Certainly, entities like to scare or worry their chosen target. The late Dr Samuel Sagan MD, founder of the Clairvision School, which specializes in entity-clearing, reports entities trying to puff themselves up with outrageous and scary claims, like "I'm going to give you cancer" over and over, or "I hate you! I'm going to kill you!"

But does this need an exorcism? No! The commotion made by the Catholic Church trying to "exorcize" entities or "demons" as they like to call them, creates more trouble than it solves. What is needed is not a confrontational approach but a gentle and compassionate dialogue. Why is it there? What does it want? What does it like most?

Given the accepted non-material nature of such entities, they are capable of nothing much—unless the person goes into agreement with the "creature" and starts a self-fulfilling prophecy! Otherwise, entities are just sad has-beens with deluded ideas of their own power.

We can negotiate terms for it leaving or prepare it for expulsion and then give it the heave-ho, with instructions to go into the light. It takes training, to do it safely and effectively, otherwise the entity can be driven deeper and really hide.

That's the only real issue and why you need to find a competent and knowledgeable entity clearer. We do it in my own Supernoetics® piloting (section 3.12). It comes up over and over and is almost routine. Otherwise I can recommend anyone trained in the ISIS technique (Inner Space Interactive Sourcing) by the Clairvision School or Samuel Sagan personally.

In case you are wondering: no, entities that have been *properly cleared* do not come back (key words in italics).

Here's a case example, edited from the Clairvision website (link in the **Valuable Resources** section in the back of the book): a twenty-four year old woman, a nurse...

What are you feeling?

I can feel something in my chest and in my abdomen. It looks like an old man, like a skeleton. I can feel his ribcage superimposed on mine. I can feel his hip bones as well.

What does it want?

I think it wants me to be his lover. It likes me because I'm young. It likes my strength and my energy. It tries to camouflage things. It tries to make me feel my body, particularly my hips. It makes me walk in a certain way, remembering my hips sexually.

What does it get out of it?

It gets the feeling of being alive. And it likes this weather [it's spring] because it's more sensual. It makes me feel the weather. There is a certain man, where I work... the skeleton is trying to manipulate me to have sex with him. Whenever I speak to that man, it modifies my voice to make it more attractive. And then in the evening it sends erotic scenes of me and that man into my mind. It pushes me to that man. It wants me to be touched by him. If the skeleton could get me to have sex with that man, it would get a sort of thrill out of it. Also it would get more power over me. It has set its mind on it, so if it achieves it it's like reinforcing its ego. And it would gain power from the sexual energy. It wants vaginal and anal sex. It would give it the feeling of extending itself to all of my body. I remember a night when I was five or six. I had a dream about destruction and I had an orgasm and I woke up. It was the skeleton that made me have an orgasm. The skeleton was lying on my body, and the dream was so powerful that the skeleton had an orgasm... Before I had my first boyfriend, it was making me feel unsure of myself. It was making me remember my body. And then I felt guilty and that gave it power over me. When I was fifteen I had my first boyfriend. I can see the skeleton was already there when I was making love, enjoying it lots.

Honestly, this stuff is only scary if you let yourself be scared. It's disturbing of course, and pathological, the woman wants this phenomenon to go away.

The Spiritual Rescue Technology Approach

David St Lawrence's way of dealing with entities is different. To begin with, he considers the obnoxious, disturbing and critical entities are often just angry or outraged, because they cannot make themselves heard or felt. That happens to any of us, here in the material world, if we are trying to communicate and yet everyone ignores us!

So a good place to start is to get into friendly communication with any "ghost" or entity. What does it really want? Ask! You'll often be surprised at the answer. Extreme stimulation or perversion seem very minor wants, compared with the deeper desire to escape enslavement to the material world. Most entities would just like to "go home". Some might ascend, some want to come around again. But being stuck as a skeleton pretending to have sex with a woman of flesh is not life!

So we help them along. Exact details of how to do this are beyond the present book, as you will appreciate. This is not a topic for have-a-go therapists. It requires training in depth.

But before leaving SRT, I should point out that the main breakthrough finding is that *most entities want to help*! They can do things. They can create for you: write music, write novels, paint, teach you hot sex, learn judo! I repeat from my Complex Of Self model, that we are all multiple entities. Get over it! Instead of suppressing it, just explore the positive possibilities.

If we are a family, live like a family.

I have some outstanding reading recommendations in the **Valuable Resources** section!

Move Ins

Not so very different is a phenomenon I have identified among certain patients I met over the years. We all (or most of us) know about the phenomenon of "walk ins". This is where an entity has the chance to enter the body, because the person is drunk, was high on drugs, had an accident or was very sick. It can lead to personality change and all the phenomena I have just been writing about.

I don't propose to deal with that separately.

But I have a growing number of cases where the person changed markedly at the point of death or near death. I believe it denotes the fact that one spiritual entity leaves (or "dies" if you like); then another takes its place. It's a sad sort of scenario, like someone running away, thinking it's all over, and someone else moves in to grab what's left.

Of course this can only take place rarely, when a person is truly sick or dying. Some people have been pronounced dead and then woken up again. But how often do you hear someone question whether it is the *same person* that awakes?

Let me give you an example, known to me: a middle-aged man, a mild-mannered academic professor has a cardiac arrest. He is "out" for several minutes but they finally revive him (or I should say revive the body). Afterwards, he has experienced a major personality change.

Of course doctors would simply attribute this to brain damage, due to hypoxia while the heart was stopped. But consider this: our quiet academic turned into a real gangster, drug running in the Caribbean. He was violent and boasted of murdering people. He even threated to kill his own son, who he believed had cheated him in some way.

I find the brain damage model completely unpersuasive for such a total transformation. It's not as if he was a confused and demented gangster. He was sharp, capable and ruthless. I think what took place is exactly what I am describing. The professor spirit left and the gangster spirit jumped in (maybe he had just been "terminated", in the middle of one of his heists).

Having read this personality shift model and hopefully grasped it, I wonder what you will make of this next story:

It was published in a British newspaper, *The Daily Mail*, 4th May 2016. A young man awoke after an anesthetic administered to let surgeons work on a broken arm. The effect of anesthetic when a person first comes round is well known—in fact it's a time of some danger, when a woman might make wild and unfounded allegations of sexual molestation. She believes it's truly happening but the misperceptions lie within her own mind.

But listen to what this young boy says. He talks like a gangster; asks his Mum to forgive him for killing people. He is told to be quiet by his concerned mother, to which he replies aggressively: 'Why you telling me to shush, lady?'

His voice and accent was very strange. It seems he didn't recognize his own mother. The youth then recounts how his 'boy Rocco' knocked a group of people out cold, leaving his mother perturbed.

She mother asks: 'Who's Rocco?' to which he says, still in an out-of-character voice, 'You know, Rocco in Dubai?' The confused youngster then confesses to his mother that he and his non-existent camel had killed people.

"I'm sorry," he said. "Don't tell my lawyer we killed people, man."

Before long his mother bursts into fits of giggles, while the youth says repeatedly: 'You laughing at me? You laughing at me, man?'

He then describes how he rode his camel through the 'wicked, wicked, wicked, wicked West' of Dubai with his 'hot-ass wife and kids' - which leaves his mother in stitches.

The boy's eyes continue to close but he swears profusely at his mother, causing her to giggle and say: "Quiet down, Honey."

There's more to the entertaining dialogue on YouTube.

OK, on one simple level this is a boy who is disoriented by a dose of anesthetic. It happens, that's true. But doesn't this sound to you like someone is in the wrong body at that time?

It set me wondering for days.

Let's close with something odd and with a peculiar spiritual element, meaning that a non-material being can be very confused about what sex it is supposed to be. That's just a body function, after all!

6.5 Gender Confusion

I'm not saying or implying that homosexuality or transgender uncertainty is a psychiatric condition. Not at all (although it was in the "official" list of psychiatric diseases until 1973, when the diagnosis was removed from the American Psychiatric Associations Diagnostic and Statistical Manual (DSM II).

Up until that time, and still today among many parties and practitioners, there are those who share the view that homosexuality is a defect, or even as morally bad, with some of these theorists being quite open about their belief that homosexuality is a social evil.

For example, psychiatrist and psychoanalyst Edmund Bergler infamously wrote in a book for general audiences, "I have no bias against homosexuals; for me they are sick people requiring medical help... Still, though I have no bias, I would say: Homosexuals are essentially disagreeable people, regardless of their pleasant or unpleasant outward manner... [their] shell is a mixture of superciliousness, fake aggression, and whimpering. Like all psychic masochists, they are subservient when confronted with a stronger person, merciless when in power, unscrupulous about trampling on a weaker person."[349] Phew! That's quite a vicious mouthful, from someone claiming to be not biased.

Freud argued that homosexuality could not be a "degenerative condition" as Richard von Krafft-Ebing maintained because, among other reasons, it was "found in people whose efficiency is unimpaired, and who are indeed distinguished by specially high intellectual development and ethical culture".[350]

It is rare to find a theory of homosexuality that does not draw upon gender beliefs that contain implicit cultural ideas about the "essential" qualities of men and women. "Real men" and "real women" are powerful cultural myths with which even heterosexuals encounter some difficulties. People express gender beliefs, their own and those of the culture in which they live, in everyday language as they either indirectly or explicitly accept and assign gendered meanings to what they and others do, think, and feel.

Gender beliefs touch upon almost every aspect of daily life, including such mundane concerns as what shoes men should wear or "deeper" questions of masculinity such as whether men should openly cry or sleep with other men. Gender beliefs are embedded in questions about what career a woman should pursue and, at another level of discourse, what it would mean if a professional woman were to forego rearing children or pursue a career more aggressively than a man.

Gender Binaries

Gender issues are usually framed around gender binaries. The most ancient and well known is the male/female binary. However there is also the 19th century binary of homosexuality/heterosexuality (or gay/straight in the 20th century) and the emerging 21st century binary of transgender/cisgender.

Such binary-based beliefs underlie mid-20th century theories that children born with anomalous genitalia had to immediately undergo unnecessary medical surgeries in order to "correct" the problem, or more truthfully, to reduce their parents' anxieties about whether they were boys or girls.[351]

Gender beliefs usually only allow for the existence of two sexes. To maintain this gender binary, most cultures traditionally insisted that every individual be assigned to the category of either man or woman at birth and that individuals conform to the category to which they have been assigned thereafter. The categories of "man" and "woman" are considered to be mutually exclusive, although there are exceptions, as in Plato's *Symposium* and some Native American cultures.[352]

The Ancient Greeks, remember, those wise father founders of our whole Western system of philosophy, politics and science, considered homosexuality quite normal and, indeed, they quite ignored any meaningful role for women, other than childbearing.

Rigid gender beliefs usually flourish in fundamentalist, religious communities where any information or alternative explanations that might challenge implicit and explicit assumptions are unwelcome. When entering the realms of gender and sexuality, it is not unusual to encounter another form of binary thinking: "morality tales" about whether certain kinds of thoughts, feelings, or behaviors are "good or bad" or, in some cases, whether they are "good or evil."[353]

Alfred Kinsey moved things forward around the middle of the 20th century, with his famous reports. After surveying thousands of people who were non-psychiatric patients, Kinsey's team found homosexuality to be more common in the general population than was generally believed, around 10%. This finding was sharply at odds with psychiatric claims of the time that homosexuality was extremely rare in the general population.[354] [355]

Additionally, honest modern research showed that many animals manifest homosexual behavior, notably the bonobos monkey, which is reckoned to be Man's closest relative in the wild. No one supposes that God or Mother Nature is twisted or abnormal. This puts a different view on things.

So herewith, we drop the supposition that homosexuality is somehow pathological.

In the late 1950s, psychologist Evelyn Hooker published a study in which she compared psychological test results of 30 gay men with 30 heterosexual controls, none of whom were psychiatric patients. Her study found no more signs of psychological disturbances in the gay male group, a finding that refuted psychiatric beliefs of her time that all gay men had severe psychological disturbances.[356]

American psychiatry mostly ignored this growing body of sex research and, in the case of Kinsey, expressed extreme hostility to findings that contradicted their own theories.

Today, we encounter gay men and women in all walks of life, often strident in the assertion of their "rights" to public display.

My wife Vivien, who meets a lot of gays in her profession (fashion design) points out there are manifestly two types of gay man: the softer, feminized and rather timid version and the very hard, often violent male, with fetishistic and bondage proclivities. The latter rather frightens the former and the two groups seem to have little in common.

But this scientific discussion is no more than a preface to what I really have to say here in this section. It is a totally novel definition of gender and gender confusion. It has nothing to do with hormones or chromosomes. It starts with the model of non-material being and specifically relates to my model of the "multiple self" or The Complex Of Self.

So first of all, if you still haven't done so, be sure to read section 3.15.

You will also need to buy into, or be very tolerant of, the idea of re-incarnation!

Certain things need to be aired and where else are you going to read what's written here below, if it doesn't come from me? No book on holistic treatment of mental health can honestly avoid what's coming next and your author is known for telling it like it is, regardless of how many people squirm in their chair when reading it.

I hope it sheds light on any confusion, that it is healing and that it sets aside all barriers and judgmental religious nonsense...

Gender and Non-Material Being

Once you really understand the complicated relationship between spirits and bodies, you will find that you have a more relaxed view of people who seem to have urges at variance with their body type. You will also have a true understanding of those people of one sex who identify as a member of the opposite sex.

The urges toward sexual activity and sexual attraction are spiritual in nature and can easily be understood once you realize that a spirit has no sex or sexual parts, but generally has a history of operating successfully in a male or female body. For the rest of this article, I will call these spirits with a successful history in bodies of a particular sex "male spirits" or "female spirits".

If a being has operated as a male successfully for many lifetimes and happens to pick up a female body in a moment of excitement or inattention, this "male spirit" may run the female body in a way that emphasizes masculine qualities and may not ever develop a true femininity. Spiritual Rescue Technology (or dealing with multiple selves in Supernoetics®) will not change his sexual orientation, but will make his life as a woman with masculine urges more comfortable.

On the other hand, if a being has operated as a female successfully for many lifetimes and happens to pick up a male body, this "female spirit" may run the male body in a way that emphasizes feminine qualities and may not ever develop a true masculinity. SRT will not change her sexual orientation, but will make her life as a man with feminine urges more comfortable.

Between these two extremes, there are a number of different situations depending on the number of spirits surrounding the body with different gender preferences. These can be helped significantly with SRT processing.

A normally masculine male (male spirit in a male body) with enough lone "female spirits" around him will find that he is attracted to male bodies in a way that he does not consider manly and he is right. His "female spirit" companions are attracted to males and will draw his attention to male bodies and may even arouse him with respect to male bodies. SRT counseling can handle these "female spirits" and get them to leave or work with the male spirit in a less distracting way. When spirits are brought into present time, they usually are able to work in harmony with the spirit running the body regardless of their sexual orientation. They become team members and contribute to the goals of the group.

A normally feminine (female spirit in a female body) with enough lone "male spirits" around her will find that she is attracted to female bodies in a way she does not consider proper and she is right. Her "male spirit" companions are attracted to females and will draw her attention to female bodies and may even arouse her with respect to female bodies. SRT counseling can handle these "male spirits" and get them to leave or work with the female spirit in a less distracting way. When spirits are brought into present time, they usually are able to work in harmony with the spirit running the body regardless of their sexual orientation. They become team members and contribute to the goals of the group.

We also encounter spirits who have run both male and female bodies for a long period of time and who have no real preference for what gender bodies they occupy. They can freely exhibit both male and female characteristics but they can suffer from not understanding or agreeing with what society expects of them. SRT counseling gives them an understanding of their true situation and will also handle any confusions of the beings surrounding this non-preferential being.

Once a being understands why it has certain urges and behaviors, it can freely choose to associate with beings with the same spiritual condition or to associate with anyone without feeling guilty for being different.

Gender uncertainty is not catching, but the spiritual uncertainty may be buried for many years until some event triggers the realization that something is wrong about the role the person has been playing. This realization can happen at any time and initiates a period of stress which may continue for the rest of the person's life. SRT counseling can ease the person into understanding who they really are and how this situation occurred.

Knowing who you really are and why you act the way you do will give you the certainty you need to live fearlessly.

Some people have decided that they want to modify their bodies to match their spiritual orientation, but this has not always been successful and some have regretted their decision to change their physical gender. Physical modification without understanding the spiritual implications will have unexpected results. Counseling will help but unless the counseling truly handles the spirits involved, spiritual problems may make life a real challenge.

If you are one who is comfortable in your gender role, this section may make it easier to understand those who have gender confusions and give you a viewpoint that enables you to help them. If someone says they identify as a member of a different sex, they are probably on the right track.

VALUABLE RESOURCES

More by Dr. Keith Scott-Mumby

For more incredible information about Holistic Psychiatry, check out www.alternative-doctor.com/yourmind for articles, videos, and more!

Supernoetics™

Punk Psychology

Diet Wise

Remember, Supernoetics® is a HUGE library of protocols, workshops, hacks, and tips that can solve just about any life situation. Punk Psychology® is only a small part of the whole; but a very handy part, nonetheless.

Go to www.PunkPsychology.net and look around. You can watch videos, download eBooks and pamphlets, sign up for some training to become a pilot and help change the world.

Or if you are struggling and want direct and immediate help, we can book you session (we call them "flights") with one of our accredited pilots. Relief will be on its way within hours. Just email Carmela at: carmela@supernoetics.com

Recommended Reading

The Myth of Mental Illness: Foundations of a Theory of Personal Conduct by Thomas S. Szasz

The Divided Self: An Existential Study in Sanity and Madness by R. Laing

The Hacking of the American Mind: The Science Behind the Corporate Takeover of Our Bodies and Brains by Robert H. Lustig

Toxic Psychiatry: Why Therapy, Empathy and Love Must Replace the Drugs, Electro-shock, and Biochemical Theories of the "New Psychiatry" by Peter Breggin, MD

Brain Disabling Treatments in Psychiatry: Drugs, Electroshock, and the Psychopharma-ceutical Complex by Peter R. Breggin, MD

Schizophrenia - The Sacred Symbol of Psychiatry by Professor Thomas S. Szasz, MD

Schizophrenia - Medical Diagnosis or Moral Verdict? By Theodore R. Sarbin, PhD and James C. Mancuso, PhD

Against Therapy by Jeffrey Masson, Ph.D.

Schiz-o-phre-nia: Straight Talk for Family and Friends by Maryellen Walsh

Surviving Schizophrenia: A Family Manual by E. Fuller Torrey, MD

Prisoners of Psychiatry by Bruce Ennis

Grain Brain by David Perlmutter

Madness: A Bipolar Life by Marya Hornbacher

The Physiology of Consciousness by Robert Keith Wallace

The Twelve Healers by Edward Bach

Loneliness: Human Nature and the Need for Social Connection by John Cacioppo

Biochemical Individuality by Roger J Williams

Brain Allergies by William H. Philpott MD and Dwight K. Kalita

The Defective Delinquent and Insane: the Relation of Focal Infections to Their Causation, Treatment and Prevention by Henry Cotton

Not All In The Mind by Richard Mackarness

The Complete Guide To Food Allergy and Intolerance by Jonathan Brostoff

Is This Your Child? Discovering and Treating Unrecognized Allergies In Children and Adults by Doris Rapp

Human Ecology and Susceptibility to the Chemical Environment by Dr. Theron Randolph

Chemical Victims by Richard Mackarness

The Yeast Connection by William Crook, MD

What Your Doctor May Not Tell You About The Menopause by John R. Lee

The Missing Diagnosis by Dr. C.Orian Truss

Forty Something Forever by Harold and Arline Brecher

Climate: The Key To Understanding Business Cycles by Professor Raymond Wheeler

Entity Possession: Freeing The Energy Body of Negative Influences by Dr. Samuel Sagan

Spiritual Rescue Technology: A Practical Solution for Changing Your Life by David St Lawrence

Soul Retrieval: Mending the Fragmented Self by Sandra Ingerman

The Relaxation Response by Dr. Herbert Benson

The Naked Spirit by Jon Whale

The Catalyst of Power by Jon Whale

Helpful Links

MindFreedom International: http://www.mindfreedom.org/

Dr. Fred Baughman: http://www.adhdfraud.net/

Psychiatric Drug Facts: https://breggin.com/brain-disabling-treatments-in-psychiatry/

Forest Bathing: www.shinrin-yoku.org

Mycoformulas: www.mycoformulas.com

Not Milk: www.notmilk.com

ADD/ADHD Support Site: www.attentiondeficit-add-adhd.com

Janie Bowthorope (Stop the Thyroid Madness): www.StopTheThyroidMadness.com

Diagnos-techs (hormone testing): www.diagnos-techs.com

Jon Whale (Whale Medical): http://www.whalemedical.com/

Dr. Greg Newson ND (ConqueringPyroluria): www.conqueringpyroluria.com

Hindawi International Scholarly Research Notices: https://www.hindawi.com/journals/isrn/2013/127365/

UCSF Researchers Control Embryonic Stem Cells With Light (free video) https://www.youtube.com/watch?v=CK7NpGQngfg

DUTCH Hormone Test: https://dutchtest.com

Erethism (Matter Hatter disease): https://en.wikipedia.org/wiki/Erethism

Lynn Woodland (exceptional human experiences): http://www.lynnwoodland.com/

Norm Shealy (Shealy Wellness): https://normshealy.com/the-sacred-rings/the-ring-of-air/

Richard Schwartz's Internal Family Systems: https://selfleadership.org/

Clairvision School (Meditation and More): http://www.clairvision.org/index.html

Beta Glucan Benefits (free PDF) www.beta-glucan-info.com/pdf/JANA2008.pdf

Open GlycoScience (free PDF) https://benthamopen.com/contents/pdf/TOGLYJ/TO-GLYJ-3-1.pdf

The Quick Environmental Exposure and Sensitivity Inventory (QEESI) (free PDF) http://familymed.uthscsa.edu/qeesi.pdf

Christopher Shade Mercury Challenge Test (free PDF): https://www.quicksilverscientific.com/images/art/PDF/ChallengeTestsForMercury20140508.pdf

Ralph Campbell, MD and Robert G. Smith, PhD: Orthomolecular Medicine News Service: http://orthomolecular.org/ (as well as some additional references you might be interested in exploring such as this article http://orthomolecular.org/library/articles/webach. shtml and the scientific journal articles below)

- Smesny S, Berger G, Rosburg T, et al. Potential use of the topical niacin skin test in early psychosis -- a combined approach using optical reflection spectroscopy and a descriptive rating scale. Psychiatr Res. 2003 May-Jun;37:237-247. https://www.ncbi.nlm.nih.gov/pubmed/12650743

- Messamore E. Niacin subsensitivity is associated with functional impairment in schizophrenia. Schizophr Res. 2012 May;137(1-3):180-4. https://www.ncbi.nlm.nih.gov/pubmed/22445461

- Lien YJ, Huang SS, Liu CM, et al. A genome-wide quantitative linkage scan of niacin skin flush response in families with schizophrenia. Schizophr Bull. 2013 Jan;39:68-76. https://www.ncbi.nlm.nih.gov/pubmed/21653277

- Nilsson BM, Holm G, Hultman CM, Ekselius L. Cognition and autonomic function in schizophrenia: inferior cognitive test performance in electrodermal and niacin skin flush non-responders. Eur Psychiatry. 2015 Jan;30:8-13. https://www.ncbi.nlm.nih.gov/pubmed/25169443

- Berger GE, Smesny S, Sch"fer MR, et al. Niacin Skin Sensitivity Is Increased in Adolescents at Ultra-High Risk for Psychosis. PLoS One. 2016 Feb 19;11(2):e0148429. https://www.ncbi.nlm.nih.gov/pubmed/26894921

- Yao JK, Dougherty GG Jr, Gautier CH, Haas GL, Condray R, Kasckow JW, Kisslinger BL, Gurklis JA, Messamore E. Prevalence and Specificity of the Abnormal Niacin Response: A Potential Endophenotype Marker in Schizophrenia. Schizophr Bull. 2016 Mar;42(2):369-376. https://www.ncbi.nlm.nih.gov/pubmed/26371338

- Sun L, Yang X, Jiang J, et al. Identification of the Niacin-Blunted Subgroup of Schizophrenia Patients from Mood Disorders and Healthy Individuals in Chinese Population. Schizophr Bull. 2017 Oct 25. https://www.ncbi.nlm.nih.gov/pubmed/29077970

- Langbein K, Schmidt U, Schack S, et al. State marker properties of niacin skin sensitivity in ultra-high risk groups for psychosis - An optical reflection spectroscopy study. Schizophr Res. 2017 Jun 8. pii: S0920-9964(17)30335-3. https://www.ncbi.nlm.nih.gov/pubmed/28602647

- Messamore E. The niacin response biomarker as a schizophrenia endophenotype: A status update. Prostaglandins Leukot Essent Fatty Acids. 2017 Jun 30. pii: S0952-3278(16)30249-6. https://www.ncbi.nlm.nih.gov/pubmed/28688777

Life Extension Magazine: http://www.lifeextension.com/

- Cytokine Test ($399 at time of writing)

- CRP-hs ($42 at time of writing)

- Protecting Against the Lethal Effects of Chronic Inflammation http://www.life-extension.com/Magazine/2003/5/report_inflam/Page-01

- Grumpy No More: Testosterone Deficiency & Depression http://www.lifeextension.com/magazine/2002/8/report_test/page-02?p=1

HEEL: www.biopathica.com

- Ignatia-homaccord – grief depression

- Nervo-Heel – reactive depression

Vaxa: www.vaxa.com

- Deprex

Passion4LifeVitamins: https://passion4lifevitamins.com/

Youngevity (MLM where I get some direct materials): https://youngevity.com/

QuickSilver Scientific: https://www.quicksilverscientific.com/

REFERENCES

1   Personal Letter from Sir Karl Popper, 1961

2   The British Journal of Psychiatry May 2012, 200 (5) 393-398; DOI: 10.1192/bjp.bp.111.104257

3   National Alliance of Mental Illness: Mental Health By The Numbers

4   The Washington Post: Facebook now has a chatbot therapist to help reduce your anxieties

5   Futurism: AI and VR Could Completely Transform How Doctors Diagnose and Treat Mental Disorders

6   JMIR Ment Health 2017;4(2):e19 doi:10.2196/mental.7785

7   MIT Technology Review: The Emerging Science of Computational Psychiatry

8   Project Gutenberg Self-Publishing Press: Bedlam Hospital

9   Breggin P. *Toxic Psychiatry*, St Martin's Press, New York, 1991

10   Hawaii *J Med Public Health*. 2012 Nov; 71(11): 326–328

11   Citizens Commission on Human Rights: Deadly Restraints: Psychiatry's 'Therapeutic' Assault

12   American Statesman: When discipline turns fatal

13   MindFreedom International

14   Wiki Medical: History of Psychosurgery

15   The Guardian: Shrinks: The Untold Story of Psychiatry by Jeffrey Lieberman review – genial and triumphalist

16   The Washington Post: This secret experiment tricked psychiatrists into diagnosing sane people as having schizophrenia

17   Association for Psychological Science: Scientific "freedom" and the Fountain of Youth

18   Daily News: When Science Turns Unscientific

19   PLOS Medicine: Why Most Published Research Findings Are False

20   Science: Panel Calls for Closer Oversight of Biomarker Tests

21   Reuters: In cancer science, many "discoveries" don't hold up

22   Economist, Oct 19th 2013

23   *New Scientist*; Volume 230, Issue 3069, 16 April 2016, Pages 38–41

24   Jon Rappoport's Blog: 2 new smoking guns: Psychiatry is a complete fraud

25   Wired: Inside the Battle to Define Mental Illness

26   The New York Times: SCIENTIST AT WORK: Allen J. Frances; Revamping Psychiatrists' Bible

27   *Brain-Disabling Treatments in Psychiatry* (2008): Drugs, Electroshock, and the Psychopharmaceutical Complex by Peter Breggin, M.D. Hardback Published by Springer Publishing Co. New 2008 Edition Revised And Updated

28   The International Journal of the Addictions: "An Outline of Hazardous Side Effects of Ritalin (Methylphenidate)" v.21(7), pp. 837-841

29   *Toxic Psychiatry*, Dr. Peter Breggin, St. Martin's Press, 1991

30   *Toxic Psychiatry*, Dr. Peter Breggin, St. Martin's Press, 1991. pp. 84-86

31   The Journal of Mind and Behaviour, Summer and Autumn 1990, Volume 11, Numbers 3 and 4 Pages 425 (179) - 464 (218)

32   A. Deutsch, *The Shame Of The States* (New York: Harcourt Brace, 1948), 41

33   "Wonder Drug of 1954?" *Time*, June 14, 1954

34   J. Swazey, *Chlorpromazine in Psychiatry* (Cambridge, MA: MIT Press, 1974), 134-135

35   F. Ayd Jr., *Discoveries in Biological Psychiatry* (Philadelphia: Lippincott, 1970), 160

36   O. Sacks, Awakenings (New York: Knopf Doubleday, 1973), p. 14).

37   https://en.wikipedia.org/wiki/Amitriptyline

38   Robert Whitaker, *Anatomy of an Epidemic Magic Bullets, Psychiatric Drugs, and the Astonishing Rise of Mental Illness in America*:
Broadway Books, Kindle edition, location 1101 of 7582

39   [*Psychiatric Drugs: An Assault on the Human Condition*, Street Spirit, Robert Whitaker interview by Terry Messman, Posted: August 20, 2005: http://thestreetspirit.org/August2005/interview.htm

40   Counter Punch Dec 29, 2015; www.counterpunch.org

41   Asberg, M., "Serotonin depression: A biochemical subgroup within the affective disorders?" Science 191(1976):478-80

42   Maas, J., "Pretreatment neurotransmitter metabolite levels and response to tricyclic antidepressant drugs," American Journal of Psychiatry 141 (1984):1159-71

43   Bowers, M., "Central dopamine turnover in schizophrenic syndromes", *Archives of General Psychiatry* 31(1974):50-54

44   Post, R., "Cerebrospinal fluid amine metabolites in acute schizophrenia", Archives of General Psychiatry 32(1975):1063-68

45   Lee, T., Seeman, P., Tourtellotte, W.W., Farley, I.J., Hornykeiwicz, O., "Binding of 31-1-neuroleptics and 3H-apomorphine in schizophrenic brains," Nature 374 (1978): 897-900

46   D. Burt, "Antischizophrenic drugs: chronic treatment elevates dopamine receptor binding in brain," Science 196 (1977): 326-27

47   M. Porceddu, "[3H]SCH 23390 binding sites increase after chronic blockade of d-1 dopamine receptors," European Journal of Pharmacology 118 (1985): 367-70

48   J. Martinot, "Striatal D2 dopaminergic receptors assessed with positron emission tomography and bromospiperone in untreated schizophrenic patients"

49   American Journal of Psychiatry 147 (1990): 44-50; L. Farde, "D2 dopamine receptors in neuroleptic-naive schizophrenic patients"

50   Archives of General Psychiatry 47 (1990): 213-19; J. Hietala, "Striatal D2 dopamine receptor characteristics in neuroleptic-naïve schizophrenic patients studied with positron emission tomography"

51   Archives of General Psychiatry 51 (1994): 116-23

52   Whitaker, R., Anatomy of an Epidemic, Kindle edition, 2016, Location 1280 of 7582

53   BMJ Open. Published online December 18, 2014

54   Able Child: New Information About Adam Lanza's Mental Health Treatment Reveals Multiple Drugs

55   Jon Rappoport's Blog: Psychiatrists drugging children for "social justice"

56   BMJ 2016;352:i1457

57   National Institute of Mental Health: Post by Former NIMH Director Thomas Insel: Are Children Overmedicated?

58   Medicine (Baltimore). 2016 Jun; 95(23): e3784

59   British Journal of Psychiatry 161, suppl. 18, (1992):145-53.

60   Cullberg, J. Acta Psychiatrica Scandinavica 83 (1991):363-72.

61   Seikkula, J. Psychotherapy Research 16 (2006):214-228.

62   Bakker, J.M., Lieverse, R., Geschwind, N., Peeters, F., Myin-Germeys, I. and Wichers, M., 2016. The Two-Sided Face of Antidepressants: The Impact of Their Use on Real-Life Affective Change during Mindfulness-Based Cognitive Therapy. Psychotherapy and Psychosomatics, 85(3), pp.180-182

63   William WK Zung. A Self-Rating Depression Scale. 12: Arch Gen Psychiatry 63-70. 1965

64   Agency for Healthcare Policy and Research. Depression in Primary Care. Vol. 1. Detection and Diagnosis. Publication 93-0550. Rockville, MD: US Dept of Health and Human Services; 1993

65   Lepine JP, Gastpar M, Mendlewicz J, et al. Depression in the community: the first pan-European study DEPRES (Depression Research in European Society). Int Clin Psychopharmacol. 1997;12:19-29.

66   Katon W, Schulberg H. Epidemiology of depression in primary care. Gen Hosp Psychiatry. 1992;14:237-247.

67   Psychosom Med. 2007;69:217-224

68   Induction of autoimmune depression in mice by anti-ribosomal P antibodies via the limbic system. Arthritis Rheum. 2007 Mar;56(3):938-48

69   Edwards R, Peet M, Shay J, Horrobin D. Omega-3 polyunsaturated fatty acid levels in the diet and in red blood cell membranes of depressed patients. J Affect Disord 1998 Mar; 48(2- 3):149-55

70   Do essential fatty acids have a role in the treatment of depression? Journal of Affective Disorders 93 (2006) 117–123

71   Psychosom Med. 2007;69:217-224

72   Feed Your Brain, Ode Magazine, Jurriaan Kamp, vol 5 issue 7, pp 40- 45

73   Phytother Res. 2014 Apr;28(4):579-85. doi: 10.1002/ptr.5025. Epub 2013 Jul 6

74   Mediterranean Diet Improves Depression - Medscape - Dec 22, 2017

75   *Journal of Nutritional Neuroscience*. Published online: 07 Dec 2017. https://doi.org/10.1080/1028415X.2017.1411320

76   *Journal Critical Reviews in Food Science and Nutrition* https://doi.org/10.1080/10408398.2017.1399860

77   Musselman DL, Miller AH, Porter MR, et al. Higher than normal plasma interleukin-6 concentrations in cancer patients with depression. *Am J Psychiatry*. 2001

78   Aug;158(8):1252-7 and Corti R, Hutter R, Badimon JJ, Fuster V. Evolving concepts in the triad of atherosclerosis, inflammation and thrombosis. *J Thromb Thrombolysis*. 2004 Feb;17(1):35-44.

79   Arch Gen Psychiatry. 2007;64:225-233, 242-249

80   American College of Cardiology 56th Annual Scientific Sessions: Abstract 1004-61. March 24 – 27, 2007

81   Bottiglieri T, Laundy M, Crellin R, Toone BK, Carney MW, Reynolds EH. Homocysteine, folate methylation, and monoamine metabolism in depression. J Neurol Neurosurg Psychiatry. 2000 Aug;69(2):228-32

82   Fava M, Borus JS, Alpert JE, Nierenberg AA, Rosenbaum JF, Bottiglieri T. Folate, vitamin B12, and homocysteine in major depressive disorder. Am J Psychiatry. 1997 Mar;154(3):426-8

83   *American Journal of Epidemiology* 1996; vol 143, no. 9 845-859

84   *Biofactors*. 2006;26(1):45-57

85   S-Adenosyl-L-Methionine (SAMe): In Depth". NCCIH. January 11, 2017

86   Ageing Res Rev. 2005 May;4(2):141-94

87   *Journal of Clinical Endocrinology & Metabolism*,1984; vol 58, pages 105-109 and Biological Psychiatry Volume 54, Issue 12, 15 December 2003, Pages 1389-1398

88   *Prog Neuropsychopharmacol Biol Psychiatry*. 2007 Mar 7; ePub, ahead of print

89   ACPM 2007 Annual Meeting: Poster 16. Presented February 22, 2007

90   Sabelli H, Fink P, Fawcett J, et al. Sustained antidepressant effects of PEA replacement. J Neuropsychiatry 1996;8:168–71

91   *Journal of Orthomolecular Psychiatry* (Regina) 5(3):199-202, 1976 and *Biological Psychiatry* 10(2):235-239, 1975

92   Diabetes Care. 2007;30:872- 877

93   Arch Intern Med. 2007;167:802-807

94   Psychosom Med 2007;69:235-241

95   Diabetes Care 2007;30:459-466

96   Hickie I, Bennett B, Mitchell P, Wilhelm K, Orlay W. Clinical and subclinical hypothyroidism inpatients with chronic and treatment-resistant depression. Aust N Z J Psychiatry 1996;30(2):246-52

97   Jackson IM. The thyroid axis and depression. Thyroid 1998;8(10):951-6

98   Joffe RT, Marriott M. Thyroid hormone levels and recurrence of major depression. Am J Psychiatry 2000;157:1689-1691

99   Archives of General Psychiatry 1993; 50(5):387-93 and Journal of Clinical Psychiatry 1993; 54(2):47-54

100 Appelhof BC, Brouwer JP, van Dyck R, Fliers E, Hoogendijk WJ, Huyser J, Schene AH, Tijssen JG, Wiersinga WM. Triiodothyronine addition to paroxetine in the treatment of major depressive disorder. J Clin Endocrinol Metab 2004:89:6271-6

101 Psychoneuroendocrinol. 2006;31(9):1029-1035

102 Cavallini G, Caracciolo S, Vitali G, Modenini F, Biagiotti G. Carnitine versus androgen administration in the treatment of sexual dysfunction, depressed mood, and fatigue associated with male aging. Urology. 2004 Apr;63(4):641-6

103 Molecular Human Reproduction 2006 12(12):749-754; doi:10.1093/molehr/gal082]. This action is probably the explanation behind premenstrual dysphoric disorder (progesterone predominates over estrogen in the latter half of the menstrual cycle)

104 Morris MC, Evans DA, Bienias JL, et al. Dietary niacin and the risk of incident Alzheimer's disease and of cognitive decline. J Neurol Neurosurg Psychiatry. 2004 Aug;75(8):1093-9

105 Clin Exp Immunol. 2003 Jan;131(1):48-52

106 High vitamin B12 level and good treatment outcome may be associated in major depressive disorder. *BMC Psychiatry* 2003, 3:17

107 *Journal of the American College of Nutrition*, Volume 19, 2000 - Issue 1. pp 68-76. Published online: 14 Jun 2013

108 Morris MS, Fava M, Jacques PF, Selhub J Rosenbert IH. Depression and folate status in the US population. Psychother Psychosom. 2003 Mar;72(2):80-7

109 Wacker WEC and Parisi AF. Magnesium Metabolism. New England Journal of Medicine. 1968;278(12):658-776.

110 Biol Psychiatry. 1985 Feb;20(2):163-71

111 Neuropsychobiology. 1999;39(2):63-70

112 King D, Mainous A 3rd, Geesey M, Woolson R. Dietary magnesium and C-reactive protein levels. J Am Coll Nutr. 2005 Jun 24(3):166-71

113 Maes M et al 1994, 1997; McLoughlin IJ et al 1990

114 Takeda A 2000

115 Nowak G et al 1999

116 J Affect Disord. 2009 Nov;118(1-3):187-95. doi: 10.1016/j.jad.2009.02.014. Epub 2009 Mar 10

117 Vasak, M. (2005), "Advances in metallothionein structure and functions", J. Trace Elem. Med. Biol., 19 (1): page 13-17

118 *Adv Mind Body Med.* 2017 Spring;31(2):4-11

119 DIET WISE, Keith Scott-Mumby MD, Mother Whale Inc. Las Vegas, 2007: ISBN 980-0-9838784-1-4

120 SB Harvey et al. Am J Psychiatry 175 (1), 28-36. 2017 Oct 03

121 *Schizophrenia - The Sacred Symbol of Psychiatry*, professor Thomas S. Szasz, MD, Syracuse University Press, 1988, p. 191)

122 *Schizophrenia - Medical Diagnosis or Moral Verdict?*, Theodore R. Sarbin, Ph.D. and James C. Mancuso, Ph.D., Pergamon Press, 1980, p. 221

123 *Against Therapy*, published in 1988, Jeffrey Masson, Ph.D., Atheneum, p. 2.

124 *Schiz-o-phre-nia: Straight Talk for Family and Friends*, published in 1985, Maryellen Walsh, Warner Books, p. 41)

125 E. Fuller Torrey, MD, *Surviving Schizophrenia: A Family Manual*, 1988. Harper & Row, p. 5

126 Bruce Ennis, *Prisoners of Psychiatry*: Harcourt Brace Jovanovich, Inc., 1972, p. 22.

127 Jack D. Barchas, M.D., et al., "Biogenic Amine Hypothesis of Schizophrenia", appearing in Psychopharmacology: From Theory to Practice, Oxford University Press, 1977, p. 100.

128 Jerrold S. Maxmen, M.D., *The New Psychiatry*, 1985 Mentor, pp. 142 & 154.

129 *Molecules of the Mind* Professor Jon Franklin, p. 114.

130 SS Key and S Matthyse. The New Harvard Guide to Psychiatry, Harvard University Press, 1988, p. 148

131 *Schizophrenia Revealed - From Neurons to Social Interaction* (W.W.Norton, New York, 2001), Michael Foster Green, Ph.D., pages 4, 6, and 95

132 Dohan FC. Hypothesis: genes and neuroactive peptides from food as cause of schizophrenia. Advances in biochemical psychopharmacology. 1980;22:535–548

133 Psychiatr Clin North Am. 2007 Sep; 30(3): 323–338. doi: 10.1016/j.psc.2007.04.007

134 Psychiatr Clin North Am. 2007 Sep; 30(3): 323–338. doi: 10.1016/j.psc.2007.04.007

135 Zandi MS. et al, (2011), J Neurol, 258, 686 – 688

136 *Orthomolecular Medicine News Service*, October 27, 2014: http://orthomolecular.org/resources/omns/v10n18.shtml

137 Gilmer, T. P., Dolder, C. R., Lacro, J. P., Folsom, D. P., Lindamer, L., Garcia, P., & Jeste, D. V. (2004). Adherence to treatment with antipsychotic medication and health care costs among Medicaid beneficiaries with schizophrenia. American Journal of Psychiatry, 161(4), 692-699. http://www.ncbi.nlm.nih.gov/pubmed/15056516

138 McGrath, J., Saha, S., Chant, D., & Welham, J. (2008). Schizophrenia: A concise overview of incidence, prevalence, and mortality. Epidemiologic Reviews, 30, 67-76. http://www.ncbi.nlm.nih.gov/pubmed/18480098

139 http://schizophreniabulletin.oxfordjournals.org/content/14/4/489.1.long

140 David Perlmutter, *Grain Brain* (Little, Brown and Company, Boston, 2013)

141 Hoffer A, Osmond H. Treatment of schizophrenia with nicotinic acid: a ten-year follow-up. Acta Psychiat Scand 1964, 40: 171-189. https://www.ncbi.nlm.nih.gov/pubmed/14235254

142 Xu XJ, Jiang GS. Niacin-respondent subset of schizophrenia -- a therapeutic review. Eur Rev Med Pharmacol Sci. 2015;19:988-997. https://www.ncbi.nlm.nih.gov/pubmed/25855923

143 Hoffer A, Saul AW, Foster HD. Niacin: The Real Story: Learn about the Wonderful Healing Properties of Niacin. Basic Health Publications, Inc; 2015. ISBN-13: 978-1591202752.

144 Hoffer A. Adventures in Psychiatry: The Scientific Memoirs of Dr. Abram Hoffer. KOS Publishing, 2005. ISBN-13: 978-0973194562

145 Gurillo, P et al (2015) Does tobacco cause psychosis? Systematic review and meta-analysis Lancet Psychiatry http://dx.doi.org/10.1016/S2215-0366(15)00152-2

146 BBC website. http://www.bbc.com/news/health-22691718

147 National Institute of Mental Health

148 Brain Sci. 2017 Oct 30;7(11). pii: E144. doi: 10.3390/brainsci7110144

149 Enhancement of hippocampal neurogenesis by lithium. J Neurochem. 2000 Oct;75(4):1729-34

150 14S,21R-Dihydroxydocosahexaenoic Acid Remedies Impaired Healing and Mesenchymal Stem Cell Functions in Diabetic WoundsJ Biol Chem 2011 286:(6) 4443-4453

151 J Thyroid Res. 2011; 2011: 306367

152 J Neuropsychiatry Clin Neurosci. 2011 Spring; 23(2): E12–E13. doi: 10.1176/appi.neuropsych.23.2.E12

153 Kessler RC, Aguilar-Gaxiola S, Alonso J, Chatterji S, Lee S, Ormel J, Ustün TB, Wang PS. The global burden of mental disorders: an update from the WHO World Mental Health (WMH) surveys. Epidemiol Psichiatr Soc 2009;18(1):23–33

154 Oxidative Medicine and Cellular Longevity. Volume 2016 (2016), Article ID 1564257, 9 pages. http://dx.doi.org/10.1155/2016/1564257

155 Bioorg Med Chem. 2009 Jan 15;17(2):867-71. doi: 10.1016/j.bmc.2008.11.034. Epub 2008 Nov 20

156 Phytother Res. 2009 Aug;23(8):1075-81. doi: 10.1002/ptr.2712

157 Modulation of mood and cognitive performance following acute administration of Melissa officinalis (lemon balm). Pharmacology Biochemistry and Behavior. Volume 72, Issue 4, July 2002, Pages 953-964

158 Neuropsychopharmacology volume 28, pages 1871–1881 (2003) doi:10.1038/sj.npp.1300230

159 Curr Pharm Des. 2006;12(35):4613-23

160 Blaylock, Russell L., *Excitoxins: The Taste that Kills*, 1994, p. 200

161 http://newsroom.ucla.edu/releases/this-is-your-brain-on-sugar-ucla-233992

162 Samuels, Adrienne, "Excitatory Amino Acids in Neurologic Disorders," The New England Journal of Medicine, 331(4): 274-5, July 28, 1994

163 Based on an article from NOHA News, Winter 1995 - The American Nutrition Association was formerly known as the Nutrition for Optimal Health Association [NOHA].

164 *The Physiology Of Consciousness,* Robert Keith Wallace (a joint publication of the Institute of Science, Technology and Public Policy and Maharishi International University Press, Iowa, USA, 1986).

165 *Applied Psychophysiology and Biofeedback*, March 2002, Volume 27, Issue 1, pp 45-98

166 https://en.wikipedia.org/wiki/Autogenic_training

167 Rivera, Jose Luis Gonzalez de (2001), Autogenic Analysis: The Tool Freud Was Looking For (PDF). *International Journal of Psychotherapy* 6 (1). Pp. 67-68

168 www.shinrin-yoku.org

169 Mother Earth News: Your Brain on Nature: Forest Bathing and Reduced Stress

170 University of Rochester: Nature Makes Us More Caring, Study Says

171 https://wakeup-world.com/2015/03/18/healing-body-and-soul-through-the-japanese-art-of-shinrin-yoku/

172 Institute of Psychiatric Services (IPS): The Mental Health Services 2016 Conference. Abstract 14. Presented October 7, 2016

173 American Academy of Neurology, news release, Feb. 23, 2011

174 Shawn D Gale, Lance David Erickson, Andrew Berrett, Bruce L Brown, Dawson W Hedges (2016). Infectious disease burden and cognitive function in young to middle-aged adults. *Brain Behavior and Immunity.* 2016 Feb;52:161-8

175 *New Scientist* 4 Jun 2016, vol 230 No 3076

176 N Engl J Med 2003; 348:2508-2516, June 19, 2003DOI: 10.1056/NEJMoa022252

177 http://www.sciencedirect.com/science/article/pii/S2352873717300598

178 *The Lancet*, 2015; DOI: 10.1016/S0140-6736(15)60461-5

179 J Tradit Complement Med. 2013 Jan-Mar; 3(1): 62–68. doi: 10.4103/2225-4110.106549

180 http://www.vitawithimmunity.com/wp-content/uploads/2014/11/VetvickaJANA2008Hi-Lites.pdf

181 https://www.sciencedirect.com/science/journal/0946672X

182 Behav Processes. 2013 Jun;96:27-35. doi: 10.1016/j.beproc.2013.02.007. Epub 2013 Feb 27

183 *Proceedings of The National Academy Of Sciences of The USA.* May 16, 2016, doi: 10.1073/pnas.1600324113

184 Serotonin in aging, late-life depression, and Alzheimer's disease: the emerging role of functional imaging. *Neuropsychopharmacology.* 1998 Jun;18(6):407-30

185 Geldenhuys WJ, Van der Schyf CJ. Role of serotonin in Alzheimer's disease: a new therapeutic target? CNS Drugs. 2011 Sep 1;25(9):765-81. doi: 10.2165/11590190-000000000-00000. Review. PubMed PMID: 21870888

186 https://www.theguardian.com/society/2013/jul/30/dementia-gardening-helping-people

187 Neural Regen Res. 2016 Apr; 11(4): 563–565. doi: 10.4103/1673-5374.180737

188 https://www.research.va.gov/currents/spring2015/spring2015-7.cfm

189 https://www.neuroscientificallychallenged.com/blog/know-your-brain-default-mode-network

190 Proc Natl Acad Sci U S A. 2001 Jan 16;98(2):676-82

191 https://www.theguardian.com/world/2002/feb/19/highereducation.research

192 The efficacy of adjunctive N-acetylcysteine in major depressive disorder: a double-blind, randomized, placebo-controlled trial. *J Clin Psychiatry.* 2014 Jun;75(6):628-36. doi: 10.4088/JCP.13m08454

193 Dev Psychobiol. 1985 Jan;18(1):59-66

194 BalestreriR., FontunaL., AstengoF. (1987). A double-blind placebo controlled evaluation of the safety and efficacy of vinpocetine in the treatment of patients with chronic vascular senile cerebral dysfunction. Journal of the American Geriatric Society, 35, 425–130

195 Lancet. 2007;369:208-216

196 Environ Health Perspect. 2006 Feb; 114(2): 156–164

197 Published online before print December 9, 2015, Neurology 10.1212/WNL.0000000000002254

198 Brain Behav. 2017 Jan; 7(1): e00598. Published online 2016 Oct 31. doi: 10.1002/brb3.598

199 Liu, G., Sterling, N. W., Kong, L., Lewis, M. M., Mailman, R. B., Chen, H., Leslie, D. and Huang, X. (2017), Statins may facilitate Parkinson's disease: Insight gained from a large, national claims database. *Mov Disord*, 32: 913–917. doi:10.1002/mds.27006

200 Barkley RA, DuPaul GJ, McMurray MB. Comprehensive evaluation of attention deficit disorder with and without hyperactivity as defined by research criteria. J Consult Clin Psychol 1990; 58: 775-789

201 Biederman J, Mick E, Faraone SV, et al. Influence of gender on attention deficit hyperactivity disorder in children referred to a psychiatric clinic. Am J Psychiatry 2002; 159: 36-42.

202 Biederman J, Faraone SV. The Massachusetts General Hospital studies of gender influences on attention-deficit/hyperactivity disorder in youth and relatives. Psychiatr Clin North Am 2004; 27: 225-232.

203 Biederman J, Petty CR, Clarke A, et al. Predictors of persistent ADHD: An 11-year follow-up study. J Psychiatr Res 2011; 45: 150-155.

204 Biederman J, Petty CR, O'Connor KB, et al. Predictors of persistence in girls with attention deficit hyperactivity disorder: results from an 11-year controlled follow-up study.

Acta Psychiatr Scand 2012; 125: 147-156. - See more at: http://www.adhd-institute.com/burden-of-adhd/epidemiology/gender/#st-hash.joKyy05q.dpuf

205 Newcorn JH, Halperin JM, Jensen PS, et al. Symptom profiles in children with ADHD: effects of comorbidity and gender. J Am Acad Child Adolesc Psychiatry 2001; 40: 137-146.

206 Egger J, Soothill J.F., Carter C.M. et al. Is migraine food allergy? A double-blind placebo-controlled trial of oligoantigenic diet treatment. Lancet 1983; 2: 865-869.

207 Egger J. Soothill J..F., Carter C.M. et al. Controlled trial of oligo antigenic treatment in the hyperkinetic syndrome. Lancet 1985; 1: 540-545

208 Newsweek 2014: http://www.newsweek.com/childrens-movies-are-rife-murder-says-science-293466

209 Scales consisting of the Conners' Parent Rating Scale-Revised and the Conners' Teacher Rating Scale-Revised, filled out by parents/caregivers and teachers, respectively. Conners CK. Development of the CRS-R. In: Conners CK, ed. Conners' Rating Scales-Revised. North Tonawanda, NY: Multi-Health Systems. 2001:83-98.

210 Journal of Restorative Medicine, Volume 2, Number 1, October 2013, pp. 14-29(16)

211 Bauer AZ, Kriebel D. Prenatal and perinatal analgesic exposure and autism: an ecological link. Environ Health. 2013;12:41. doi: 10.1186/1476-069X-12-41.

212 US Observer: http://www.usobserver.com/archive/july-10/the-truth-about-ritalin.html

213 World Week Daily: http://www.wnd.com/2013/04/radical-increase-in-kids-prescribed-ritalin/

214 Richard Scarnati, "An Outline of Hazardous Side Effects of Ritalin (Methylphenidate)", International Journal of the Addictions; Volume 21, Issue 7, 1986, pages 837-841

215 Lonsdale D, Shamberger R: Red cell transketo-lase as an indicator of nutritional deficiency. Am. J. Clin. Nutr. 33(2):205-11, 1980

216 Matsunami N, Hadley D, Hensel CH, Christensen GB, Kim C, et al. (2013) "Identification of Rare Recurrent Copy Number Variants in High-Risk Autism Families and Their Prevalence in a Large ASD Population," PLOS ONE 8(1): e52239. doi:10.1371/journal.pone.0052239

217 http://content.time.com/time/magazine/article/0,9171,986282,00.html

218 Mednick, S. A., W. F. Gabrielli Jr., and B. Hutchings, "Genetic influences in criminal convictions: Evidence from an adoption cohort," Science 224:891-94, 1984

219 Cloninger, C. R., S. Sigvardsson, M. Bohman, and A. L. von Knorring, "Predisposition to petty criminality in Swedish adoptees. II. cross-fostering analysis of gene-environment interaction," Archives of General Psychiatry 39:1242-47,1982

220 Walsh, W, J., "Chemical Classification of Violent Criminals," Report No. HRI-104-3, 37th Annual meeting of the American Chemical Society, San Diego, 1985

221 William J. Walsh, PhD, President, Health Research Institute at: http://americannutritionassociation.org/newsletter/chemical-imbalences-criminal-violence

222 Nutrients. 2014 Nov 26;6(12):5405-18, doi: 10.3390/nu6125405

223 Lawrence F. Omega-3, junk food and the link between violence and what we eat. The Guardian, October 17, 2006

224 Gesch CB, Hammond SM, Hampson SE, Eves A, Crowder MJ. Influence of supplementary vitamins, minerals and essential fatty acids on the antisocial behaviour of young adult prisoners. Randomised, placebo-controlled trial. British J Psychiatry 2002. 181, 22-28. Full text: http://bjp.rcpsych.org/content/181/1/22.long

225 Boucher M, Bryan S, Dukes S. Deficiency or dementia? Exploring B12 deficiency after urostomy. Br J Nurs. 2015 Jun 11-24;24(11):594-7. doi: 10.12968/bjon.2015.24.11.594.

226 Schoenthaler SJ, Bier ID. The effect of vitamin-mineral supplementation on juvenile delinquency among American schoolchildren: a randomized, double-blind placebo-controlled trial. J Altern Complement Med. 2000 Feb;6(1):7-17. http://www.elkinsappsych.com/uploads/8/4/3/5/8435157/omega-3__violence-article.pdf

227 Gropper SS, Smith JL. Advanced Nutrition and Human Metabolism, 6th Ed. Wadsworth, 2013. ISBN-13 9781133104056

228 Gesch B. Adolescence: Does good nutrition = good behaviour? Nutr Health. 22(1): 55-65. Published online 2014 Feb 4. doi: 10.1177/0260|106013519552 http://www.ncbi.nlm.nih.gov/pmc/articles/PMC4817227/

229 Interview given for Health Daily (Medical News), 2012

230 Herbert Benson Interview with *The Washington Post*

231 'Small Dose' Exercise Guards Against Depression - Medscape - Oct 10, 2017

232 Am J Psychiatry. Published online October 3, 2017

233 THE BLOG 06/11/2013 01:45 pm ET Updated Aug 11, 2013

234 New Scientist. 14 Oct 2017, pp. 30-33. Volume 2136 No 3147

235 Social Psychological and Personality Science, 2014, Vol. 5(5) 526-533

236 The varieties of contemplative experience: A mixed-methods study of meditation-related challenges in Western Buddhists. PLOS One, May 24, 2017https://doi.org/10.1371/journal.pone.0176239

237 Eur Neurol. 2009;62(5):316-20. doi: 10.1159/000235945

238 N Engl J Med 1986; 315:1519-1524December 11, 1986DOI: 10.1056/NEJM198612113152405

239 Journal of Epidemiology and Community Health (DOI: 10.1136/jech.2005.041541

240 A neural link between generosity and happiness. *Nature Communications*;11 Jul 2017

241 Nelson, S. K., Layous, K., Cole, S. W., & Lyubomirsky, S. (2016, April 21). Do Unto Others or Treat Yourself? The Effects of Prosocial and Self-Focused Behavior on Psychological Flourishing. Emotion. Advance online publication. http://dx.doi.org/10.1037/emo0000178

242 https://www.hearing-voices.org/about-voices/famous-people/

243 http://www.intervoiceonline.org/about-intervoice/founders-welcome

244 https://www.statnews.com/2017/07/13/hearing-voices-mental-illness/

245 https://en.wikipedia.org/wiki/Cognitive_dissonance

246 Circulation. 2007;116:1845-1854, originally published October 15, 2007

247 Roger J. Williams. Biochemical Individuality. Keats, New Canaan, CT; 1956, page xv

248 Roger J. Williams. Biochemical Individuality. Keats, New Canaan, CT; 1956, page 2

249 William H. Philpott MD and Dwight K. Kalita, *Brain Allergies. The Psychonutrient Connection*. (Keats Publishing Inc., New Canaan, CT. 1980, pp. 120-121

250 Soledad Cepeda, M., Stang, P., & Makadia R. (2016) Depression Is Associated With High Levels of C-Reactive Protein and Low Levels of Fractional Exhaled Nitric Oxide: Results From the 2007-2012 National Health and Nutrition Examination Surveys. J Clin Psychiatry. 1666-71

251 Sophie E. Holmes, Rainer Hinz, Silke Conen, Catherine J. Gregory, Julian C. Matthews, Jose M. Anton-Rodriguez, Alexander Gerhard, Peter S. Talbot. Elevated Translocator Protein in Anterior Cingulate in Major Depression and a Role for in Suicidal Thinking: A Positron Emission Tomography Study. Biological Psychiatry, 2017; DOI: 10.1016/j.biopsych.2017.08.005252   http://www.npr.org/sections/health-shots/2015/10/25/451169292/could-depression-be-caused-by-an-infection

253 Biology of Mood & Anxiety Disorders20144:10. https://doi.org/10.1186/2045-5380-4-10

254 JAMA Psychiatry. 2013;70(8):812-820. doi:10.1001/jamapsychiatry.2013.1111

255 Wotton CJ, Goldacre MJ. Associations between specific autoimmune diseases

and subsequent dementia: retrospective record-linkage cohort study, UK [published online March 1, 2017]. J Epidemiol Community Health. doi:10.1136/jech-2016-207809

256 http://www.npr.org/sections/health-shots/2015/10/25/451169292/could-depression-be-caused-by-an-infection

257 Brain, Behavior, and Immunity. Available online 6 May 2018 https://doi.org/10.1016/j.bbi.2018.05.006

258 Altern Ther Health Med. 2015 Aug;21 Suppl 3:18-26

259 [Curr Med Chem. 2011;18(17):2630-7. Aluminum vaccine adjuvants: are they safe?]

260 New York Times April 18, 2012

261 Journal of Cognitive Neuroscience November 2017; 29(11): 1895-1907

262 NeuroImage. Volume 166, 1 February 2018, Pages 230-238

263 Lao CD, Ruffin MTt, Normolle D, et al. Dose escalation of a curcuminoid formulation. BMC Complement Altern Med. 2006;6:10

264 Prevalence of people reporting sensitivities to chemicals in a population-based survey. Am J Epidemiol. 1999 Jul 1;150(1):1-12

265 https://www.ncbi.nlm.nih.gov/books/NBK268889/

266 Indian J Occup Environ Med. 2008 Aug; 12(2): 61–64

267 Ann Fam Med. 2012 Jul; 10(4): 357–365. doi: 10.1370/afm.1346

268 Dampness and mold in the home and depression: an examination of mold-related illness and perceived control of one's home

as possible depression pathways. Am J Public Health. 2007 Oct;97(10):1893-9

269 Psychology Today (online Aug 3, 2017)

270 https://en.wikipedia.org/wiki/Air_ioniser

271 Truss, C.O. 1978. Tissue injury induced by Candida albicans: Mental and neurologic manifestations. The Journal of Orthomolecular Psychiatry 7: pp 17–37

272 Proceedings of the Royal Society of Medicine Symposium of Intestinal Toxaemia, 1911

273 Bond Stow, M.D., on autointoxication and Lactobacillus bulgaricus – Medical Record Journal of Medicine and Surgery, 1914

274 Gut Pathog. 2013; 5: 5. Published online 2013 Mar 18. doi: 10.1186/1757-4749-5-5

275 Clin Psychopharmacol Neurosci. 2016 May; 14(2): 131–147. Published online 2016 May 31

276 https://www.ncbi.nlm.nih.gov/pmc/articles/PMC3897394/

277 Think Twice: How the Gut's "Second Brain" Influences Mood and Well-Being, Scientific American, Feb 12, 2010

278 J Psychiatry Neurosci. 2017 Mar; 42(2): 75–77

279 Herter CA, Kendall AI. The influence of dietary alterations on the types of intestinal flora. J Biol Chem. 1910;7:203–236

280 Journal Critical Reviews in Food Science and Nutrition https://doi.org/10.1080/10408398.2017.1399860

281 J Psychiatry Neurosci. 2017 Mar; 42(2): 75–77

282 Kaplan BJ, Rucklidge JJ, Romijn R, McLeod K. The emerging field of nutritional

mental health: inflammation, the microbiome, oxidative stress, and mitochondrial function. Clin Psychol Sci. 2015 doi: 10.1177/2167702614555413

283 Jacka FN, Mykletun A, Berk M, Bjelland I, Tell GS. The association between habitual diet quality and the common mental disorders in community-dwelling adults: the Hordaland Health study. Psychosom Med. 2011;73:483–490. doi: 10.1097/PSY.0b013e318222831a

284 Jacka FN, Pasco JA, Mykletun A, Williams LJ, Hodge AM, O'Reilly SL, et al. Association of Western and traditional diets with depression and anxiety in women. Am J Psychiatry. 2010;167:305–311. doi: 10.1176/appi.ajp.2009.09060881

285 Lee J, Pase M, Pipingas A, Raubenheimer J, Thurgood M, Villalon L, et al. Switching to a 10-day Mediterranean-style diet improves mood and cardiovascular function in a controlled crossover study. Nutrition. 2015;31:647–652. doi: 10.1016/j.nut.2014.10.008

286 Scand J Gastroenterol. 2006 Apr;41(4):408-19

287 Hoffer A & Mahon M: The presence of unidentified substances in the urine of psychiatric patients. *J. Neuropsychiatry* 2; 331-362: 1961

288 *Mental Illness and Schizophrenia. The Nutrition Connection.* Carl C Pfeiffer, Thorson's, Wellingborough, UK. 1987 (edited by Patrick Holford BSc)

289 *Diabetes Care*, Volume 30, Number 6, June 2007. Pp. 1437-1441

290 Effects of growth hormone on glucose metabolism. *Hormone Research*. 1991;36 Suppl 1:32-5

291 Intranasal Oxytocin Mechanisms Can Be Better Understood, but Its Effects on Social Cognition and Behavior Are Not to Be Sniffed At/ Leng, Gareth; Ludwig, Mike. In: *Biological Psychiatry*, 15.04.2016

292 Striepens N, Kendrick KM, Hanking V, Landgraf R, Wüllner U, Maier W, & Hurlemann R (2013). Elevated cerebrospinal fluid and blood concentrations of oxytocin following its intranasal administration in humans. Scientific reports, 3 PMID: 24310737

293 Hypothyroidism Presenting as Psychosis: Myxedema Madness Revisited. *Prim Care Companion J Clin Psychiatry*. 2003; 5(6): 260–266

294 PNAS USA, vol. 113 no. 41, 11633–11638, doi: 10.1073/pnas.1608085113

295 https://www.niddk.nih.gov/health-information/endocrine-diseases/adrenal-insufficiency-addisons-disease

296 Spencer RL, Hutchison KE (1999). "Alcohol, aging, and the stress response". Alcohol Research & Health. 23 (4): 272–83

297 *Psychological Bulletin*. 133 (1): 25–45]

298 The role of the glucocorticoids in developing resilience to stress and addiction. Front. Psychiatry, 01 August 2013 | https://doi.org/10.3389/fpsyt.2013.00068

299 http://www.ema.europa.eu/docs/en_GB/document_library/Scientific_guideline/2009/09/WC500003646.pdf

300 https://www.livescience.com/42198-what-is-oxytocin.html accessed: Oct 30, 2017, 10.00 am PDT

301 Psychol Sci. 2007 Nov;18(11):965-70

302 https://www.livescience.com/42198-what-is-oxytocin.html accessed: Oct 30, 2017, 10.00 am PDT

303 Proceedings of The National Acadmey of Sciences. vol. 107 no. 50, 21371–21375, doi: 10.1073/pnas.1012669107

304 Wenk GL. Neuropathologic changes in Alzheimer's disease: potential targets for treatment. J Clin Psychiatry. 2006;67 Suppl 33-7

305 Schmidt PJ et al 2005

306 Psychopharmacology (Berl). 2005 Oct 18;:1-11 Psychobiology Research Group, School of Neurology, Neurobiology and Psychiatry, University of Newcastle upon Tyne, Newcastle upon Tyne, UK

307 Crit Rev Toxicol. 1995;25(1):1-24

308 Fisher Acros Organics: Fair Lawn, NJ, Mar. 7, 2007. http//:fsimage.fishersci.com/msds/96252.htm (accessed June 15, 2010)

309 Wedeen, R. P. Were the hatters of New Jersey "mad"? Am. J. Ind. Med. 1989, 16, 225-233

310 Needleman, H (2009). "Low level lead exposure: history and discovery". Annals of Epidemiology. 19 (4): 235–.

311 Payne, M (2008). "Lead in drinking water". Canadian Medical Association Journal. 179 (3): 253–4. doi:10.1503/cmaj.071483. PMC 2474873 Freely accessible. PMID 18663205

312 Int J Environ Res Public Health. 2009 May; 6(5): 1609–1619

313 J Trace Elem Med Biol. 2017 Mar;40:30-36. doi: 10.1016/j.jtemb.2016.12.001. Epub 2016 Dec 9

314 Brown JS. Psychiatric Issues in Toxic Exposures. 2007 Psychiatr Clin N Am 30 837-854

315 Microbes and Mental Illness Symposium; American Psychiatric Association Institute for Psychiatric Services; October 2000. Available at: http://psychservices. psychiatryonline. org/cgi/content/full/52/1/37#SEC4. Accessed October 24, 2007/

316 Lyme Disease, Comorbid Tick-Borne Diseases, and Neuropsychiatric Disorders. Psychiatric Times, Dec 01, 2007

317 Atypical behavioral and psychiatric symptoms: Neurosyphilis should always be considered. Autops Case Rep. 2015 Jul-Sep; 5(3): 43–47

318 Lyme Disease, Comorbid Tick-Borne Diseases, and Neuropsychiatric Disorders. Psychiatric Times, Dec 01, 2007

319 Stricker RB, Burrascano JJ, Harris NS, et al. Coinfection with Borrelia burgdorferi and Babesia microti: bad or worse? J Infect Dis. 2006;193:901-902

320 Centers for Disease Control: https://www.cdc.gov/lyme/treatment/index.html

321 Cameron D, Gaito A, Harris N, et al; The International Lyme and Associated Diseases Society. Evidence-based guidelines for the management of Lyme disease. Available at: www.ilads.org/files/ILADS_Guidelines.pdf. Accessed October 17, 2007

322 Karolinska Institute, news release, Dec. 7, 2012

323 GABAergic Signaling Is Linked to a Hypermigratory Phenotype in Dendritic Cells Infected by Toxoplasma gondii. PLOS Pathogens. December 6, 2012https://doi.org/10.1371/journal.ppat.1003051

324 How Your Cat Is Making You Crazy. Kathleen Mcauliffe. *The Atlantic*. March 2012 issue

325 Homeopathic remedy made from *Toxoplasma gondii* reduces the number of bradyzoites in mice infected by the protozoan. *European Journal of Integrative Medicine*. Volume 7, Issue 5, October 2015, Pages 517-524

326 Becker et al, later followed by similar results published by Friedman et al (1963)

327 RW Kay, Geomagnetic storms: association with incidence of depression as measured by hospital admission. The British Journal of Psychiatry. 1994, 164: 403-409

328 Natural Hazards, November 2012, Volume 64, Issue 2, pp 1447-1459. Space weather hazards and their impact on human cardio-health state parameters on Earth. H. Mavromichalaki, M. Papailiou, S. Dimitrova, E. S. Babayev, P. Loucas

329 Stoupel E., Effect of geomagnetic activity on cardiovascular parameters, Journal of Clinical and Basic Cardiology 1999; 2 (Issue 1), 34-40

330 Kuleshova, V.P., S.A. Pulinets, E.S. Sazanova, A.M. Kharchenko (1998). Biotropic effects of geomagnetic storms and their seasonal variations, Biofizika, Vol. 46, Issue 5, September - October 2001, pp. 930-934

331 G. De Matteis, M Vellante, A Marrelli, U Villante, P Santalucia, P Tuzi, M Prencipe (1994). Geomagnetic Activity, Humidity, Temperature and Headache: Is, There Any Correlation? Headache: The Journal of Head and Face Pain 34 (1), 41–43

332 Lyall Watson, Supernature, Hodder and Stoughton, London, 1973, pp. 51- 53

333 Robine, Jean-Marie; Cheung, Siu Lan K.; Le Roy, Sophie; Van Oyen, Herman; Griffiths, Clare; Michel, Jean-Pierre; Herrmann,

François Richard (2008). "Death toll exceeded 70,000 in Europe during the summer of 2003". Comptes Rendus Biologies. 331 (2): 171–178

334 "Valores extremos – Agencia Estatal de Meteorología – AEMET. Gobierno de España" (in Spanish). Aemet.es. Archived from the original on 17 March 2010. Retrieved 15 March 2010

335 https://www.hindawi.com/journals/isrn/2013/127365/

336 Phytother Res. 2002 Nov;16(7):639-45

337 J Altern Complement Med. 2010 Jul;16(7):753-9. doi: 10.1089/acm.2009.0342

338 Does Bacopa monnieri improve memory performance in older persons? Results of a randomized, placebo-controlled, double-blind trial. *J Altern Complement Med*. 2010 Jul;16(7):753-9. doi: 10.1089/acm.2009.0342.

339 Holmquist L, Stuchbury G, Berbaum K, et al. Lipoic acid as a novel treatment for Alzheimer's disease and related dementias. Pharmacol Ther. 2007 Jan;113(1):154-64

340 Panigrahi M, Sadguna Y, Shivakumar BR, et al. alpha-Lipoic acid protects against reperfusion injury following cerebral ischemia in rats. Brain Res. 1996 Apr 22;717(1-2):184-8

341 http://www.lifeextension.com/magazine/2007/10/nu_lipoic_acid/page-01

342 https://en.wikipedia.org/wiki/Mystical_psychosis

343 DSM-IV, 1994

344 Dodds, E. (1951). *The Greeks and the irrational*. Berkeley: University of California Press

345 Maslow, Abraham (1968). *Toward a Psycholo-gy of Being*. New York, NY: Van Nostrand-Rein-hold

346 The Mystica, 29, 438-439

347 Ingerman S, *Soul Retrieval: Mending The Frag-mented Self*, Harper San Francisco, 1991, p. 17

348 Ingerman S, *Soul Retrieval: Mending The Frag-mented Self*, Harper San Francisco, 1991, p. 23

349 Bergler E. *Homosexuality: Disease or Way of Life*. Hill & Wang; New York, NY, USA: 1956, pp. 28–29.

350 Freud S. *Three Essays on the Theory of Sexual-ity*. Hogarth Press; London, UK: 1953 [1905]. pp. 123–246. Standard Edition Volume 7, p. 139

351 Drescher J. From bisexuality to intersexuali-ty: Rethinking gender categories. Contemp. Psychoanal. 2007;43:204–228

352 Williams W. *The Spirit and the Flesh: Sexual Diversity in American Indian Culture*. Beacon Press; Boston, MA, USA: 1986

353 Drescher J. Queer diagnoses: Parallels and contrasts in the history of homosexual-ity, gender variance, and the diagnostic and statistical manual. *Arch. Sex. Behav.* 2010;39:427–460

354 Kinsey A.C., Pomeroy W.B., Martin C.E.. *Sexual Behavior in the Human Male*. W.B. Saunders; Philadelphia, PA, USA: 1948.

355 Kinsey A., Pomeroy W., Martin C., Gebhard P. *Sexual Behavior in the Human Female*. Saun-ders; Philadelphia, PA, USA: 1953

356 Hooker E.A. The adjustment of the male overt homosexual. J. Proj. Tech. 1957;21:18–31. doi: 10.1080/08853126.1957.10380742

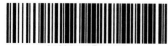

Made in the USA
Middletown, DE
08 February 2019